Springhouse
Certification Review

CRITICAL CARE
NURSING

Springhouse Certification Review

CRITICAL CARE NURSING

Springhouse Corporation
Springhouse, Pennsylvania

Staff

Senior Publisher
Minnie B. Rose, RN, BSN, MEd

Art Director
John Hubbard

Acquisitions Editors
Patricia Kardish Fischer, RN, BSN; Maryann Foley, RN, BSN

Editors
Diane Labus, David Moreau, Karen Zimmermann

Copy Editor
Diane M. Armento

Designers
Stephanie Peters (senior associate art director), Lesley Weissman-Cook, Donald G. Knauss

Manufacturing
Deborah Meiris (director), T.A. Landis

Editorial Assistants
Louise Quinn, Betsy K. Snyder

Printed in the United States of America.
CCRN1-030896

ℛ A member of the Reed Elsevier plc group

Library of Congress Cataloging-in-Publication Data
Springhouse certification review: critical care nursing
   p. cm.
  Includes bibliographical references and index.
  1. Intensive care nursing—Outlines, syllabi, etc.
2. Intensive care nursing—Examinations, questions, etc.
I. Springhouse Corporation. II. Title: Critical care nursing.
  [DNLM: 1. Critical Care—nurses' instruction. 2. Critical Illness—nursing—examination questions. 3. Critical Care—examination questions.   WY 18.2 S769 1996]
RT120.I5S67 1996
610.73'61—dc20
DNLM/DLC   95-35911
ISBN 0-87434-782-3 (alk. paper)   CIP

Contents

Section I: Body Systems Review

Section II: Sample Test

Contributors and Reviewers

CONTRIBUTORS

Susan Breda Galea, RN, MSN, CCRN
Critical Care Nurse, Surgical ICU
University of Pennsylvania
Philadelphia

Martha Kennedy, RN, BSN, CCRN
Critical Care Instructor
The Johns Hopkins Oncology Center
Baltimore

JoAnne Konick-McMahan, RN, MSN, CCRN
Clinical Lecturer
Adult Health and Illness Graduate Program
University of Pennsylvania
Philadelphia;
Medical ICU Nurse
Hospital of the University of Pennsylvania
Philadelphia

Anna Owen, RN, BSN, MA, CCRN, CNRN
Critical Care Consultant
Staff Nurse
Surgical ICU
St. Francis Medical Center
Monroe, La.

Cathy Sellergren, RN, MSN, CCRN
Pulmonary Case Manager
Hinsdale Hospital
Hinsdale, Ill.

Joanne Farley Serembus, RN, MSN, CCRN
Medical-Surgical Nursing Instructor
School of Nursing
Roxborough Memorial Hospital
Philadelphia

Brenda K. Shelton, RN, MS, CCRN, OCN
Clinical Nurse Specialist
The Johns Hopkins Oncology Center
Baltimore

Gloria Sonnesso, RN, MSN
Clinical Education Consultant
Nellcor, Inc.
Pleasanton, Calif.

Patricia L. Vaska, RN, MSN, CCRN
Cardiovascular Surgery Clinical Nurse Specialist
Sioux Valley Hospital
Sioux Falls, S.D.

Susan Heidenwolf Weaver, RN, MSN, CCRN, CNA
Assistant Director of Nursing
St. Clares-Riverside Medical Center
Denville, N.J.;
ICU Staff Nurse
Morristown Memorial Hospital
Morristown, N.J.

Kathy M. Witta, RN, MSN, CCRN
Pulmonary Clinical Nurse Specialist
Pulmonary Associates
Wilmington, Del.;
Per Diem Staff Nurse
Intermediate Medical Care Unit
Hospital of the University of Pennsylvania
Philadelphia

Patti R. Zuzelo, RN, MSN
Program Coordinator
School of Nursing
Roxborough Memorial Hospital
Philadelphia

REVIEWERS

Sondra G. Ferguson, RN, MSN, CS, CCRN
Clinical Nurse Specialist for Critical Care
Department of Veteran Affairs
Veterans Administration Medical Center
Lexington, Ky.

Ellie Franges, RN, MSN, CCRN, CNRN
Neuroscience Coordinator
Sacred Heart Hospital
Allentown, Pa.

Susan Breda Galea, RN, MSN, CCRN
Critical Care Nurse, Surgical ICU
University of Pennsylvania
Philadelphia

Sharon Lehmann, RN, MS, CCRN, CNSN
Surgical ICU Nurse
University of Minnesota Hospital
Minneapolis

Foreword

Critical care nurses have been practicing in the throes of change for the past 2 decades. With major advances in medicine and technology increasing the demand for higher levels of nursing skill and knowledge, and with fast-paced changes occurring in health care financing and delivery, today's critical care nurses must play a vital role on the health care team. They are required to manage each patient's constantly changing plan of care with an in-depth understanding of varied assessment findings, complex disease processes, and high-tech treatments.

To meet these challenges, the nurse must demonstrate competence and currency in all aspects of critical care. One of the best ways to do this is to pass the CCRN certification examination. This nationally recognized examination validates an experienced nurse's specialized knowledge and judgment for practice as a critical care nurse. Passing this rigorous test signifies professional achievement and helps ensure high-quality nursing care.

If you are preparing to take the CCRN exam, *Springhouse Certification Review: Critical Care Nursing* can be your most valuable study tool. Designed according to the CCRN certification examination blueprint, this book readies you for the exam in two important ways. First, its review chapters provide in-depth coverage of all the major topics on the exam. Second, its nearly 1,000 questions sharpen your test-taking skills in the best possible way—by giving you practice with multiple-choice questions *in the exact style and content as those used on the CCRN exam.*

Section I, Body Systems Review, offers eight comprehensive chapters that address all areas covered by the CCRN exam: cardiovascular, respiratory, neurologic, renal, gastrointestinal, endocrine, hematologic and immunologic, and multisystem patient care problems. To provide maximum coverage of the major topic areas, the questions in Section I reflect the *approximate* percentage of the nursing process steps and cognitive levels as specified in the CCRN blueprint. This section's well-organized, clear, concise style makes the information easy to review, and its numerous patient scenarios stimulate critical thinking. Each chapter in Section I includes dozens of practice questions. As an aid to self-testing and instant feedback, these questions appear on the left, rationales for correct and incorrect answers appear on the right, and a card is included so you can cover the answers if desired.

Section II, Sample Test, provides a comprehensive exam to simulate the test-taking experience, with 200 questions covering all eight subject areas in the CCRN examination. Furthermore, all questions in Section II reflect the *exact percentages* specified in the CCRN blueprint for nursing process steps (assessment 32%, planning 15%, implementation 40%, and evaluation 13%) and cognitive levels (knowledge/comprehension 36%, application/analysis 39%, and synthesis/evaluation 25%). A blank answer sheet also is provided for your use, followed by answers and rationales for correct and incorrect responses.

Additionally, the reader will find helpful appendices on critical laboratory values and hemodynamic monitoring, a generous list of current references to allow further review, and a comprehensive index for rapid access to essential information.

Many critical care nursing experts, including educators and clinicians, have contributed to *Springhouse Certification Review: Critical Care Nursing*. Their collective decades of experience have been distilled into the most current and accurate review book for CCRN certification. This book not only provides everything you need to pass the CCRN examination but also will likely become one of the most trusted references on your bookshelf.

Barbara A. Erickson, RN, PhD, CCRN
Clinical Nurse Specialist
Case Manager Critical Care
Western Reserve Care System
Youngstown, Ohio

CARDIOVASCULAR SYSTEM

CHAPTER 1

Cardiovascular System

Questions 1 to 4 refer to the following information:
A 74-year-old female patient is admitted to the coronary care unit to rule out a myocardial infarction (MI). The initial assessment reveals:

- blood pressure, 100/76 mm Hg
- heart rate, 110 beats/minute
- respiratory rate, 18 breaths/minute
- skin, cool but dry
- lungs, clear bilaterally
- no murmurs, rubs, or extra heart sounds
- no edema.

When asked to quantify her chest pain on a 10-point scale, with 1 being the least and 10 being the worst pain, the patient rates her substernal chest pain as 6. ECG monitoring indicates sinus tachycardia with occasional premature ventricular contractions (PVCs) and occasional premature atrial contractions. A 12-lead ECG reveals ST-segment elevation in leads II, III, and aV_F.

---

1. The first responsibility of the nurse caring for this patient is to:

A. Explain the unit routine to alleviate anxiety

B. Relieve chest pain by administering supplemental oxygen and sublingual nitroglycerin

C. Complete a head-to-toe assessment

D. Administer a lidocaine infusion to eliminate the PVCs

CORRECT ANSWER—B. The primary goal in managing a patient with MI is to preserve the myocardium. Because chest pain is directly related to the ischemic myocardium, relief of such pain signals the return of oxygen to the affected muscle. Although relieving anxiety also is important, the nurse should do more than simply explain the unit routine. A complete and thorough physical assessment can be done when the patient is free of pain. Lidocaine may be given for PVCs with R-on-T phenomenon, couplets, or multifocal PVCs.

Nursing process step: Implementation
Cognitive level: Analysis

2. Approximately 10 minutes after a nitroglycerin I.V. infusion is begun at 100 mcg/minute, the patient's blood pressure drops to 80/60 mm Hg and she complains of dizziness and nausea. Which of the following actions should the nurse take?
   A. Place the patient in Trendelenburg's position
   B. Attempt a fluid challenge
   C. Decrease the nitroglycerin I.V. infusion to 50 mcg/minute
   D. Administer morphine sulfate

CORRECT ANSWER—C. With any symptomatic patient experiencing decreased blood pressure, the blood pressure is treated first. In this case, although the drop in pressure is severe enough to elicit symptoms, it is not yet considered life-threatening. The patient's nitroglycerin dose should be decreased to treat the vasodilation. However, the nurse must remember that rapid discontinuation of a nitroglycerin infusion can elicit coronary artery spasm or pulmonary congestion, which could lead to devastating consequences in a cardiac patient. Trendelenburg's position is no longer used to treat patients with hypotension because it contributes to venous congestion and can impede heart pumping. It also can cause cerebral congestion, which can lead to hypoxia. The position used to treat hypotension would be with the legs elevated and the head of the bed flat. A fluid challenge generally is contraindicated in most cardiac patients because of the increased risk of congestive heart failure. Morphine sulfate is indicated to relieve pain and anxiety and can produce coronary and pulmonary dilation; it would be administered judiciously, if at all, to a hypotensive patient.
Nursing process step: Implementation
Cognitive level: Application

3. Suspecting right ventricular involvement, the nurse could examine the 12-lead ECG using the following lead placement:
   A. Left precordial leads
   B. Right precordial leads
   C. Limb leads
   D. Augmented vector leads

CORRECT ANSWER—B. This patient is exhibiting symptoms of acute MI, and the primary 12-lead ECG changes are occurring to the inferior wall of the left ventricle. In any inferior wall MI, the patient should be assessed for involvement of the right ventricle (RV). A standard 12-lead ECG cannot be used to diagnose RV infarctions because the right ventricle is covered by the left ventricle, thereby obscuring electrical signals from the right side. Placing precordial leads to the right side of the chest allows the electrical signals from the RV to be seen. Suggested lead placement is V_4R and V_6R.
Nursing process step: Evaluation
Cognitive level: Analysis

4. On confirmation of a right ventricular MI, the nurse would anticipate the following treatment plan:
A. Administer fluids to maintain a pulmonary capillary wedge pressure greater than 15 mm Hg
B. Infuse I.V. nitroglycerin to keep the patient pain-free
C. Administer nitroprusside to reduce afterload
D. Administer furosemide to prevent congestive heart failure

CORRECT ANSWER—A.   The primary goals in the treatment of right ventricular MI are to improve cardiac output and to salvage muscle. Right ventricular stroke volume must be increased to maintain adequate cardiac output. According to the Frank-Starling law, the addition of fluid volume stretches the muscle fibers to produce a greater output. The purpose of this higher output is to overcome the pressure gradient between the right and left ventricles, thus forcing a right-to-left flow of blood. Nitroglycerin, a preload reduction agent, is used to dilate the coronary arteries. Because the patient requires an increased preload, the fluids would need to be administered before or concomitantly with nitroglycerin to maintain cardiac output and increase coronary perfusion. Nitroprusside, which would decrease the patient's systemic vascular resistance, and furosemide, which could decrease the patient's preload, are not indicated in this case.
Nursing process step: Planning
Cognitive level: Application

5. Which measurement would be most helpful in assessing the fluid balance of a patient exhibiting symptoms associated with acute left-sided heart failure?
A. Arterial oxygen saturation
B. Pulmonary artery pressure
C. Cardiac output
D. Mean right atrial pressure

CORRECT ANSWER—D.   In a normal ventricle, the mean right atrial pressure correlates with right ventricular filling pressure. In this situation, the right side of the heart has not yet been affected, and pressures on the right should be close to normal. To evaluate the patient's fluid status, the nurse should observe for trends in the right atrial pressure along with trends in cardiac output, pulmonary artery pressure, and pulmonary capillary wedge pressure. Arterial oxygen saturation indicates the level of hypoxemia that may result from acute left heart failure, but it is not an indicator of fluid balance. Cardiac output measurements indicate the heart's ability to effectively pump blood. Although these measurements are affected by fluid status, they are not an indicator of the patient's volume status.
Nursing process step: Assessment
Cognitive level: Evaluation

6. The nurse caring for a patient with infective mitral endocarditis monitors the ECG for evidence of the abscess's invasion into the atrioventricular (AV) node. Which rhythm is indicative of this occurrence?
A. Atrial fibrillation
B. Ventricular fibrillation
C. Heart blocks
D. Junctional rhythms

CORRECT ANSWER—C. A dangerous sequelae of infective mitral endocarditis is heart blocks, which indicate invasion of the AV node and permanent destruction of the conductive tissues. The other rhythms are not related to AV node invasion by the abscess.
Nursing process step: Evaluation
Cognitive level: Evaluation

7. The critical care nurse would suspect which medication as precipitating torsades du pointes?
A. Procainamide
B. Diltiazem
C. Atenolol
D. Bretylium

CORRECT ANSWER—A. Procainamide and, less commonly, quinidine can be proarrhythmic and precipitate the type of ventricular tachycardia known as torsades du pointes. Diltiazem, atenolol, and bretylium are not associated with torsades du pointes.
Nursing process step: Evaluation
Cognitive level: Analysis

8. The nurse correctly instructs a patient with peripheral vascular disease that stress reduction techniques:
A. Are helpful only because they assist in smoking cessation
B. Are helpful because stress stimulates the release of vasoconstricting catecholamines
C. Are helpful because they distract the patient from focusing on claudication pain
D. Have not proved useful in patients with peripheral vascular disease

CORRECT ANSWER—B. The stress-induced release of vasoactive catecholamines, such as epinephrine, causes vasoconstriction, which directly aggravates peripheral vascular disease by intensifying the ischemic burden of the affected tissues. Vasoconstriction also indirectly aggravates atherogenesis by inducing hypertension. Stress-reduction techniques make it easier for patients to avoid bad habits, such as smoking; however, this is not the only reason why they are useful. Claudication is a signal of muscle ischemia and should not be ignored.
Nursing process step: Implementation
Cognitive level: Application

9. Which of the following reasons best explains why the nurse should exercise caution in the fluid resuscitation of a patient with a cardiac contusion?
A. The patient is at risk for ventricular rupture
B. The patient may have preexisting ischemic heart disease
C. Blood pressure is not a reliable indicator of fluid volume status in a trauma patient
D. Myocardial depression is common after cardiac contusion

CORRECT ANSWER—D. Bruising of the heart, as occurs with cardiac contusion, causes myocardial dysfunction and often depresses contractility. Although the patient is at risk for rupture of the free wall of the ventricle, this would require massive fluid resuscitation. Blood pressure is a reliable indicator of fluid volume in trauma patients, although tachycardia is not. Preexisting ischemic disease is not as likely to occur as myocardial depression in this situation.
Nursing process step: Implementation
Cognitive level: Application

10. Which type of monitoring is most useful for a patient with postpartum cardiomyopathy?
A. Pulmonary artery catheterization
B. Arterial blood gas studies
C. Pulse oximetry
D. Arterial line monitoring

CORRECT ANSWER—A. This patient would be expected to have elevated pulmonary artery pressures and reduced cardiac output. Thus, therapy would be aimed at optimizing these hemodynamic parameters to improve the patient's overall condition. Arterial blood gas studies, pulse oximetry, and an arterial line are useful adjunctive techniques but would not determine the effects of therapy to as great a degree as a pulmonary artery catheter.
Nursing process step: Assessment
Cognitive level: Comprehension

Questions 11 to 13 refer to the following information:
A 27-year-old female patient with acute renal tubular necrosis has a new onset of uremia and a blood urea nitrogen (BUN) level of 84 mg/dl. She has been diagnosed with acute uremic pericarditis.

11. Which signs and symptoms are related to the patient's pericarditis?
A. Fever, chest discomfort, and elevated erythrocyte sedimentation rate
B. Low urine output secondary to left ventricular dysfunction
C. Lethargy, anorexia, and congestive heart failure
D. Pitting edema, chest discomfort, and nonspecific ST-segment elevation

CORRECT ANSWER—A. The classic signs and symptoms of pericarditis include fever, positional chest discomfort, nonspecific ST-segment elevation, elevated erythrocyte sedimentation rate, and pericardial friction rub. All the other symptoms may result from acute renal failure.
Nursing process step: Evaluation
Cognitive level: Comprehension

12. Which medication would best treat this patient's pericarditis?
A. Ibuprofen
B. Steroids
C. Acetaminophen
D. Nifedipine

CORRECT ANSWER—B. Anti-inflammatory agents, such as steroids, are the treatment of choice for pericarditis. Ibuprofen, however, can worsen renal function and would be contraindicated in a patient with acute renal failure. Acetaminophen is an antipyretic analgesic and nifedipine is a calcium channel blocker; neither would be used to treat a patient with pericarditis.
Nursing process step: Planning
Cognitive level: Application

13. The nurse monitors the patient for cardiac tamponade secondary to acute pericarditis and observes closely for:

A. Pulsus paradoxus, hypertension, and low central venous pressure

B. Pulsus alternans, hypotension, and distended neck veins

C. Pulsus paradoxus, hypotension, and distended neck veins

D. Pulsus alternans, hypertension, and high central venous pressure

CORRECT ANSWER—C. The classic signs of cardiac tamponade are pulsus paradoxus secondary to impaired venous return, hypotension secondary to decreased preload and mechanical compression of the heart, and distended neck veins secondary to buildup of venous blood before entering the right atrium. Pulsus alternans occurs with severe left ventricular dysfunction. If monitored, central venous pressure would be elevated.
Nursing process step: Evaluation
Cognitive level: Evaluation

14. Which of the following can cause hypovolemic shock?

A. Allergic reaction to medications

B. Third-space shifting of fluid into the abdominal cavity

C. Sepsis

D. Profound bradycardia

CORRECT ANSWER—B. The extravasation of plasma fluids into the abdominal cavity can cause significant loss of circulating volume and result in hypovolemic shock. Allergic reactions can cause anaphylactic shock. Release of endotoxins in sepsis results in peripheral vasodilation and septic shock. Profound bradycardia can lead to circulatory collapse and cardiogenic shock.
Nursing process step: Assessment
Cognitive level: Comprehension

15. The most common site of aneurysm formation is in the:

A. Abdominal aorta, just below the renal arteries

B. Ascending aorta, around the aortic arch

C. Descending aorta, beyond the subclavian arteries

D. Aortic arch, around the ascending and descending aorta

CORRECT ANSWER—A. About 75% of aneurysms occur in the abdominal aorta, just below the renal arteries (Debakey type I aneurysms). Options B and D are characteristic of Debakey type II aneurysms, whereas option C is indicative of Debakey type III aneurysms.
Nursing process step: Assessment
Cognitive level: Comprehension

16. Which of the following can cause mitral regurgitation (insufficiency)?

A. Tumor

B. Left atrial thrombus

C. Bacterial vegetation

D. Atherosclerosis

CORRECT ANSWER—C. Mitral valve regurgitation may be caused by rheumatic heart disease, endocarditis, prolapse, dilation of the left ventricle, calcification, trauma, dysfunction of a mitral valve prosthesis, or rupture of the papillary muscle.
Nursing process step: Assessment
Cognitive level: Knowledge

17. The nurse caring for a patient in cardiogenic shock should prepare for the insertion of any of the following *except:*
A. Transvenous pacing wires
B. Femoral intra-arterial line
C. Left atrial catheter
D. Pulmonary artery catheter

CORRECT ANSWER—A. Transvenous pacing wires are indicated only for identified arrhythmias requiring the restoration of adequate heart rate. The following serial measurements need to be made in all cases of cardiogenic shock: pulmonary capillary wedge pressure, pulmonary artery end-diastolic pressure, right atrial pressure, intra-arterial pressure, and urine output. Left atrial pressure measurements are useful, and often the insertion of such a line will be performed in the operating room or the cardiac catheterization laboratory.
Nursing process step: Planning
Cognitive level: Analysis

18. A male patient is admitted to the intensive care unit with a blood pressure of 180/90 mm Hg by cuff. He explains that he has been taking blood pressure medication since 1985 but that he often stops taking the pills because they cost too much. The nurse realizes that this patient has:
A. Malignant hypertension
B. Secondary hypertension
C. Essential hypertension
D. Hypertensive crisis

CORRECT ANSWER—C. Arterial hypertension can be categorized as essential (also known as primary) hypertension, in which the course is slow but progressive over a period of 10 to 20 years, or as secondary hypertension, which results from various conditions that impair blood pressure regulation, such as renal, endocrine, vascular, and neurologic disorders. Malignant hypertension is a fulminating form of hypertension common to both primary and secondary types. Malignant hypertension is characterized by marked diastolic hypertension and is accompanied by severe vascular damage, which can lead to death within 1 year if left untreated. A hypertensive crisis—when mean arterial pressure (MAP) exceeds 150 mm Hg—is manifested by headache, irritability, vision loss, and coma. The formula for calculating MAP uses systolic blood pressure (SBP) and diastolic blood pressure (DBP) values:

$$\frac{SBP + 2\,(DBP)}{3}$$

For this patient, MAP = 190 mm Hg + 2(90 mm Hg) divided by 3, which equals 120 mm Hg. He is not in hypertensive crisis.
Nursing process step: Assessment
Cognitive level: Evaluation

19. What measurement can best be used to monitor the respiratory status of a patient with pulmonary edema?
   A. Arterial blood gas analysis
   B. Pulse oximetry
   C. Skin color assessment
   D. Lung sounds

CORRECT ANSWER—A. Blood gas analysis is the best measure for determining the extent of the hypoxia caused by pulmonary edema and for monitoring the effects of therapy. Although any of the options can be used to detect pulmonary changes, assessment of skin color and assessment of the lung fields often are subject to interpretation by practitioners. The use of pulse oximetry, especially in the case of severe vasoconstriction as is present in pulmonary edema, is unreliable.
Nursing process step: Assessment
Cognitive level: Analysis

20. Which development occurs during the early stage of hypovolemic shock?
   A. Hypotension
   B. Decreased secretion of antidiuretic hormone (ADH)
   C. Profound tachycardia
   D. Shunting of blood flow away from the skin

CORRECT ANSWER—D. The body shunts blood away from nonessential organs, including the skin, fat, and skeletal muscle, during the early stage of shock. Secretion of ADH, renin, and aldosterone is increased, thus assisting in maintaining blood pressure. Profound tachycardia does not occur until the later stages of hypovolemic shock.
Nursing process step: Assessment
Cognitive level: Comprehension

21. The nurse is caring for a patient with an automatic implantable cardioverter defibrillator (AICD). The patient develops symptomatic ventricular tachycardia that does not convert with AICD discharge. The nurse would:
   A. Deactivate the AICD and apply external countershock
   B. Contact the electrophysiologist to adjust the AICD sensitivity
   C. Apply external countershock without regard to deactivation of the device
   D. Institute cardiopulmonary resuscitation without external countershock

CORRECT ANSWER—C. Standard emergency procedures should always be used for a patient with an AICD if the device discharge does not terminate the rhythm. Deactivation of the device and consultation with the electrophysiologist can be done after the patient has been stabilized. External countershock will not damage the internal device; however, external countershock may be more effective if anterior/posterior paddles are used.
Nursing process step: Implementation
Cognitive level: Application

22. Which of the following is not a nursing priority during thrombolytic agent administration?
   A. Monitoring for arrhythmias and changes in vital signs
   B. Teaching the patient and family about myocardial infarction
   C. Providing emotional support and reassurance
   D. Frequently observing for bleeding

CORRECT ANSWER—**B.** The most common complication of thrombolytic agent therapy is bleeding. Other complications include arrhythmias and changes in vital signs. Anxiety and fear are common reactions in patients with an acute myocardial infarction. Although teaching is always an important aspect of patient care, it does not take precedence in emergencies. Brief but clear explanations during treatment are appropriate, not discussions on coronary artery disease and thrombolytic agent therapy.
Nursing process step: Planning
Cognitive level: Application

23. The nurse is admitting a patient with a diagnosis of unstable angina to the cardiac care unit. The physician orders a 12-lead ECG after the patient describes his substernal chest pain as 4 on a scale of 1 to 10, with 10 being the worst pain. Which ECG change is indicative of coronary artery ischemia?
   A. ST-segment elevation
   B. Significant Q waves
   C. Inverted T waves
   D. Peaked, tented T waves

CORRECT ANSWER—**C.** Although there are several possible ECG changes associated with myocardial ischemia, the most predominant changes include ST-segment depression and T-wave inversion due to repolarization difficulties in the affected areas of muscle. ST-segment elevation indicates myocardial injury, and the presence of significant Q waves indicates myocardial infarction; conduction delays also can cause Q waves. Peaked, tented T waves are common in patients with hyperkalemia.
Nursing process step: Assessment
Cognitive level: Knowledge

24. Afterload can be indirectly measured by:
   A. Pulmonary vascular resistance (PVR)
   B. Systemic vascular resistance (SVR)
   C. Left atrial pressure
   D. Cardiac output

CORRECT ANSWER—**B.** Afterload is the resistance against which the left ventricle must eject its volume of blood during left ventricular contraction. This resistance is produced by the vessel wall (aorta) and the volume of blood already in the vascular system. Afterload is difficult to measure. It can be indirectly determined by calculating the SVR, which takes into account the cardiac output and the right ventricular pressure as a measure of the volume of blood already in the vascular system. To calculate SVR, subtract central venous pressure (CVP) from mean arterial blood pressure (MAP); then divide the result by cardiac output (CO). PVR is the resistance in the pulmonary vascular bed against which the right ventricle must pump blood. In pulmonary hypertension, PVR is elevated. Neither PVR nor left atrial pressure indirectly measures afterload.
Nursing process step: Implementation
Cognitive level: Comprehension

25. Dressler syndrome, also called postcardiotomy syndrome or post-myocardial infarction syndrome, is best treated with:
A. Indomethacin
B. Antibiotics
C. Dobutamine
D. Amphotericin B

CORRECT ANSWER—**A.** Dressler syndrome, often called chronic pericarditis, occurs 1 to 6 weeks after a myocardial infarction and may be due to an immune response to the infarction. It also can occur after open heart surgery. Symptoms include fever, pericardial pain, pleuritis, and, occasionally, pneumonitis. Treatment options include aspirin, indomethacin, and steroids to reduce the inflammation.
Nursing process step: Implementation
Cognitive level: Comprehension

26. The nurse would obtain serum levels of which electrolytes in a patient with frequent episodes of ventricular tachycardia?
A. Calcium and magnesium
B. Potassium and calcium
C. Magnesium and potassium
D. Potassium and sodium

CORRECT ANSWER—**C.** Hypomagnesemia as well as hypokalemia and hyperkalemia are common causes of ventricular tachycardia. Calcium imbalances cause changes in the QT interval and ST segment. Alterations in sodium level do not cause rhythm disturbances.
Nursing process step: Implementation
Cognitive level: Analysis

27. Restrictive cardiomyopathy is characterized by:
A. Systolic dysfunction
B. Diastolic dysfunction
C. Septal hypertrophy
D. Jugular vein distention

CORRECT ANSWER—**B.** The abnormal cardiac stiffness in restrictive cardiomyopathy causes diastolic dysfunction and, subsequently, a prolonged left ventricular relaxation period. Septal hypertrophy is a hallmark of hypertrophic cardiomyopathy. Jugular vein distention may be noted in the late stages of restrictive cardiomyopathy, but it is more likely to be associated with dilated (congestive) cardiomyopathy.
Nursing process step: Assessment
Cognitive level: Comprehension

Questions 28 to 30 refer to the following information:
A 77-year-old man arrives at the emergency department complaining of severe back pain and symptoms of shock. He is diagnosed as having a leaking abdominal aortic aneurysm and is taken to the operating room for an emergency aneurysm resection. The patient receives 12 units of packed red blood cells, 10 units of fresh frozen plasma, and 16 units of pooled platelets, and 7 liters of a crystalloid solution. After surgery, he is transported to the intensive care unit, intubated, and fully ventilated with a pulmonary artery catheter and a mechanical ventilator. He is receiving an I.V. infusion of dopamine at a rate of 11 mcg/kg/minute.

28. During the initial postoperative assessment of this patient, the nurse would focus on:
A. Assessing fluid volume status
B. Auscultating breath sounds
C. Observing for signs and symptoms of infection
D. Assessing neurologic status

CORRECT ANSWER—A. Postoperatively, a patient who has had a ruptured abdominal aortic aneurysm will experience third-space fluid shifting from the intravascular space to the interstitial space, resulting in massive fluid shifts and hypotension. Therefore, the nurse would initially assess the patient's fluid volume status. Subsequently, the nurse would assess breath sounds and neurologic status, ensuring that the patient is not in impending circulatory collapse. Infection generally does not occur in the early postoperative period.
Nursing process step: Assessment
Cognitive level: Analysis

29. The patient becomes hypotensive, and the nurse observes that the pulmonary capillary wedge pressure (PCWP) is 3 mm Hg. Which intervention is most appropriate?
A. Increase the rate of the dopamine I.V. infusion until the blood pressure rises
B. Add an epinephrine I.V. infusion to maintain a systolic blood pressure of 90 mm Hg
C. Place the patient in Trendelenburg's position
D. Administer fluid in the form of a colloid or crystalloid solution

CORRECT ANSWER—D. The low PCWP indicates intravascular volume depletion and the need for fluids. The addition of vasoactive drugs (dopamine or epinephrine) will constrict the vascular bed but will not augment tissue perfusion. Although Trendelenburg's position would increase blood pressure in the upper part of the body, the volume depletion would persist.
Nursing process step: Implementation
Cognitive level: Application

30. Which finding would be *least* helpful in identifying intravascular depletion?
A. Tachycardia
B. High systemic vascular resistance (SVR)
C. Oliguria
D. Low SVR

CORRECT ANSWER—D. Low SVR is seen in high-output cardiac disorders, such as septic shock. Tachycardia is a compensatory mechanism for low cardiac output, which could be secondary to intravascular depletion. High SVR results from compensatory vasoconstriction, which occurs with hypovolemia. Oliguria results from low renal blood flow caused by reduced cardiac output.
Nursing process step: Evaluation
Cognitive level: Evaluation

31. Which diagnostic method would provide the most useful information about a patient with dilated (congestive) cardiomyopathy?
   A. Multiple-gated acquisition (MUGA) scan
   B. Intra-arterial line
   C. Central venous pressure monitoring
   D. 12-lead ECG

CORRECT ANSWER—A. A MUGA scan provides data on the ability of the right and left sides of the heart to pump adequately. It also provides information on the ejection fractions of the right and left ventricles. An arterial line provides only a more accurate method of measuring blood pressure, while a central venous pressure line provides information only on right atrial filling pressure. A 12-lead ECG would not indicate the severity of the cardiomyopathy, nor would it be useful in selecting appropriate medical therapy for the patient.
Nursing process step: Evaluation
Cognitive level: Comprehension

32. Funduscopic findings for a patient with malignant hypertension may include:
   A. Papilledema
   B. Retinal exudate
   C. Retinal hemorrhage
   D. All of the above

CORRECT ANSWER—D. A patient with malignant hypertension has a diastolic blood pressure greater than 120 mm Hg and some advanced funduscopic changes, including retinal exudate, retinal hemorrhage, and, commonly, papilledema.
Nursing process step: Assessment
Cognitive level: Evaluation

33. Which consequence is clinically significant in a patient with atrial fibrillation?
   A. Heart sounds cannot be evaluated
   B. The atrial component of cardiac output (atrial kick) is lost
   C. Blood pressure may increase
   D. No clinically significant consequences occur

CORRECT ANSWER—B. In atrial fibrillation, multiple chaotic depolarizations occur at different atrial sites, producing a rapid, irregular series of atrial impulses. The atrial rate is indeterminate with varying numbers of atrial fibrillatory waves occurring between ventricular contractions. Atrial fibrillation results in a loss of atrial contraction, or atrial kick, and may cause a clinically significant decrease in the patient's cardiac output, which can lead to hypotension. Heart sounds can still be evaluated; however, the S_4 sound is not heard because of the loss of atrial contraction.
Nursing process step: Evaluation
Cognitive level: Comprehension

34. The nurse would suspect early pericarditis following myocardial infarction with the development of which group of symptoms?

A. Exertional chest pain, pericardial friction rub, and diffuse ST-segment elevation

B. Positional chest pain, pericardial friction rub, and diffuse ST-segment elevation

C. Positional chest pain, pleural friction rub, and dyspnea

D. Exertional chest pain, pericardial friction rub, and persistent fever

CORRECT ANSWER—B. Early pericarditis is associated with positional chest pain that worsens on inspiration, transient pericardial friction rub, and diffuse ST-segment elevation without pathologic Q waves. Pulmonary symptoms (pleural friction rub and dyspnea) are not associated with pericarditis. Exertional chest pain is associated with myocardial ischemia. Persistent fever may be associated with late pericarditis.

Nursing process step: Assessment

Cognitive level: Evaluation

35. The most important reason for the nurse to encourage a patient with peripheral vascular disease to initiate a walking program is because this form of exercise:

A. Reduces stress

B. Aids in weight reduction

C. Increases high-density lipoprotein level

D. Promotes collateral circulation

CORRECT ANSWER—D. Regular walking is the best way to promote collateral circulation, which becomes a critical source of blood supply to limbs with compromised blood flow distal to a stenotic lesion. Regular exercise also aids in stress reduction, weight reduction, and increases the formation of high-density lipoproteins—all of which are helpful for a patient with peripheral vascular disease. However, these changes do not have as significant an effect on the patient's condition as the development of collateral circulation.

Nursing process step: Implementation

Cognitive level: Comprehension

36. Which of the following arrhythmias is not typically seen as a result of coronary artery reperfusion with a thrombolytic agent?

A. Ventricular tachycardia

B. Premature ventricular contractions

C. Accelerated idioventricular rhythm

D. Atrial fibrillation

CORRECT ANSWER—D. The most common arrhythmias associated with reperfusion are ventricular tachycardia, sinus bradycardia, accelerated idioventricular rhythm, and premature ventricular contractions.

Nursing process step: Assessment

Cognitive level: Comprehension

37. Which hemodynamic value is elevated in cardiogenic shock and indicative of left-sided heart failure?

A. Right atrial pressure
B. Central venous pressure
C. Right ventricular end-diastolic pressure
D. Pulmonary artery systolic and diastolic pressures

CORRECT ANSWER—D. Blood backs up into the pulmonary circulation because the failing left side of the heart cannot move blood forward into the circulation. Right atrial pressure and central venous pressure are elevated in end-stage left-sided heart failure that has progressed to right-sided heart failure. Low cardiac output and compensatory sympathetic stimulation usually are associated with an increased end-diastolic pressure in both the right and left ventricles, which is indicative of congestive heart failure. These increased pressures may be associated with clinical signs of either right- or left-sided heart failure.
Nursing process step: Assessment
Cognitive level: Application

38. Nursing interventions for a patient in hypertensive crisis may include:

A. Teaching about blood pressure medication
B. Maintaining a calming environment
C. Restricting visitors
D. Encouraging patient activity, as tolerated

CORRECT ANSWER—B. Nursing interventions during a hypertensive crisis include reassuring the patient and family and maintaining a calming environment. Teaching about blood pressure medication or anything else is inappropriate because of the patient's condition. In many cases, restricting visitors will increase the patient's anxiety. However, this should be assessed for each individual patient and family. The patient should remain calm and do as little as possible; the nurse should provide care for the patient as needed.
Nursing process step: Implementation
Cognitive level: Application

39. A patient has an automatic implantable cardioverter defibrillator (AICD) in place. During an episode of pulseless ventricular tachycardia, the AICD fires but does not terminate the arrhythmia. The nurse should prepare to:

A. Administer lidocaine intravenously
B. Cardiovert at 100 joules
C. Defibrillate at 100 joules
D. Defibrillate at 200 joules or higher

CORRECT ANSWER—D. Because the AICD has fired, the nurse should proceed with external defibrillation following advanced cardiac life support (ACLS) protocol. An energy level of 300 to 360 joules may be used because defibrillation has already been attempted by the AICD, and impedance levels have been lowered. Lidocaine is used after epinephrine has been administered; both drugs are used after attempts at defibrillation have been unsuccessful. Cardioversion is not indicated because the patient has pulseless ventricular tachycardia.
Nursing process step: Implementation
Cognitive level: Application

40. Which organism is the most common causative agent of bacterial endocarditis?
   A. *Aspergillus* species
   B. *Candida albicans*
   C. *Staphylococcus aureus*
   D. *Escherichia coli*

CORRECT ANSWER—C. Staphylococci and group A nonhemolytic streptococci are the most common causative organisms of bacterial endocarditis. *Aspergillus* and *Candida* species are the most common causative organisms of fungal endocarditis. *Escherichia coli* rarely causes bacterial endocarditis.
Nursing process step: Assessment
Cognitive level: Knowledge

41. The nurse is providing postoperative care for a patient who has undergone cardiac surgery and has atrial and ventricular epicardial wires in place. The patient develops atrial fibrillation with a ventricular response of 30 beats/minute. Which type of pacemaker should the nurse attach?
   A. Atrioventricular sequential pacemaker, asynchronous mode
   B. Atrial pacemaker, asynchronous mode
   C. Ventricular pacemaker, demand mode
   D. Ventricular pacemaker, asynchronous mode

CORRECT ANSWER—C. A patient in atrial fibrillation does not have normal communication between the atrium and the ventricle. Although some atrial electrical activity occurs, it is insufficient to produce a full atrial contraction along with its ensuing atrial kick, thereby resulting in decreased cardiac output. Thus, a ventricular pacemaker is the correct choice. Ventricular pacemakers usually are set in the demand mode for patients with intrinsic rhythms because of the risk of a pacemaker spike occurring on the T wave, which produces R-on-T phenomenon and possibly malignant ventricular rhythms. Atrioventricular sequential pacemakers require intact atrial activity and are not used in atrial fibrillation.
Nursing process step: Implementation
Cognitive level: Application

42. The nurse observes a patient with an acute occlusion of the anterior tibial artery lying in bed with the affected leg hanging over the bedside. The best action is to:
   A. Allow the patient to maintain this position because it improves arterial blood flow to the distal tissues
   B. Encourage the patient to elevate the leg because this position reduces edema
   C. Encourage the patient to elevate the leg because this position enhances blood flow from both the arterial and venous systems
   D. Explain to the patient that the position does not affect the delivery of arterial blood

CORRECT ANSWER—A. The dependent position is a compensatory behavior that may improve arterial blood flow to the distal tissues through gravity, thereby decreasing pain and increasing oxygen delivery. Elevating the leg has the opposite effect on arterial flow, reducing the delivery of blood to affected tissues. Edema can be reduced by elevating the limb, but this is not of primary importance in a patient with an acute arterial occlusion.
Nursing process step: Implementation
Cognitive level: Evaluation

43. The best approach for preventing hypovolemic shock in a patient with severe burns is to:
A. Administer dopamine
B. Apply medical antishock trousers (MAST suit)
C. Infuse I.V. fluids
D. Infuse fresh frozen plasma

CORRECT ANSWER—C. During the early postburn period, large amounts of plasma fluid extravasate into the interstitial spaces. Restoring the fluid loss is necessary to prevent hypovolemic shock; this is best accomplished with crystalloid and colloid solutions, such as albumin. Fresh frozen plasma is expensive and carries the risk of disease transmission. A MAST suit would be applied to treat, not prevent, shock. Dopamine causes vasoconstriction and elevates blood pressure, but it does not prevent the development of hypovolemia in burn patients.
Nursing process step: Implementation
Cognitive level: Application

44. After an exploratory laparotomy, a patient with normal sinus tachycardia develops sustained supraventricular tachycardia (SVT). The nurse would anticipate all of the following to occur except:
A. Hypotension
B. Increased myocardial oxygen demand
C. Seizures
D. Ischemia

CORRECT ANSWER—C. A patient with SVT typically does not have seizures unless the tachycardia is severe enough to cause cardiopulmonary arrest and subsequent hypoxia. The fast heart rate generated by SVT usually decreases cardiac output by decreasing ventricular filling time. SVT also increases myocardial oxygen demand while coronary perfusion is diminishing. This may cause ischemia and precipitate angina pectoris, hypotension, palpitations, dizziness, or syncope.
Nursing process step: Assessment
Cognitive level: Comprehension

Questions 45 to 48 refer to the following information:
A 74-year-old male patient is admitted to the intensive care unit with a tearing, knifelike pain in his chest and between his shoulders. Assessment reveals a right-arm blood pressure of 210/96 mm Hg, sinus tachycardia with a rate 120 beats/minute, and a respiratory rate of 28 breaths/minute. The patient's medical history includes tobacco use, chronic obstructive pulmonary disease (COPD), hypertension, and coronary artery disease that has been medically treated. His admitting diagnosis is thoracic aortic dissection.

45. During the initial assessment, the nurse would expect to note all of the following *except:*

A. Diastolic murmur indicative of aortic regurgitation

B. Oliguria with elevated blood urea nitrogen (BUN) and creatinine levels

C. Normal or low hematocrit and hemoglobin values

D. Lower left-arm blood pressure reading (146/82 mm Hg)

CORRECT ANSWER—B. Although the patient may exhibit acute oliguria, elevations of the BUN and creatinine levels would indicate acute intrarenal or postrenal failure or chronic renal failure, which are unlikely in this situation. This patient is more likely to have an elevated BUN level and a normal creatinine level, indicative of prerenal failure secondary to hypoperfusion of the kidneys. If the dissection extends into the aortic valve annulus, a diastolic murmur would be noted because of aortic regurgitation. Initial blood levels for a patient with this condition typically are normal; however, the levels can drop as blood shunts into the false lumen of the dissection. A blood pressure differential may exist between the two arms if the dissection begins at or near the left subclavian artery.
Nursing process step: Assessment
Cognitive level: Comprehension

46. Which medication would the nurse expect to administer early in this patient's treatment?

A. Propranolol (Inderal)

B. Nitroprusside sodium (Nipride)

C. Dopamine I.V. infusion at a rate of 6 mcg/kg/minute

D. I.M. meperidine (Demerol)

CORRECT ANSWER—B. Reducing the patient's blood pressure to limit the extent of the dissection is of paramount importance. Thus, nitroprusside sodium is an appropriate medication. Propranolol, a beta blocker, is contraindicated in patients with COPD. The vasoactive effects of dopamine at this dosage would increase the patient's blood pressure and the strength of the cardiac contraction, possibly extending the dissection. Because I.M. analgesics, such as meperidine, may not be completely absorbed in a patient with impending circulatory collapse, the I.V. route of administration is best.
Nursing process step: Planning
Cognitive level: Application

47. Which nursing intervention has top priority for this patient?

A. Insert an indwelling urinary (Foley) catheter and monitor urine output

B. Administer medications to reduce blood pressure

C. Prepare the patient for a chest computed tomography (CT) scan

D. Obtain an ECG

CORRECT ANSWER—B. Rapid reduction of blood pressure is necessary to limit the extent of the dissection. Urine output must be monitored, but it is not a top priority at this time. A chest CT scan and an ECG may be necessary for diagnosis but are not therapeutic priorities.
Nursing process step: Implementation
Cognitive level: Application

48. After surgical repair of the patient's thoracic aortic dissection, the nurse would:

A. Implement active range-of-motion exercises of the upper and lower extremities as soon as the patient is stable

B. Obtain an overhead trapeze for the bed to encourage the patient's independence and activity

C. Promote pulmonary hygiene measures to prevent pneumonia

D. Instruct the patient and family members about long-term anticoagulant therapy

CORRECT ANSWER—C. After thoracotomy, a patient is prone to atelectasis and left basilar lung changes. Therefore, the nurse should promote pulmonary hygiene measures to prevent pneumonia. Active range-of-motion exercises of the arms and use of an overhead trapeze can disrupt thoracic surgical closure and should be avoided until complete healing occurs. Routine long-term anticoagulant therapy generally is not prescribed unless the patient has undergone aortic valve replacement along with the aortic repair. **Nursing process step:** Implementation **Cognitive level:** Application

49. Which substance is the most common toxic causative agent for dilated (congestive) cardiomyopathy?

A. Alcohol

B. Marijuana

C. Cocaine

D. Lead

CORRECT ANSWER—A. Alcohol consumption can lead to severe cardiomyopathy as a result of direct toxic effects, nutritional deficits connected with thiamine deficiency, or toxic additives in alcohol preparations. Marijuana use and lead ingestion are not known to cause cardiomyopathy. Cocaine can cause severe hypertension and lead to coronary artery disease, but it is not directly linked to cardiomyopathy. **Nursing process step:** Assessment **Cognitive level:** Knowledge

50. Which treatment would be the best therapy for a stable patient with digitalis toxicity?

A. Activated charcoal

B. Time and symptomatic treatment

C. Hemodialysis

D. Atropine

CORRECT ANSWER—B. Stable patients with digitalis toxicity are best treated with time while their kidneys excrete the metabolites and with symptomatic treatment for the rhythm disturbances or nausea resulting from the toxicity. Activated charcoal is effective only if the patient has taken an overdose of digitalis and a large amount of unabsorbed drug is in the GI tract, before serum level is elevated. Hemodialysis is reserved for patients who are extremely unstable despite symptomatic treatment or who have inadequate renal function to excrete the drug. Atropine might be used to treat the bradycardia that results from digitalis toxicity, but it is not necessarily used to treat the toxicity itself. **Nursing process step:** Planning **Cognitive level:** Comprehension

51. Nursing care of a patient with an ischemic lower extremity includes:
A. Applying alcohol rubs to the affected area to toughen the skin
B. Using heating pads to enhance vasodilation
C. Applying antiembolism stockings to prevent venous thrombosis
D. Using a foot cradle and sheepskin to prevent mechanical trauma from bedclothes

CORRECT ANSWER—D. The nursing goals for a patient with ischemic vascular disease include prevention of mechanical, thermal, and chemical trauma. Alcohol dries the skin and exacerbates open cracks. Because patients with poor circulation are at high risk for burns and frostbite, heat and cold packs are contraindicated. Antiembolism stockings also are contraindicated because they can constrict arterial blood flow.
Nursing process step: Implementation
Cognitive level: Application

52. The survival rate following cardiac rupture is better in patients who have experienced:
A. Left ventricular tears
B. Right ventricular tears
C. Atrial tears
D. No other associated injuries

CORRECT ANSWER—C. Although survival after cardiac rupture is rare, patients with atrial tears may have an improved chance of survival because of the low pressure in the atrial chambers and, consequently, less blood loss. Nevertheless, immediate surgical repair is required.
Nursing process step: Evaluation
Cognitive level: Comprehension

53. Which of the following is the best long-term therapy for a patient with alcoholic cardiomyopathy?
A. Digoxin
B. Nifedipine
C. Alcohol abstinence
D. Low-salt diet

CORRECT ANSWER—C. A patient with alcoholic cardiomyopathy who receives acute therapy and completely abstains from alcohol has an excellent long-term outlook as long as heart failure has not set in. Digoxin, nifedipine, and a low-sodium diet are adjunctive therapies required during acute treatment of this condition.
Nursing process step: Implementation
Cognitive level: Analysis

54. Which therapy is usually considered inappropriate for the treatment of asystole?
A. Isoproterenol
B. Atropine
C. Epinephrine
D. Temporary pacing

CORRECT ANSWER—A. The only indications for isoproterenol in the advanced cardiac life support (ACLS) protocol are refractory torsades de pointes, symptomatic atrioventricular blockages not responsive to atropine while a pacemaker is being prepared for insertion, and immediate temporary control of symptomatic bradycardia in patients with denervated hearts. Atropine, a vagolytic agent, is given to patients with asystole whose rhythm does not respond to epinephrine. As a last resort in refractory asystole, the physician may attempt to insert a transvenous pacemaker to pace the heart.
Nursing process step: Implementation
Cognitive level: Application

55. When a patient is started on oral or I.V. diltiazem (Cardizem), the nurse should monitor for which potential complication?
A. Flushing
B. Heart failure
C. Renal failure
D. Hypertension

CORRECT ANSWER—B. The chief side effects of diltiazem are hypotension, atrioventricular blocks (atrioventricular node conduction and refractoriness are prolonged), congestive heart failure (diltiazem is a negative inotropic agent), and elevated liver enzyme levels. Other reactions that have been reported include flushing, nocturia, and polyuria, but not renal failure. Although flushing may occur, it is an adverse reaction, not a potential complication. Heart failure is a life-threatening reaction.
Nursing process step: Evaluation
Cognitive level: Comprehension

56. A patient admitted to the cardiac care unit with a diagnosis of acute myocardial infarction (MI) is being treated with I.V. lidocaine for frequent bursts of ventricular tachycardia. The patient continues to experience frequent premature ventricular contractions (PVCs) and bouts of ventricular tachycardia. The nurse should respond by:
A. Continuing to administer I.V. lidocaine to treat the PVCs
B. Doing nothing because PVCs are expected after acute MI
C. Switching the patient from lidocaine to procainamide
D. Administering I.V. potassium chloride

CORRECT ANSWER—C. In a patient with acute MI, PVCs are common and the potential for sustained ventricular tachycardia or ventricular fibrillation exists. Therefore, it is appropriate to treat these arrhythmias initially with lidocaine, then switch to a second antiarrhythmic agent, such as procainamide, if the lidocaine is not suppressing the arrhythmia. PVCs may indicate hypokalemia. In a patient with MI, the nurse must monitor carefully for hypokalemia to avoid potentially lethal sequelae. However, the nurse at the bedside would need to evaluate the patient's potassium level before administering I.V. potassium chloride.
Nursing process step: Evaluation
Cognitive level: Application

57. An initial compensatory mechanism in cardiogenic shock is:
A. Decreased heart rate
B. Increased heart rate
C. Increased cardiac output above baseline
D. Decreased stroke volume

CORRECT ANSWER—B. In cardiogenic shock, the decreased strength of the heart causes reduced stroke volume and, consequently, decreased cardiac output. The resulting decrease in blood pressure stimulates compensatory mechanisms. As a result of sympathetic stimulation, heart rate increases. In addition, myocardial contractility increases in an attempt to return cardiac output to normal level.
Nursing process step: Assessment
Cognitive level: Comprehension

58. The goal of oxygen therapy is to achieve a partial pressure of oxygen in arterial blood (PaO2) value of:
A. 40 to 60 mm Hg
B. 60 to 80 mm Hg
C. 70 to 100 mm Hg
D. More than 100 mm Hg

CORRECT ANSWER—**C.** The goal of oxygen therapy is to maintain PaO_2 between 70 and 100 mm Hg. The PaO_2 level in a healthy adult is between 80 and 100 mm Hg but becomes slightly lower with age. A PaO_2 less than 60 mm Hg may indicate dangerous hypoxia. A PaO_2 higher than 120 mm Hg is not necessary to perfuse end-organs (kidneys, heart, brain, and eyes), and oxygen toxicity can develop at a PaO_2 level above 150 mm Hg.
Nursing process step: Planning
Cognitive level: Application

59. The nurse in the intensive care unit is admitting a patient with a stab wound to the chest. Cardiac tamponade is suspected. Assessment of cardiac tamponade includes all of the following *except:*
A. Auscultatory finding of a small, quiet heart
B. Pulsus paradoxus
C. Low right atrial filling pressures
D. High right atrial filling pressures

CORRECT ANSWER—**C.** Cardiac tamponade occurs when the pericardial lining surrounding the myocardium is disrupted and excess fluid accumulates within the pericardial space. The excess fluid compresses the pumping action of the heart and impairs diastolic filling and cardiac function. Thus, a patient with cardiac tamponade exhibits high right atrial filling pressures because of the heart's inability to pump, pulsus paradoxus because of the decreased venous return with inspiration, and muffled heart sounds resulting from fluid accumulation in the pericardial space.
Nursing process step: Assessment
Cognitive level: Application

60. Aortic aneurysms are most likely to rupture:
A. In cigarette smokers
B. When the aneurysm is 6 cm or more in diameter
C. During periods of prolonged hypotension
D. When serum triglyceride level exceeds 300 mg/dl and low-density lipoprotein (LDL) level exceeds 180 mg/dl

CORRECT ANSWER—**B.** The incidence of aortic rupture is directly related to the size of the aneurysm. Thus, the risk of rupture increases significantly when the diameter exceeds 6 cm. Cigarette smoking and mixed hyperlipidemia (serum triglyceride level of 300 mg/dl and LDL level of 180 mg/dl) are risk factors for aneurysm formation. Hypertension, not hypotension, promotes aneurysm formation and rupture by causing endothelial injury and degeneration of the medial wall lining.
Nursing process step: Assessment
Cognitive level: Comprehension

61. Which finding is an early clinical indicator of hypovolemia?
   A. Postural hypotension
   B. Decreased blood urea nitrogen (BUN) level
   C. Hyperthermia
   D. Tachypnea

CORRECT ANSWER—A. A difference of more than 15 mm Hg between sitting and supine systolic blood pressure readings indicates postural hypotension, which commonly is caused by hypovolemia, inadequate vasoconstrictor mechanisms, or autonomic insufficiency. An elevated BUN level may indicate dehydration. Hyperthermia and tachypnea are late signs of hypovolemia.
Nursing process step: Assessment
Cognitive level: Evaluation

62. Valvular lesions of infective endocarditis are most likely to be isolated on:
   A. Both sides of the damaged valve
   B. The high-pressure side of the damaged valve
   C. The low-pressure side of the damaged valve
   D. The valve annulus

CORRECT ANSWER—C. Platelets adhere to the damaged endothelial surfaces of the damaged valve. The natural adhesiveness of platelets causes a platelet-fibrin mass that provides a protective haven for infective organisms. The platelet-fibrin mass is most protected and hence most likely to exist on the low-pressure side of the valve.
Nursing process step: Assessment
Cognitive level: Comprehension

63. Which statement about pericardial friction rub associated with pericarditis is true?
   A. It is independent of respiration
   B. It is independent of the cardiac cycle
   C. It is caused by inflammatory exudate
   D. It is caused by ventricular hypertrophy

CORRECT ANSWER—C. Pericardial friction rub results from inflammatory exudate, a fluid, and is affected by both the respiratory and cardiac cycles. Ventricular hypertrophy does not cause pericardial friction rub.
Nursing process step: Assessment
Cognitive level: Comprehension

Questions 64 to 66 refer to the following information:
A 33-year-old multiparous woman delivered a healthy boy 3 weeks ago. During the past 2 months, she has had shortness of breath, palpations, ankle edema, and fatigue, but attributed these symptoms to her late stage of pregnancy. When her symptoms worsened over the past few days, she arrived at the emergency department with the following findings: extreme shortness of breath, bilateral rales, atrial fibrillation with a ventricular response of 144 beats/minute, and hypotension manifested by a blood pressure of 84/56 mm Hg.

---

64. The patient is placed on a heart transplant list. In preparing the patient for a transplant, the nurse would:
A. Make every effort to limit invasive monitoring to prevent infection
B. Provide emotional support and education for the patient and her family
C. Transfuse the patient with packed red blood cells to optimize her oxygen-carrying capacity
D. Initiate parenteral nutrition

CORRECT ANSWER—**B.** The patient and her family most likely are in a state of shock and have multiple concerns about the outcome and the patient's ability to care for her new baby. Invasive monitoring is required during the acute phases of illness to optimize the patient's hemodynamic status until her symptoms improve. Efforts to limit blood transfusion are appropriate to prevent activation of antibodies that could preclude a good donor-recipient match. Good nutrition is imperative, but use of the GI tract is the best way to prevent infection because an I.V. access site could provide a port of entry for infection.
Nursing process step: Implementation
Cognitive level: Application

65. Which medications would the nurse anticipate administering to this patient initially?
A. Dopamine, nitroprusside sodium, and propranolol
B. Dopamine, digoxin, and verapamil
C. Dopamine, nitroprusside sodium, digoxin, and furosemide
D. Furosemide and procainamide

CORRECT ANSWER—**C.** Dopamine and nitroprusside sodium would be administered to increase contractility and improve blood pressure. Digoxin slows the heart rate, improves contractility, and may convert the atrial fibrillation. Furosemide would be administered as needed to reduce preload, maintain adequate urine output, and reduce peripheral and pulmonary edema. Nitroprusside sodium also may be useful in reducing afterload. Beta blockers, such as propranolol, decrease contractility and could be harmful. Verapamil and procainamide might be useful if the atrial fibrillation does not convert, but they would not be first-line agents. Verapamil may be added later as chronic therapy for afterload reduction.
Nursing process step: Planning
Cognitive level: Analysis

66. What hemodynamic response to pharmacologic therapy would the nurse consider beneficial for this patient?
A. Increase in pulmonary artery systolic pressure with a decrease in systemic vascular resistance (SVR)
B. Increase in arterial systolic pressure with an increase in SVR
C. Decrease in pulmonary artery systolic pressure with a decrease in SVR
D. Increase in pulmonary artery diastolic pressure with an increase in SVR

CORRECT ANSWER—**C.** A decrease in pulmonary artery systolic pressure with a concomitant decrease in SVR indicates adequate unloading therapy that would result in a subsequent decrease in the workload of the left ventricle and improved cardiac output. Any increase in pulmonary artery pressures indicates increased preload, which could suggest left ventricular distention and aggravated pulmonary edema. An increase in SVR (afterload) would increase the workload of the left ventricle.
Nursing process step: Evaluation
Cognitive level: Evaluation

67. The nurse caring for a patient with an acutely ischemic leg would closely monitor all cardiovascular parameters because:

A. It is routine procedure in critical care units to monitor ECGs and vital signs closely

B. The patient is at high risk for shock due to lactic acidosis secondary to the ischemic extremity

C. Patients with ischemic extremities often are hypovolemic because of fluid sequestration in the affected limb

D. Nearly half of the patients with symptomatic peripheral vascular disease have clinically detectable coronary artery disease, cerebrovascular disease, or hypertension

CORRECT ANSWER—D. Nearly half of all patients with symptomatic peripheral vascular disease have significant arterial disease elsewhere in their bodies because the disease is systemic and chronic. Data from the Framingham Heart Study suggest that the incidence of coronary disease is 2.4 times greater in men and 1.4 times greater in women with peripheral vascular disease compared to those without peripheral vascular disease (Sytkowkski, P., Kannel, W., and D'Agostino, R., "Changes in risk factors and the decline in mortality from cardiovascular disease." The Framingham Heart Study. *New England Journal of Medicine*, June 7, 1990.). Unit procedure should not dictate the reason why nurses implement monitoring techniques. Lactic acidosis may be a consequence of lactate release from acutely ischemic tissues. Although common in patients with shock, the presence of lactate does not cause shock. Dehydration can predispose patients to further hemoconcentration, but ischemic extremities do not sequester fluid.
Nursing process step: Assessment
Cognitive level: Application

Questions 68 and 69 refer to the following information:
A 56-year-old female patient is admitted to the cardiac care unit (CCU) with a diagnosis of unstable angina. She has a 2-year history of angina and states that she frequently uses Mylanta at home for heartburn but obtains no relief.

---

68. Which information is most pertinent for the patient to know before being sent to the cardiac catheterization laboratory?

A. Morbidity statistics related to arteriography

B. Lifestyle changes necessary because of unstable angina

C. Potential complications of cardiac catheterization

D. Preoperative and postoperative procedure care

CORRECT ANSWER—D. Patient teaching is an important aspect of care in any situation. For this patient, it would be most pertinent for her to know what to expect before and after the procedure. The nurse should not focus on statistics or complications; the physician will describe these when the patient's consent is obtained. Because the nurse cannot accurately project the patient's outcome at discharge, predicting any lifestyle changes is impossible at this point.
Nursing process step: Implementation
Cognitive level: Synthesis

69. The patient undergoes coronary angioplasty of the left anterior descending artery. When transferring the patient from the CCU to a telemetry unit, the nurse should make sure the patient knows:

A. The amount of fat she can consume in her diet
B. The level of activity she can achieve at home
C. The importance of reporting any discomforts promptly to nurses on the telemetry unit
D. The need to store sublingual nitroglycerin away from bright light

CORRECT ANSWER—C. The CCU nurse should ensure that the patient is aware of the importance of reporting any physical discomforts to the staff of the telemetry unit. The nurse on the step-down telemetry unit will provide the patient with discharge instructions, including information about diet, activity level, and medication.
Nursing process step: Planning
Cognitive level: Application

70. Which rhythm can be considered a form of supraventricular tachycardia (SVT)?

A. Second-degree atrioventricular (AV) block, Mobitz type I
B. Ventricular tachycardia
C. Atrial tachycardia
D. First-degree AV block

CORRECT ANSWER—C. In SVT, the heart rate is rapid, the QRS complexes are normal, and P waves often are not identifiable. The term *supraventricular* also suggests that the pacemaker is above the ventricles, somewhere in the atria or AV junction. Ventricular tachycardia originates in the ventricles. First-degree and second-degree (Mobitz type I) AV blocks usually are not tachycardic; they typically are associated with atrial heart rates between 60 and 100 beats/minute.
Nursing process step: Assessment
Cognitive level: Comprehension

Questions 71 to 74 refer to the following information:
A 68-year-old female patient is admitted to the hospital with crushing chest pain. A sample of her cardiac rhythm strip is pictured below.

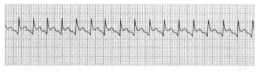

---

71. How would the nurse assess this rhythm?

A. Sinus tachycardia with peaked T wave
B. Sinus tachycardia with inverted T wave
C. Sinus tachycardia with ST-segment elevation
D. Sinus tachycardia with ST-segment depression

CORRECT ANSWER—C. P waves are 1:1 with the QRS complex, the rate is approximately 170 beats/minute, and the ST segment is elevated, indicating an acute ischemic process.
Nursing process step: Assessment
Cognitive level: Analysis

72. Which medications would the nurse expect to administer to this patient?
  A. Oxygen, metoprolol, digoxin, and morphine
  B. Oxygen, digoxin, morphine, and nitroglycerin
  C. Oxygen, morphine, nitroglycerin, and lidocaine
  D. Oxygen, metoprolol, morphine, and nitroglycerin

CORRECT ANSWER—D. Nitroglycerin dilates the coronary arteries, enhancing the myocardial oxygen supply. Morphine controls pain, and both morphine and nitroglycerin produce venous dilation, which decreases venous return to the heart and consequently decreases the workload of the heart. Metoprolol slows the heart rate and decreases myocardial oxygen consumption. Oxygen increases the available oxygen supply. Digoxin is not a first-line drug in patients with acute ischemia because it can increase myocardial oxygen consumption. Lidocaine should be used only as needed to treat ventricular arrhythmias.
Nursing process step: Planning
Cognitive level: Application

73. The physician has ordered tissue plasminogen activator (TPA) for the patient. Knowledge about this medication would prompt the nurse to:
  A. Closely monitor the patient for an allergic response to the drug
  B. Ensure that the patient has a central vascular access line for administration of TPA
  C. Limit venipunctures during the administration of TPA
  D. Implement a teaching plan for the patient and family regarding thrombolytic agent therapy before administering TPA

CORRECT ANSWER—C. Patients receiving any type of thrombolytic agent are at high risk for bleeding complications. For this reason, invasive procedures, such as venipuncture, should be limited as much as possible during administration of thrombolytic drugs. Allergic responses are common after streptokinase infusion, but rare after infusion of TPA. Teaching the patient and family members about the therapy is important, but should be done after TPA is administered. TPA is not caustic to veins and therefore does not require central vascular access line (although it may be preferred).
Nursing process step: Implementation
Cognitive level: Knowledge

74. The critical care nurse would consider TPA therapy effective after observing which ECG changes in the patient's rhythm?
  A. Decreased heart rate
  B. Development of reperfusion arrhythmias
  C. Return of the ST segment to baseline
  D. Depression of the ST segment

CORRECT ANSWER—C. ST-segment elevation is a sign of acute ischemia, and its return to baseline indicates that the myocardium is receiving an adequate oxygen supply. Decreased heart rate may result from the effects of other medications or as a consequence of the decreased myocardial ischemia; however, it is not evidence of effective thrombolysis. Reperfusion arrhythmias may occur during or after administration of the thrombolytic agent, but they also are not evidence of effective thrombolysis. Depression of the ST segment occurs with a posterior wall infarct.
Nursing process step: Evaluation
Cognitive level: Evaluation

75. Mediastinal widening on the chest X-ray film of a multiple trauma patient suggests:
A. Diaphragmatic hernia
B. Pneumothorax
C. Hemothorax
D. Aortic disruption

CORRECT ANSWER—D. The aortic arch is highly visible in the mediastinal shadow on a chest X-ray film, and widening suggests aortic disruption. A further workup is warranted in this situation. A diaphragmatic hernia is suspected when the patient has associated abdominal trauma and the abdominal contents are transposed onto the chest X-ray film. Pneumothorax is identified by separation of the lung markings from the chest wall on the X-ray film. Hemothorax is distinguished by a fluid density on the affected side on the chest X-ray film.
Nursing process step: Assessment
Cognitive level: Evaluation

76. The activity level for a patient with cardiomyopathy should be:
A. Limited to strict bed rest until a transplant becomes available
B. Directed at helping the patient maintain independent activities of daily living
C. Based on the patient's tolerance to incremental increases in exertion
D. Limited to passive range-of-motion exercises

CORRECT ANSWER—C. Efforts should be made early to prevent deconditioning during the patient's course of treatment. Progression of activities should be based on vital signs, ECG rhythm, and emotional tolerance. Strict bed rest or minimal activity (passive range of motion) promotes detrimental skeletal and cardiopulmonary deterioration. Independent activities of daily living may not be possible for a patient with end-stage cardiomyopathy.
Nursing process step: Implementation
Cognitive level: Application

77. When assisting the physician during pericardiocentesis, the nurse would:
A. Monitor the ECG for ST-segment elevation, which indicates that the needle has made contact with the epicardium
B. Assess the character of the fluid, noting that pericardial fluid should clot rapidly
C. Assist in aspirating at least 200 ml of blood from the pericardial sac to provide symptom relief
D. Instruct the patient that the procedure rarely needs to be repeated

CORRECT ANSWER—A. An injury pattern on the ECG suggests that the needle has gone through the pericardium and epicardium and should be withdrawn. Pericardial fluid usually is partly blood and contains inflammatory exudate. Unlike ventricular blood, it generally does not clot rapidly. The removal of 25 to 100 ml of fluid from the pericardium often provides significant relief of symptoms. Depending on the cause of pericardial fluid, pericardiocentesis may need to be repeated; a drainage catheter sometimes is placed on subsequent attempts. If these procedures are unsuccessful and the pericarditis is chronic, pericardiectomy may be performed.
Nursing process step: Implementation
Cognitive level: Application

78. A 34-year-old cancer patient arrives at the emergency department complaining of orthostatic hypotension and vomiting for the past 3 days. What should the nurse do first?
A. Administer an antiemetic to stop the vomiting
B. Obtain cultures and administer antibiotics to combat probable sepsis
C. Start a dopamine I.V. infusion to maintain a systolic blood pressure above 90 mm Hg
D. Infuse I.V. fluids to treat hypovolemia

CORRECT ANSWER—**D.** The patient probably is hypovolemic because of the loss of large amounts of fluid resulting from vomiting; it is unlikely that he has been able to replace the fluid loss orally. The patient probably will need lactated Ringer's solution with potassium chloride to combat his low fluid status. Antiemetics also should be administered, but this is not the first action the nurse would take. The patient may have sepsis as a result of immunosuppressant therapy, but the decision to obtain cultures and administer antibiotics should be based on more than just orthostatic hypotension. Dopamine would be appropriate only after the patient has been adequately hydrated and still is hypotensive.
Nursing process step: Planning
Cognitive level: Application

Questions 79 to 83 refer to the following information:
A 26-year-old female patient is admitted to the intensive care unit (ICU) with bacterial endocarditis. At the time of admission, she has a fever of 103.6° F (39.8° C), a blood pressure of 94/62 mm Hg, supraventricular tachycardia (SVT) with 162 beats/minute, and a respiratory rate of 22 breaths/minute. Her physical examination reveals dyspnea, rales throughout all lung fields, hematuria, splenomegaly, and a systolic murmur over the mitral valve.

---

79. What is the best diagnostic test for identifying the cardiac manifestations of this patient's endocarditis?
A. Right- and left-heart catheterization
B. ECG
C. Echocardiogram
D. Nuclear stress test

CORRECT ANSWER—**C.** The echocardiogram is a noninvasive diagnostic test that provides the health care team with a precise image of the cardiac valves and myocardial function. Cardiac catheterization also provides helpful information about the heart valves, cardiac function, and coronary anatomy; however, this procedure places the patient at risk for disruption of valvular vegetation and embolization. An ECG provides information about cardiac rhythm, ischemia, and axis deviation, but would not offer specific information about the endocarditis. The nuclear stress test would provide information only about ischemic areas of the heart and would not be useful in this patient.
Nursing process step: Assessment
Cognitive level: Comprehension

80. During the first few hours of the patient's ICU stay, the nurse would:
  A. Administer I.V. antibiotics, then obtain blood cultures
  B. Prepare the patient for mitral valve replacement
  C. Assist with insertion of a Hickman catheter for long-term antibiotic administration
  D. Obtain blood cultures, then administer I.V. antibiotics

CORRECT ANSWER—D. The patient requires broad-spectrum antibiotics until the blood culture results are available. Cultures should always be obtained before antibiotic therapy is started to avoid false-negative results. The patient probably will need a mitral valve replacement. However, this procedure should be performed several months later, after the blood has been sterilized and the patient is not actively infected; an active infection would increase the patient's risk of surgical complications. Extended antibiotic administration via a Hickman or another long-term central catheter should be in the patient's discharge plan, not part of an initial intervention.
Nursing process step: Implementation
Cognitive level: Application

81. The nurse would anticipate which laboratory finding in this patient?
  A. Elevated hematocrit
  B. Low number of immature granulocytes
  C. Elevated erythrocyte sedimentation rate
  D. Elevated creatinine level

CORRECT ANSWER—C. An elevated erythrocyte sedimentation rate is a nonspecific indication of inflammation. Because the patient has an active infection, the nurse would expect an elevated erythrocyte sedimentation rate. Hematocrit and hemoglobin values would be low or normal, not elevated. The white blood cell differential count would show a normal or high number of immature cells. The creatinine level probably would be normal, unless the patient had a renal artery embolization that caused renal ischemia, which might be indicated by hematuria.
Nursing process step: Assessment
Cognitive level: Comprehension

82. The teaching plan for this patient would include information about:
  A. Birth control methods, including oral contraceptives, diaphragms, and intrauterine devices
  B. Daily prophylactic antibiotic therapy
  C. Routine oral hygiene and the need to avoid dental floss
  D. Prophylactic antibiotic therapy for certain invasive procedures

CORRECT ANSWER—D. The patient will require prophylactic antibiotics for certain invasive procedures, such as dental procedures, but she must be instructed to limit the duration of the prophylaxis to prevent microbial resistance. Intrauterine devices are contraindicated in patients with diseased valves and those with valve replacements because the devices are a potential source of infection. Use of dental floss and good oral hygiene should be encouraged to prevent endocarditis secondary to gingival disease. However, endocarditis can result from a cut in the gum incurred during flossing.
Nursing process step: Implementation
Cognitive level: Application

83. The most effective initial therapy for this patient would include:

A. Esmolol hydrochloride to treat supraventricular tachycardia (SVT)

B. Dopamine to treat hypotension

C. Mannitol to treat hematuria

D. Acetaminophen to treat fever

CORRECT ANSWER—**A.** The patient's heart rate of 162 beats/minute is higher than the nurse would expect as a result of fever; if the rate is not controlled, the patient's condition can worsen. Esmolol hydrochloride is an ultra-short-acting beta-adrenergic blocker used to control heart rate in patients with SVT. Dopamine would be administered if the patient's blood pressure dropped further, but 94/62 mm Hg is an adequate blood pressure for a young woman. Mannitol could be administered if hematuria were severe and acetaminophen could be given if the patient were uncomfortable from the fever; however, these are not the best treatments in this situation.

Nursing process step: Implementation

Cognitive level: Analysis

84. The nurse should be prepared to manage complications after abdominal aneurysm resection. Which of the following complications is most common postoperatively?

A. Renal failure

B. Hemorrhage and shock

C. Graft occlusion

D. Enteric fistula

CORRECT ANSWER—**B.** Hemorrhage and shock are the most common complications after abdominal aneurysm resection. Renal failure can occur as a result of shock or from injury to the renal arteries during surgery. Graft occlusion and enteric fistula formation are rare complications of abdominal aortic aneurysm repair.

Nursing process step: Evaluation

Cognitive level: Evaluation

85. The nurse should be alert for aortic aneurysm formation in which group of young adults?

A. Tall, lanky adolescents with sternal abnormalities

B. Cocaine abusers

C. Obese youths

D. Young athletes with a history of multiple orthopedic injuries

CORRECT ANSWER—**A.** The physical prototype of long extremities, tall stature, and sternal deformities corresponds with Marfan syndrome, a connective tissue disorder linked to degeneration of the elastic fibers in the aortic media and subsequent dissection of the aorta. Although cocaine abuse is associated with a high incidence of sudden death and premature coronary disease, it is not related to aortic aneurysm. Obesity can be associated with hypertension and hyperlipidemia, which are risk factors for aneurysm formation later in life. However, obesity is not directly linked to aneurysm formation. Orthopedic injuries are not associated with aortic aneurysm.

Nursing process step: Assessment

Cognitive level: Knowledge

86. Chest pain associated with aortic stenosis can be caused by:
   A. Underlying coronary artery disease
   B. Disproportionate oxygen supply versus demand
   C. Prolapsed valve leaflets
   D. Both A and B

CORRECT ANSWER—**D.** Approximately 50% of patients with aortic stenosis develop chest pain (angina). The causes of this pain may be related to underlying coronary artery disease or an imbalance in the oxygen supply to the myocardium and the oxygen demands of the body. Oxygen supply to the heart can be influenced by coronary artery anatomy, diastolic time, diastolic filling pressures, and the ability to extract oxygen by the tissues. Oxygen demands can be increased by increases in heart rate, afterload, preload, and contractility. Aortic stenosis occurs when the valve leaflets are calcified and stiff; prolapsed valve leaflets occur in aortic insufficiency.
Nursing process step: Assessment
Cognitive level: Application

87. The nurse caring for a patient in cardiogenic shock would expect the arterial blood gas analysis to reveal which imbalance?
   A. Respiratory acidosis
   B. Metabolic alkalosis
   C. Respiratory alkalosis
   D. Metabolic acidosis

CORRECT ANSWER—**D.** Cardiogenic shock occurs when the heart fails to pump and tissue perfusion is impaired. With impaired tissue perfusion, anaerobic metabolism occurs and lactic acid production leads to metabolic acidosis. As a respiratory compensatory mechanism in this acid-base state, a patient who is not mechanically ventilated will attempt to rid the body of excess acid in the form of carbon dioxide, with an increased rate and depth of respirations. This may lead to a compensatory respiratory alkalosis, but this is secondary to the body's response to metabolic acidosis. Respiratory acidosis is seen in conditions in which hypoventilation occurs, such as in pulmonary failure and oversedation. Metabolic alkalosis is seen in conditions in which a loss of hydrochloric acid occurs, such as in vomiting.
Nursing process step: Assessment
Cognitive level: Comprehension

88. Which of the following is a major complication associated with thrombolytic agent therapy?
   A. Extension of the infarct
   B. Presence of pulmonary emboli
   C. Bleeding
   D. Coronary artery rupture

CORRECT ANSWER—**C.** Bleeding is a major complication of thrombolytic agent therapy. Frequent monitoring of laboratory values (partial thromboplastin time, thrombin time, fibrinogen, fibrinogen split products, and hemoglobin) should be done. The patient's neurologic status also should be monitored; even though the risk of cerebral bleeding is low, the damage can be extensive. The nurse should avoid all needle punctures and frequently assess all potential bleeding sites, especially I.V. access sites. The nurse should also assess for internal bleeding (lower back pain, abdominal distention, guaiac-positive drainage or output, decreased pulses, and headache or confusion). Extension of the infarct, pulmonary emboli, and coronary artery rupture are not complications of thrombolytic agent therapy. The area of a myocardial infarction may increase, and coronary artery rupture most often is associated with invasive procedures. Thrombolytics dissolve all clots, including emboli.
Nursing process step: Assessment
Cognitive level: Knowledge

89. The nurse would observe which rhythm disturbances in a patient with digitalis toxicity?
   A. Atrial fibrillation
   B. Second-degree atrioventricular heart block, Mobitz type II
   C. Ventricular fibrillation
   D. All of the above

CORRECT ANSWER—**D.** Virtually any heart rhythm can be produced by digitalis toxicity, including sinoatrial blocks, paroxysmal atrial tachycardia, atrioventricular (AV) blocks, tachycardia with AV dissociation, ventricular ectopy, ventricular tachycardia, ventricular fibrillation, and atrial fibrillation.
Nursing process step: Assessment
Cognitive level: Evaluation

90. Which of the following procedures would be used to differentiate restrictive pericarditis from constrictive pericarditis?
   A. Echocardiogram
   B. Multiple-gated acquisition (MUGA) scan
   C. Endomyocardial biopsy
   D. Electrophysiologic studies

CORRECT ANSWER—C. The primary indication for an endomyocardial biopsy is to monitor a patient for rejection after a cardiac transplant. This procedure also can be used to detect myocarditis, as well as cardiac toxicity in patients receiving chemotherapy. An endomyocardial biopsy also may be helpful in differentiating restrictive pericarditis from constrictive pericarditis. An echocardiogram is used to study structural abnormalities and blood flow dynamics. A MUGA scan provides information about the ability of the right and left sides of the heart to pump adequately and about the ejection fractions of both the right and left ventricles. Electrophysiologic studies are used to evaluate the electrical activity of the heart and any related pathophysiology.
Nursing process step: Implementation
Cognitive level: Analysis

91. A patient with aortic stenosis may exhibit clinical symptoms associated with:
   A. Peripheral edema
   B. Angina
   C. Palpitations
   D. Headache

CORRECT ANSWER—B. Clinical symptoms associated with aortic stenosis include angina, arrhythmia, myocardial infarction, syncope, fatigue, cough, exertional dyspnea, orthopnea, paroxysmal nocturnal dyspnea, pulmonary edema, faint peripheral pulses, exercise intolerance, and systolic murmur.
Nursing process step: Assessment
Cognitive level: Evaluation

92. I.V. fluids are given to a patient in cardiogenic shock to correct hypovolemia. The nurse, while monitoring the volume of fluid being infused, would notify the physician if the patient develops:
   A. Central venous pressure of 0 to 6 mm Hg
   B. Pulmonary capillary wedge pressure of 15 mm Hg
   C. Clinical signs of pulmonary congestion
   D. PaO_2 of 70 mm Hg

CORRECT ANSWER—C. If the initial pulmonary capillary wedge pressure is between 15 and 18 mm Hg, an I.V. fluid challenge should be done. Further administration of fluids depends on increases in the wedge pressure, changes in blood pressure, and the presence or absence of clinical signs of pulmonary congestion. Pulmonary congestion rarely occurs when the wedge pressure is less than 18 mm Hg. Moderate congestion occurs with wedge pressures between 20 and 25 mm Hg; severe congestion, between 25 and 30 mm Hg; and pulmonary edema, above 30 mm Hg. A central venous pressure between 0 and 6 mm Hg indicates hypovolemia, and a PaO_2 of 70 mm Hg is the goal.
Nursing process step: Implementation
Cognitive level: Application

93. Which nursing intervention is inappropriate for a patient admitted to the cardiac care unit with a diagnosis of unstable angina?
  A. Establishing a patent I.V. line
  B. Administering supplemental oxygen
  C. Maintaining nothing-by-mouth (NPO) status
  D. Providing a calming environment

CORRECT ANSWER—C. Treatment goals for a patient with angina focus on balancing oxygen supply and demand. Maintaining a patient on NPO status does nothing to improve the oxygen balance. Establishing a patent I.V. line is important for administering medications and may be needed in an emergency. Administering oxygen is appropriate because the patient will have increased myocardial oxygen consumption and demands. Providing a calming environment helps alleviate anxiety, which can increase the heart rate and further increase myocardial oxygen needs.
Nursing process step: Implementation
Cognitive level: Application

Questions 94 to 96 refer to the following information:
A 44-year-old male patient is admitted to the cardiac care unit (CCU) to rule out myocardial infarction. He reports that he became nauseated, short of breath, and dizzy after eating a fairly large lunch and that this was enough to cause significant discomfort and a call to the paramedics. The nurse's initial assessment reveals:
  • skin: pale, gray, and diaphoretic
  • vital signs: blood pressure, 98/62 mm Hg; heart rate, 90 beats/minute and irregular; respiratory rate, 24 breaths/minute
  • lungs: scattered rales and rhonchi
  • heart sounds: S_1, S_2, and S_3, but no murmur or rub
  • 12-lead ECG: sinus tachycardia with multifocal premature ventricular contractions, ST-segment elevations in leads V_1 to V_4, and reciprocal changes in leads II, III, and aV_F
  • cardiac enzymes: aspartate aminotransferase (AST), 25 IU/liter; total creatine kinase (CK), 529 units/liter; and total lactate dehydrogenase (LD), 237 units/liter.

---

94. Which clinical finding is most common in patients with acute heart failure?
  A. S_3 gallop
  B. Sinus bradycardia
  C. Fever
  D. Ascites

CORRECT ANSWER—A. Heart sounds in severe forms of congestive heart failure often are obscured by rales in the lung fields. The pulmonic component of the second heart sound tends to be accentuated, and an S_3 gallop commonly is present. In acute heart failure, the low blood pressure resulting from low cardiac output triggers receptors to increase sympathetic nervous stimulation, and heart rate increases as a compensatory response. Ascites is a clinical finding of right-sided congestive heart failure. Fever is not associated with heart failure.
Nursing process step: Assessment
Cognitive level: Evaluation

95. In a patient with compensated heart failure, the CCU nurse would expect to discover all of the following *except:*
A. Arterial oxygen saturation of 97%
B. Acute prerenal failure
C. Mean right atrial pressure of 10 mm Hg
D. Elevated catecholamine level

CORRECT ANSWER—B. The body responds to heart failure with three compensatory mechanisms. The first compensatory mechanism is activation of the autonomic nervous system, which increases the level of circulating catecholamines and the retention of sodium and water. The second compensatory mechanism causes myocardial hypertrophy, which increases filling pressure, as evidenced by a mean right atrial pressure of 10 mm Hg (normal right atrial pressure is 2 to 8 mm Hg). The third compensatory mechanism causes more 2,3-diphosphoglycerate to circulate, which increases oxygen delivery to the tissues, as indicated by an arterial oxygen saturation of 97%. Failure of the heart to pump sufficient blood for adequate kidney function results in decompensation. A patient with heart failure who is not compensating sufficiently will not be adequately perfusing vital organs, such as the kidneys. Thus, acute prerenal failure can occur secondary to hypoperfusion.
Nursing process step: Assessment
Cognitive level: Analysis

96. The most likely cause of this patient's heart failure is:
A. Hypertension
B. Chronic obstructive pulmonary disease (COPD)
C. Acute myocardial infarction (MI)
D. Mitral regurgitation

CORRECT ANSWER—C. From the nurse's assessment of the precipitating events leading to the patient's admission to the CCU and the subsequent changes in cardiac enzymes and 12-lead ECG, the most probable cause of the acute heart failure is left ventricular failure secondary to acute MI. The most common cause of congestive heart failure (CHF) is decreased left ventricular function following MI. With a blood pressure of 98/62 mm Hg, the patient is not hypertensive. Patients with COPD commonly experience shortness of breath and tachypnea. This patient has a respiratory rate of 24 breaths/minute. Also, patients with COPD usually display signs of right ventricular failure because the right heart has difficulty pumping blood through the diseased lungs. Although mitral regurgitation can lead to CHF, a loud systolic murmur would be present in such a case.
Nursing process step: Assessment
Cognitive level: Analysis

97. Which narcotic is indicated for a patient with acute heart failure?
  A. Codeine sulfate
  B. Midazolam (Versed)
  C. Meperidine (Demerol)
  D. Morphine sulfate

CORRECT ANSWER—D. Morphine sulfate is considered the narcotic agent of choice in cardiac patients because it not only relieves pain and anxiety but also decreases preload because of its vasodilating effects. The sedative-hypnotic midazolam (Versed) is used cautiously in patients with acute heart failure because it can cause variations in blood pressure. Codeine sulfate is used to treat mild to moderate pain but is 10 times less potent than morphine sulfate. Neither codeine nor meperidine decreases preload, which is a benefit of morphine sulfate.
Nursing process step: Implementation
Cognitive level: Comprehension

98. Vasodilators are among the drugs used to control blood pressure during a hypertensive crisis. This group of medications includes:
  A. Methyldopa (Aldomet)
  B. Captopril (Capoten)
  C. Nitroprusside sodium (Nipride)
  D. Ethacrynic acid (Edecrin)

CORRECT ANSWER—C. I.V. vasodilators are used to manage hypertensive crises because of their rapid onset of action and because they are titratable. These agents include nitroprusside, trimethaphan, diazoxide, hydralazine, and nitroglycerin. The antihypertensive agent methyldopa has a peak action 2 to 4 hours after administration. Captopril, an antihypertensive of the renin-angiotensin antagonist class, has a half-life of 6 to 7 hours. Thus, methyldopa and captopril are unsuitable for treating a hypertensive crisis. Ethacrynic acid is a loop diuretic used to treat pulmonary edema.
Nursing process step: Implementation
Cognitive level: Knowledge

99. A patient with mitral valve stenosis develops atrial fibrillation while hospitalized. The treatment plan should include:
  A. Anticoagulant therapy
  B. Antiarrhythmic therapy
  C. Beta-blocker therapy
  D. Both A and B

CORRECT ANSWER—D. A patient with an atrial arrhythmia must be monitored for systemic embolization caused by blood clots forming in the atria. The patient should receive anticoagulant therapy and an atrial antiarrhythmic agent to control the atrial fibrillation and attempt to convert the arrhythmia to a normal sinus rhythm. Beta blockers primarily are indicated for control of recurrent ventricular tachycardia and recurrent ventricular fibrillation.
Nursing process step: Planning
Cognitive level: Application

100. The nurse typically would assess for all of the following signs and symptoms of dissecting abdominal aortic aneurysm *except:*
A. Hypotension
B. Severe abdominal pain
C. Cool, mottled lower extremities
D. Dyspnea

CORRECT ANSWER—**D.** Dyspnea is more likely to be associated with an aortic arch aneurysm impinging on the pulmonary structures than with a dissecting abdominal aortic aneurysm. Hypotension, severe abdominal pain, and cool, mottled legs are the cardinal signs of dissecting abdominal aortic aneurysm.
Nursing process step: Assessment
Cognitive level: Knowledge

101. The nurse should be alert for complications associated with embolic phenomena in which group of patients regardless of their disease stage?
A. Patients with dilated (congestive) cardiomyopathy
B. Patients with hypertrophic cardiomyopathy
C. Patients with restrictive cardiomyopathy
D. Patients with myocarditis

CORRECT ANSWER—**A.** Patients with dilated cardiomyopathy develop reduced ventricular ejection with elevations in the left ventricular end-diastolic pressure and subsequent decreases in the ejection fraction. This predisposes these patients to mural thrombi that can break loose and become embolisms. Patients with hypertrophic cardiomyopathy usually have hyperdynamic left ventricle and high ejection fractions. Patients with restrictive cardiomyopathy and those with myocarditis can develop congestive heart failure with the potential for thrombus formation, but this occurs late in the course of the disease and is not as common as with dilated cardiomyopathy.
Nursing process step: Planning
Cognitive level: Evaluation

Questions 102 to 107 refer to the following information:
A 67-year-old female patient underwent coronary artery bypass surgery 1 hour ago and is now in the intensive care unit (ICU). She has lost 350 ml of blood from her mediastinal tubes since her admission to the ICU. Her blood pressure is 168/84 mm Hg and her heart rate is 144 beats/minute. Respirations are controlled by mechanical ventilation. The patient has a pulmonary artery catheter in place, and her readings are 21/8 mm Hg, with a wedge pressure of 6 mm Hg.

102. Which assessment parameter is most important to monitor over the course of the next hour?
A. Central venous pressure
B. Pulse rate
C. Pulmonary artery pressure
D. Amount of chest tube drainage

CORRECT ANSWER—**D.** During the first postoperative hour, 350 ml of blood drained from the mediastinal tubes. If the drainage continues at this rate, surgical exploration may be necessary to identify and stop any possible source of bleeding. Although vital signs and pulmonary artery pressures must be monitored, they are less important than the amount of chest tube drainage in determining the patient's fluid status.
Nursing process step: Assessment
Cognitive level: Analysis

103. Which finding would the nurse expect to see on the patient's chest X-ray film?
A. Widened mediastinum
B. Pulmonary edema
C. Bibasilar pleural effusions
D. Pulmonary infiltrates

CORRECT ANSWER—**A.** In this situation, a widened mediastinum would indicate cardiac tamponade resulting from postoperative hemorrhage. The other findings would not be expected during the immediate postoperative period.
Nursing process step: Assessment
Cognitive level: Comprehension

104. Which medication would the nurse expect to administer first?
A. Nitroprusside sodium
B. Dopamine hydrochloride
C. Digoxin
D. Verapamil

CORRECT ANSWER—**A.** The patient's blood pressure must be reduced to maintain the patency of the coronary artery graft and to decrease the rate of blood loss. Because the patient is not hypotensive, dopamine is not indicated. The tachycardia the patient is experiencing probably is secondary to hemorrhage, so digoxin and verapamil should not be administered until the underlying problem is addressed.
Nursing process step: Planning
Cognitive level: Application

105. Which adjustment might the nurse make to the mechanical ventilator to help reduce the bleeding?
A. Increase the rate
B. Increase the positive end-expiratory pressure
C. Increase the tidal volume
D. Increase the inspired oxygen concentration

CORRECT ANSWER—**B.** Positive end-expiratory pressure may help reduce mediastinal bleeding by applying a mechanical tamponade to the bleeding chest. The other interventions would not affect the bleeding.
Nursing process step: Implementation
Cognitive level: Application

106. The nurse increases the positive end-expiratory pressure (PEEP) to 10 cm H_2O, and the cardiac index falls to 1.6 liters/minute. What is the best explanation for this decrease?
A. The large amount of blood loss caused a decrease in the stroke volume and a subsequent decrease in cardiac output
B. The tachycardia caused a decrease in the filling pressures and a subsequent decrease in cardiac output
C. The PEEP caused a decrease in venous return and a subsequent decrease in cardiac output
D. The PEEP caused a pneumothorax and a subsequent decrease in cardiac output

CORRECT ANSWER—**C.** A high PEEP will decrease venous return to the right side of the heart and subsequently decrease cardiac output. This effect is pronounced in hypovolemic patients. Although the other explanations are possible, they are not likely to be the cause of the reduced cardiac output because the cardiac index decreased after the PEEP was increased.
Nursing process step: Evaluation
Cognitive level: Analysis

107. What nursing intervention would best treat this patient's low cardiac index?
A. Administering I.V. fluids
B. Turning off PEEP
C. Administering dopamine
D. Inserting a chest tube

CORRECT ANSWER—A. Restoring the circulating blood volume reduces the effect of PEEP on venous return and cardiac output. Because PEEP offers the therapeutic benefit of reducing the rate of mediastinal blood loss, it should be continued if the patient can tolerate it. Dopamine would only serve to vasoconstrict and further aggravate the tachycardia. It also would not increase the cardiac index because circulating blood volume needs to be replaced first. Chest tube insertion is indicated only if there is clinical or radiographic evidence of a pneumothorax.
Nursing process step: Implementation
Cognitive level: Application

108. The nurse caring for a patient with a history of rheumatic fever should be aware that:
A. Rheumatic fever occurs as a result of untreated streptococcal fevers in 30% of the population
B. Rheumatic fever places the patient at risk for acute bacterial endocarditis
C. Acute rheumatic fever usually attacks the myofibrils of the heart and can cause cardiomyopathy
D. The incidence of rheumatic fever is increasing in the United States

CORRECT ANSWER—B. Rheumatic fever is a systemic connective tissue disease that damages collagen tissues, including the heart valves. It develops in 1% to 3% of patients with untreated streptococcal infections. The incidence of rheumatic fever has steadily declined with the availability of penicillin. Rheumatic carditis, affecting the pericardium, myocardium, and endocardium, can result from rheumatic fever, but it is less common than collagen tissue involvement.
Nursing process step: Evaluation
Cognitive level: Knowledge

109. Which of the following is a potentially life-threatening complication of blunt chest trauma in a patient who previously has undergone coronary artery bypass surgery?
A. Sternal fracture
B. Disruption of the anastomosis
C. Cardiac contusion
D. Pneumothorax

CORRECT ANSWER—B. Because coronary artery bypass grafts often have a prominent position in the chest, they are at risk for laceration or disruption of the anastomosis. This rare but life-threatening condition can result in death from cardiac tamponade or myocardial ischemia. Sternal fracture, cardiac contusion, and pneumothorax are potential complications of blunt chest trauma but are not considered life-threatening.
Nursing process step: Planning
Cognitive level: Analysis

Questions 110 to 112 refer to the following information:
A 44-year-old male patient is admitted to the critical care unit after right femoral-tibial bypass grafting. The nurse notes that the patient's total cholesterol is 188 mg/dl, with a high level of low-density lipoprotein (LDL) cholesterol and a low level of high-density lipoprotein (HDL) cholesterol. The patient's history includes tobacco use, hypertension, and type II diabetes, which is controlled with oral agents.

110. The nurse assesses the patient's history as it relates to his lipid profile. Which conclusion is correct?
A. The patient's lipid profile is not contributing to his peripheral vascular disease because his total cholesterol level is low
B. The patient's lipid profile may be protective because he has a high level of "good cholesterol" and a low level of "bad cholesterol"
C. The patient's lipid profile may be contributing to his disease because he has a high level of "bad cholesterol" and a low level of "good cholesterol"
D. The patient's lipid profile is incomplete; without a triglyceride level, the nurse cannot draw a conclusion

CORRECT ANSWER—C. LDL cholesterol ("bad cholesterol") has been implicated in atherogenesis. In patients with known arterial disease, the LDL level should be less than 100 mg/dl. HDL lipoprotein cholesterol ("good cholesterol") protects against atherogenesis; at a level above 60 mg/dl, it is even considered a negative risk factor. Total cholesterol is the least important component of the lipid profile. Triglycerides have recently been associated with atherogenesis, and a level would be helpful; however, its absence does not preclude assessment of the patient's lipid profile.
Nursing process step: Assessment
Cognitive level: Evaluation

111. When planning discharge instructions for this patient, the nurse would expect to include information about:
A. Low-cholesterol diet and need for follow-up visit to monitor lipid profile 2 to 3 months after discharge
B. Low-cholesterol diet and cholesterol-reducing medications
C. Low-cholesterol diet, exercise program, and need for follow-up visit to monitor lipid profile 2 to 3 months after discharge
D. Low-cholesterol diet, alcohol abstinence, and need for follow-up visit to monitor lipid profile 2 to 3 months after discharge

CORRECT ANSWER—C. Initial treatment for elevated cholesterol level includes an exercise program, a low-cholesterol diet, and monitoring of the lipid profile 2 to 3 months after discharge. Cholesterol-reducing agents should be added to treatment regimen only if diet alone fails to control the hyperlipidemia. Aerobic exercise increases the HDL level, and studies suggest that ingestion of 3 to 4 ounces of alcohol per day also can increase HDL. However, the triglyceride level may increase with excess alcohol intake. Close follow-up is imperative in all patients with hyperlipidemia.
Nursing process step: Planning
Cognitive level: Synthesis

112. Which medications would the nurse most likely administer to this patient?
A. Aspirin, propranolol, and vitamin E
B. Aspirin, nifedipine, and vitamin E
C. Warfarin sodium, nifedipine, and vitamin K
D. Warfarin sodium, enalapril, and vitamin K

CORRECT ANSWER—**B.** All patients with arterial vascular disease should receive one aspirin tablet per day for its antiplatelet effects. Nifedipine, a calcium channel blocker, is a good choice in a hypertensive patient with peripheral vascular disease because it relaxes arterial smooth muscle, which decreases blood pressure and improves peripheral vascular status. Enalapril also is an appropriate antihypertensive agent for this patient. The antioxidant vitamin E may help prevent atherosclerosis, among other diseases. Warfarin sodium is not a first-line drug in patients with peripheral vascular disease but might be added if problems occur with reocclusion. Vitamin K is an antidote for warfarin sodium and would not be administered concurrently. Beta blockers, such as propranolol, generally are contraindicated in diabetic patients because they can mask signs and symptoms of hypoglycemia.
Nursing process step: Implementation
Cognitive level: Application

113. The nurse should anticipate which immediate treatment for a patient experiencing pulseless ventricular tachycardia?
A. Transcutaneous pacing
B. Intravenous bolus of lidocaine 100 mg
C. Transvenous pacing
D. Electrical countershock

CORRECT ANSWER—**D.** Electrical countershock via defibrillation is the treatment of choice for eradicating pulseless ventricular tachycardia. Research has shown that survival rates for patients with ventricular fibrillation and pulseless ventricular tachycardia depend on early recognition and immediate defibrillation. Pharmacologic intervention is initiated after defibrillation has been unsuccessful and I.V. access has been established. Pacing is not indicated for this arrhythmia. However, if the patient converted to a symptomatic sinus bradycardia, pacing would be initiated.
Nursing process step: Planning
Cognitive level: Knowledge

114. The nurse might administer the following I.V. vasodilator to lower systemic vascular resistance (decreasing afterload) and increase venous capacitance (decreasing preload):
A. Captopril
B. Nitroprusside sodium
C. Amrinone lactate
D. Dobutamine hydrochloride

CORRECT ANSWER—B. Nitroprusside and nitroglycerin cause venous vasodilation and reduce preload and afterload. Nitroprusside generally is used when the patient is hypertensive; nitroglycerin has a more pronounced effect on the venous system at lower dosages. Captopril is an angiotensin-converting enzyme inhibitor used to treat hypertension and congestive heart failure. Amrinone lactate is a positive inotropic agent that causes direct smooth-muscle relaxation and could decrease systemic vascular resistance. Dobutamine hydrochloride stimulates beta-receptor cells in the heart to increase myocardial contractility and stroke volume, resulting in increased cardiac output.
Nursing process step: Implementation
Cognitive level: Comprehension

115. The nurse records a patient's history and discovers several risk factors for coronary artery disease. Which cardiac risk factors are considered controllable?
A. Diabetes, hypercholesterolemia, and heredity
B. Diabetes, age, and gender
C. Age, gender, and heredity
D. Diabetes, hypercholesterolemia, and hypertension

CORRECT ANSWER—D. Uncontrollable risk factors for coronary artery disease include gender, age, and heredity. Controllable risk factors include hypertension, hypercholesterolemia, obesity, lack of exercise, smoking, diabetes, stress, alcohol abuse, and use of contraceptives.
Nursing process step: Assessment
Cognitive level: Comprehension

116. An increase in the creatine kinase-MB isozyme (CK-MB) can be caused by:
A. Cerebral bleeding
B. I.M. injection
C. Myocardial necrosis
D. Skeletal muscle damage due to a recent fall

CORRECT ANSWER—C. An increase in CK-MB is related to myocardial necrosis. An increase in total creatine kinase (CK) might occur for several reasons, including skeletal muscle damage, which can be caused by I.M. injections or falls; brain injury, such as cerebral bleeding; muscular or neuromuscular disease; vigorous exercise; trauma; or surgery.
Nursing process step: Evaluation
Cognitive level: Analysis

117. The nurse would expect which findings in a patient with a potassium level of 2.3 mEq/liter?
A. Flattened T wave and presence of a Q wave
B. Peaked T wave and prolonged QT segment
C. Flattened T wave and presence of a U wave
D. Inverted T wave and prolonged PR interval

CORRECT ANSWER—C. Hypokalemia produces flattening and eventual inversion of the T wave. A U wave also occurs and becomes increasingly prominent as the potassium level decreases. Increasing ventricular ectopy also is seen on the ECG of a hypokalemic patient. Q waves are a sign of transmural myocardial infarction. Peaked T waves occur in hyperkalemia. Prolonged QT segment occurs in hypocalcemia. Prolonged PR interval is not associated with electrolyte imbalances.
Nursing process step: Assessment
Cognitive level: Evaluation

118. The nurse would advise a patient with an axillary-femoral bypass graft to:
A. Avoid standing for prolonged periods
B. Avoid tight belts around the waist
C. Avoid reclining and instead sit in a chair for prolonged periods
D. Avoid upper extremity exercises

CORRECT ANSWER—B. Tight belts around the waist can occlude the axillary-femoral bypass; the patient should use suspenders instead. Prolonged sitting can kink the femoral portion of the graft. Prolonged standing and upper extremity exercises need not be avoided.
Nursing process step: Implementation
Cognitive level: Application

119. An intraventricular conduction disturbance occurs when:
A. The QRS complex equals or is greater than 0.10 second
B. The QRS complex narrows to less than 0.06 second
C. The PR interval lengthens
D. Supraventricular tachycardia (SVT) develops

CORRECT ANSWER—A. Intraventricular conduction disturbances are caused by complete or partial blockage of an electrical impulse in an area of the bundle branch-Purkinje conduction system. This causes the abnormal widening of the QRS complex of 0.10 second or greater. A normal QRS complex has a duration of .06 to .10 second; a value greater than .10 is considered an intraventricular conduction disturbance, and a value greater than .12 often is termed a bundle branch block. Atrioventricular junction blocks are indicated by prolonged PR intervals. SVTs are representative of a fast rate originating above the ventricles; they do not cause widened QRS complexes and are not intraventricular conduction disturbances.
Nursing process step: Assessment
Cognitive level: Knowledge

120. A patient with a diagnosis of heart failure is being transferred from the intensive care unit to a general unit. The heart failure resulted from a recent anterior wall myocardial infarction. Which symptom should the patient be instructed to report immediately to the medical team?
   A. Frequent urination
   B. Shortness of breath
   C. Nausea
   D. Diarrhea

CORRECT ANSWER—B. An anterior infarction primarily damages the left ventricle. Thus, the symptoms of heart failure are related to the left side of the heart. Shortness of breath, palpitations, and diaphoresis are symptoms that the patient should report immediately.
Nursing process step: Implementation
Cognitive level: Application

121. During the immediate postoperative period, the nurse observes bradycardia in a patient who has undergone carotid endarterectomy. The nurse correctly concludes that the bradycardia may result from:
   A. Intraoperative stimulation of the carotid sinus
   B. Intraoperative stimulation of the carotid bodies
   C. Postoperative hemorrhage
   D. Postoperative hypotension

CORRECT ANSWER—A. Stimulation of the carotid sinus causes bradycardia and is a common postoperative finding in patients who have undergone carotid endarterectomy. The carotid bodies are chemoreceptors that respond to changes in arterial oxygen tension and pH by affecting the respiratory rate. Both postoperative hypotension and hemorrhage would be expected to cause tachycardia.
Nursing process step: Evaluation
Cognitive level: Analysis

122. The nurse is caring for a patient in normal sinus rhythm who is being monitored in leads I and II. The nurse suddenly observes tall, peaked T waves in both leads. What action should be taken first, based on this finding?
   A. Obtain a 12-lead ECG
   B. Obtain a potassium level
   C. Obtain a magnesium level
   D. Obtain a calcium level

CORRECT ANSWER—B. Hyperkalemia is associated with tall, peaked T waves, widened QRS complexes, and wide, flat P waves. Patients with a low magnesium level often develop ventricular arrhythmias. Alterations in the calcium level are associated with changes in the QT interval and ST segment. A 12-lead ECG may be obtained to further document the change in rhythm; however, this action would not take precedence over obtaining the potassium level.
Nursing process step: Implementation
Cognitive level: Analysis

123. A 55-year-old patient who underwent a coronary artery bypass graft and has no signs of valvular disease is admitted to the surgical intensive care unit. The physician asks the nurse to report if the patient's pulmonary capillary wedge pressure is above normal. The nurse knows that a normal pulmonary capillary wedge pressure ranges from:
   A. 0 to 6 mm Hg
   B. 0 to 10 mm Hg
   C. 4 to 12 mm Hg
   D. 14 to 20 mm Hg

CORRECT ANSWER—C. The pulmonary capillary wedge pressure is equal to the left atrial pressure when mitral stenosis is absent. Thus, it is a sensitive indicator of the presence of pulmonary congestion and left-sided heart failure. A normal mean wedge pressure is 9 mm Hg but can range from 4 to 12 mm Hg.
Nursing process step: Assessment
Cognitive level: Knowledge

124. The nurse would anticipate the insertion of which of the following as an intervention for a patient experiencing chest pain unrelieved by a nitroglycerin I.V. infusion?
A. Intra-arterial line
B. Intra-aortic balloon pump
C. Pulmonary artery catheter
D. Ventricular assist device

CORRECT ANSWER—B. The intra-aortic balloon pump (IABP) restores the balance of oxygen supply and demand by increasing the coronary perfusion pressure and decreasing cardiac workload. If conventional modes of treatment fail to reverse the ischemia, the IABP can help salvage the remaining viable muscle. An intra-arterial line and pulmonary artery catheter also may be inserted in this patient. However, these devices only provide information regarding treatment; they do not specifically assist the heart. A ventricular assist device is indicated only after unsuccessful treatment with IABP.
Nursing process step: Planning
Cognitive level: Knowledge

125. Which bed rest position is indicated for a patient with pulmonary edema?
A. Trendelenburg's position
B. High-Fowler's position
C. Left lateral position
D. Supine position

CORRECT ANSWER—B. Placing the patient in an upright position, such as the high-Fowler's position, increases lung volume and vital capacity and decreases venous return and the work of breathing. Trendelenburg's position and the supine position increase venous return, decrease lung capacity, and increase the work of breathing. The left lateral position will not help the patient increase lung capacity or volume and may increase the work of breathing.
Nursing process step: Implementation
Cognitive level: Application

126. At what point should a 12-lead ECG be obtained for a patient complaining of chest pain?
A. After I.V. nitroglycerin is administered
B. After the third sublingual nitroglycerin tablet is given
C. Before any medical interventions are initiated
D. After the chest pain is relieved

CORRECT ANSWER—C. Any ECG changes caused by ischemia should be recorded before medical interventions are instituted. Once the pain is treated medically, changes on the ECG may alter or become undetectable. A 12-lead ECG provides information on the location of the ischemia, which is important for determining the urgency of the situation.
Nursing process step: Implementation
Cognitive level: Application

127. The normal dosage range for I.V. nitroprusside
sodium is:
A. 0.5 to 10 mcg/kg/minute
B. 0.5 to 10 mg/minute
C. 0.5 to 10 mg/kg/minute
D. 0.5 to 10 mcg/minute

CORRECT ANSWER—A. The normal dosage for
I.V. nitroprusside is 0.5 to 10 mcg/kg/minute.
Excessive dosage or rapid infusion (greater than
15 mcg/kg/minute) can cause cyanide toxicity.
For patients who have been receiving nitroprusside for more than 72 hours and for those receiving large doses of this drug, serum thiocyanate
level must be monitored. Serum thiocyanate level greater than 100 mcg/ml is associated with
toxicity, as evidenced by hypotension, metabolic
acidosis, dyspnea, headache, loss or change of
consciousness, ataxia, and vomiting.
Nursing process step: Planning
Cognitive level: Knowledge

128. Cardiogenic shock can be caused by any of the
following conditions *except:*
A. Acute cerebrovascular accident
B. Massive pulmonary embolism
C. Pneumonia
D. Aortic aneurysm

CORRECT ANSWER—C. Cardiogenic shock can result from massive pulmonary embolism, acute
dissecting aneurysm of the aorta, acute cerebrovascular accident, diabetic ketoacidosis, sepsis,
and the effects of hypotensive drugs. Although
pneumonia places a cardiac patient at risk for decompensated heart failure, it would not be the
sole precipitating factor for cardiogenic shock.
Nursing process step: Assessment
Cognitive level: Comprehension

Questions 129 to 132 refer to the following information:
A 17-year-old male collapses during a basketball game. Paramedics on the scene observe ventricular
tachycardia. The patient is successfully defibrillated, with normal sinus rhythm and stable vital signs,
and taken to the intensive care unit.

129. After an echocardiogram, the patient is diagnosed with cardiomyopathy. Which type of cardiomyopathy is most likely in this patient?
A. Ischemic cardiomyopathy
B. Dilated (congestive) cardiomyopathy
C. Restrictive cardiomyopathy
D. Hypertrophic cardiomyopathy

CORRECT ANSWER—D. The leading cause of sudden cardiac death in young athletes is hypertrophic cardiomyopathy. Ischemic cardiomyopathy
results from severe coronary artery disease. A patient with restrictive cardiomyopathy has a low
cardiac output, especially with vigorous exertion, and is unlikely to be involved in competitive sports. Similarly, a patient with dilated cardiomyopathy is unlikely to be involved in sports.
Nursing process step: Assessment
Cognitive level: Evaluation

130. Which class of drugs is contraindicated in this patient?

A. Beta blockers
B. Positive inotropic agents
C. Calcium channel blockers
D. Angiotensin-converting enzyme inhibitors

CORRECT ANSWER—B. A patient with hypertrophic cardiomyopathy has a hypertrophied ventricular septum that distorts the alignment of the papillary muscles, causing the anterior mitral leaflet to be abnormally pulled toward the septum. This causes an obstruction in ventricular outflow that is exaggerated by anything that increases myocardial contractility, such as positive inotropic agents, or decreases left ventricular volume, such as nitrates or diuretics. Beta blockers are the drug of choice in patients with hypertrophic cardiomyopathy because they decrease myocardial contractility, thus relieving the outflow tract obstruction. Calcium channel blockers can be used in these patients to decrease contractility. Angiotensin-converting enzyme inhibitors are of little benefit in these patients, and could worsen symptoms; however, they are not contraindicated.
Nursing process step: Implementation
Cognitive level: Analysis

131. During teaching sessions with the patient and his family, the nurse should explain that the:

A. Patient can continue to play basketball if he complies with his medication regimen
B. Patient can take up weight lifting
C. Patient's siblings should be evaluated for hypertrophic cardiomyopathy
D. Patient's life expectancy will be shortened because of his disorder

CORRECT ANSWER—C. Hypertrophic cardiomyopathy may be genetically transmitted, passed on as an autosomal dominant trait. The condition typically is asymptomatic; therefore, siblings of a patient with this disorder should be evaluated. Sports that increase myocardial contractility, such as basketball and weight lifting, are contraindicated, even if the patient complies with the medication regimen. (The American College of Cardiology has determined which sports are safe for patients with various cardiac abnormalities; this information is available to health care professionals through published media.) The patient will not necessarily have a shortened life expectancy if he follows medical advice regarding activity and medications.
Nursing process step: Implementation
Cognitive level: Analysis

132. In a patient with hypertrophic cardiomyopathy, the nurse would expect to auscultate a murmur during which phase of the cardiac cycle?

A. Early diastole
B. Systole
C. Entire cardiac cycle
D. Late diastole

CORRECT ANSWER—B. The murmur associated with hypertrophic cardiomyopathy is a systolic ejection murmur heard over the mitral area. It results from systolic anterior motion of the mitral leaflets and outflow tract obstruction.
Nursing process step: Assessment
Cognitive level: Comprehension

133. The nurse would anticipate which diagnostic tests for a patient admitted with a left arm that is cold, painful, pulseless, and cyanotic?
A. Upper extremity angiogram, venous Doppler ultrasonography, and cardiac catheterization
B. Arterial Doppler ultrasonography, cardiac catheterization, and echocardiogram
C. Upper extremity angiogram, arterial Doppler ultrasonography, and cardiac catheterization
D. Upper extremity angiogram, arterial Doppler ultrasonography, and echocardiogram

CORRECT ANSWER—**D.** Pain, cold, pulselessness, and pallor or cyanosis are classic signs and symptoms of arterial occlusion. An arterial Doppler ultrasonography would be used to detect the arterial occlusion. An upper extremity angiogram would be performed if the Doppler ultrasonography revealed such an occlusion. An echocardiogram would be obtained to search for clots in the left atrium. A large percentage of patients with acute arterial occlusion suffer an embolism in the heart secondary to atrial fibrillation. Venous Doppler ultrasonography may or may not be performed after the arterial studies are completed. However, the patient in this situation does not display signs of venous congestion. Based on the available information, cardiac catheterization is not indicated.
Nursing process step: Planning
Cognitive level: Comprehension

134. A venous catheter can be placed at which site before administration of a thrombolytic agent?
A. Internal jugular vein
B. Femoral vein
C. Subclavian vein
D. External jugular vein

CORRECT ANSWER—**B.** All noncompressible venous insertion sites should be avoided. When the catheter is removed or needs to be removed because of bleeding problems, the nurse must apply pressure to the vein. The femoral vein, as well as the brachial vein, can be easily compressed. Pressure to any bleeding area should be maintained for at least 30 minutes and the site frequently assessed thereafter for both external and internal bleeding.
Nursing process step: Implementation
Cognitive level: Comprehension

135. The nurse would anticipate the physician ordering which noninvasive diagnostic procedure to assess both the heart and lungs of a patient with heart failure?
A. Gated cardiac blood pool imaging with multiple-gated acquisition (MUGA) scan
B. Echocardiography
C. Chest radiography
D. Cardiac catheterization

CORRECT ANSWER—C. The only noninvasive test that can detect changes in both the heart and lungs is chest radiography. Evidence of pulmonary congestion and cardiac enlargement can be detected and monitored daily by examining the chest X-ray film. Cardiac catheterization is an invasive test used to reveal abnormalities of the heart and measure pulmonary pressures. Gated cardiac blood pool imaging with MUGA scan is a radionuclide technique used to assess ventricular performance. The MUGA scan measures ejection fraction and can be useful in evaluating left ventricular wall motion. Echocardiography is a diagnostic procedure used to study the structure and motion of the heart via noninvasive ultrasonic waves.
Nursing process step: Planning
Cognitive level: Comprehension

136. The nurse would anticipate which procedure for a patient with unstable angina?
A. Percutaneous transluminal angioplasty
B. Coronary artery bypass grafting
C. Coronary arteriography
D. Pyrophosphate (PYP) nuclear scan

CORRECT ANSWER—C. Although coronary angioplasty or bypass grafting may be done during the hospitalization of a patient with unstable angina, the patient must first be evaluated with coronary arteriography or cardiac catheterization. A PYP scan is a nuclear medicine test that evaluates whether myocardial necrosis has occurred in a patient for whom a diagnosis of myocardial infarction is questionable.
Nursing process step: Planning
Cognitive level: Analysis

137. When a patient with unstable angina complains of pain, the nurse's priority is to take all of the following actions *except:*
A. Perform a 12-lead ECG
B. Administer sublingual nitroglycerin
C. Administer oxygen by nasal cannula
D. Review the cardiac enzyme results

CORRECT ANSWER—D. The nursing priority is to relieve the patient's pain as quickly as possible using nitrates and oxygen therapy. A 12-lead ECG is performed before treatment with nitrates to record any ECG changes caused by the ischemic myocardium. Because muscle necrosis can occur in the first 10 to 15 minutes of an ischemic event, reviewing the results of cardiac enzyme tests would not alter the course of treatment for this patient.
Nursing process: Implementation
Cognitive level: Application

138. All of the following statements about normal QT intervals are true *except:*

A. QT intervals vary with heart rate, gender, and age

B. QT intervals typically last 0.36 to 0.44 second

C. QT intervals can be affected by serum drug levels

D. QT intervals often are difficult to measure

CORRECT ANSWER—D. The QT interval is measured from the beginning of the QRS complex to the point at which the T wave returns to the baseline. Although the QT interval sometimes is difficult to measure accurately because the precise end of the T wave is obscure, it is important to be aware of any changes in the QT interval. Class I antiarrhythmics, such as procainamide, increase the refractory period of the heart and decrease conduction time. At adequate drug serum levels, the QT interval lengthens with the prolonged refractory time. Toxic levels of these drugs often can be evidenced by a QT interval that is greater than half the R-R interval. Other drugs and conditions that affect the QT interval are quinidine, bradycardia, hypokalemia, and hypomagnesemia.
Nursing process step: Assessment
Cognitive level: Comprehension

139. Which treatment may be used for a patient with a pulse who develops stable ventricular tachycardia?

A. Nothing if the patient is asymptomatic

B. Lidocaine I.V. push

C. Defibrillation

D. Precordial thump

CORRECT ANSWER—B. A patient in ventricular tachycardia should never remain untreated. The first-line therapy is lidocaine I.V. push (IVP). If lidocaine is unsuccessful, procainamide, bretylium, and electrical cardioversion may be tried. While the lidocaine is being prepared, the patient may perform Valsalva's maneuver to attempt to terminate the arrhythmia. A conscious patient should not receive a precordial thump or defibrillation.
Nursing process step: Planning
Cognitive level: Application

140. A hypertensive emergency is a situation in which the:

A. Systolic blood pressure is greater than 200 mm Hg

B. Systolic blood pressure is greater than 220 mm Hg

C. Diastolic blood pressure is less than 120 mm Hg

D. Diastolic blood pressure is greater than 120 mm Hg

CORRECT ANSWER—D. A hypertensive emergency is a situation in which the blood pressure must be lowered within 1 hour to prevent serious end-organ (kidneys, heart, brain, and eyes) damage and possible death. Such an emergency arises when the diastolic blood pressure is 120 mm Hg or higher. A hypertensive urgency is a situation in which the blood pressure should be controlled within 24 hours. Sometimes it is not possible to differentiate between the two conditions.
Nursing process step: Assessment
Cognitive level: Knowledge

Questions 141 to 144 refer to the following information:
A 29-year-old male patient is admitted to the trauma unit after a motor vehicle accident. He was not wearing a seat belt. Injuries include multiple rib fractures and blunt chest and abdominal trauma. He is profoundly short of breath and hypotensive. A pulmonary artery (PA) catheter and arterial line are inserted.

141. The nurse observes bright red blood in the syringe when aspirating from the distal port of the PA catheter. Based on this observation as well as the clinical examination, the nurse suspects the patient has suffered:
A. Rupture of the free wall of the ventricle
B. Traumatic ventricular septal defect
C. Coronary artery laceration
D. Aortic dissection

CORRECT ANSWER—B. A left-to-right shunting created by a traumatic ventricular septal defect causes high oxygen saturations in the right ventricle and pulmonary artery. The conditions listed in the other options would cause massive hemorrhage into the chest but would not affect oxygen saturation in the pulmonary artery.
Nursing process step: Assessment
Cognitive level: Analysis

142. The patient is hemodynamically stable after volume resuscitation. Which test would the nurse expect the patient to undergo to ensure a positive diagnosis?
A. Cardiac catheterization with ventriculography
B. Echocardiography
C. Computed tomography (CT) scan of the chest
D. Aortography

CORRECT ANSWER—A. Ventriculography is the only diagnostic method that can absolutely distinguish even a small ventricular septal defect (VSD). Echocardiography is useful in identifying larger VSDs, but this test often misses smaller lesions. A CT scan of the chest or aortography are of limited use in diagnosing VSD.
Nursing process step: Planning
Cognitive level: Comprehension

143. Therapeutic modalities that would be used until the patient can be taken to surgery include:
A. Mechanical ventilation and ventricular assist device
B. Mechanical ventilation and intra-aortic balloon counterpulsation
C. Intra-aortic balloon counterpulsation and temporary pacemaker
D. Mechanical ventilation and temporary pacemaker

CORRECT ANSWER—B. Mechanical ventilation will help relieve the patient's respiratory distress. Intra-aortic balloon counterpulsation can be used as a temporary measure to unload the left ventricle, thus decreasing left-to-right shunting and relieving the pulmonary edema that often accompanies a ventricular septal defect. A ventricular assist device or temporary pacemaker are not indicated for the patient's current condition.
Nursing process step: Implementation
Cognitive level: Analysis

144. The nurse would conclude that the patient's left ventricle is adequately unloading based on:
A. Decrease in pulmonary artery wedge pressure (PAWP) and increase in right atrial pressure
B. Decrease in PAWP and decrease in cardiac output
C. Increase in PAWP and increase in cardiac output
D. Decrease in PAWP and decrease in right atrial pressure

CORRECT ANSWER—D. Adequate unloading of the left ventricle in a patient with a ventricular septal defect can be achieved via medications, such as nitroprusside, or mechanically by an intra-aortic balloon pump. Adequate unloading is demonstrated by a decrease in all pulmonary artery pressures, a decrease in right atrial pressure, and improvement of cardiac output.
Nursing process step: Evaluation
Cognitive level: Comprehension

145. Which nursing intervention is most important before a patient undergoes elective surgery for abdominal aortic aneurysm resection?
A. Assess the patient's peripheral pulses to establish baseline for postoperative comparison
B. Instruct the patient and family about the postoperative intensive care unit regimen
C. Provide necessary respiratory treatments to optimize the patient's pulmonary function
D. Implement measures to reduce the patient's anxiety

CORRECT ANSWER—C. To ensure quick extubation and prevent postoperative pulmonary complications, preoperative respiratory care must be performed in many patients, especially those who smoke. All of the other responses are important, but they are not as critical.
Nursing process step: Implementation
Cognitive level: Synthesis

146. Of the following medications, which would provide the most benefit to a patient with dilated (congestive) cardiomyopathy who is awaiting a transplant?
A. Procainamide hydrochloride
B. Diltiazem hydrochloride
C. Dobutamine hydrochloride
D. Dopamine hydrochloride I.V. at a rate of 15 mcg/kg/minute

CORRECT ANSWER—C. Dobutamine is the most beneficial agent for a patient with dilated cardiomyopathy because it increases the contractility of the failing ventricle. Other beneficial forms of therapy include vasodilators and angiotensin-converting enzyme inhibitors. Calcium channel blockers, such as diltiazem hydrochloride, decrease contractility and are contraindicated in a patient with a failing heart. Dopamine at predominantly alpha-range doses (greater than 10 mcg/kg/minute) would provide peripheral vasoconstriction, thus increasing afterload and worsening cardiac output. Antiarrhythmic agents, such as procainamide, would be used to treat associated arrhythmias, not the cardiomyopathy itself.
Nursing process step: Implementation
Cognitive level: Application

147. A patient in cardiogenic shock has an intra-aortic balloon pump (IABP) inserted. The nurse caring for this patient will monitor for which complication directly associated with this therapy?
A. Thrombus formation
B. Hypoxemia
C. Pneumonia
D. Pressure ulcers

CORRECT ANSWER—A. An IABP is a counterpulsation device that provides a temporary cardiac assist in patients with refractory left ventricular failure. This device is used to increase coronary artery perfusion and reduce the workload of the heart. Complications directly associated with IABP include aortic dissection, infection, bleeding, and possible thrombus formation with distal extremity ischemia. Complications associated with the immobility imposed by the IABP include pressure ulcers and pneumonia. A patient should become less hypoxic because of the effects of the IABP improve the balance between oxygen delivery and oxygen consumption.
Nursing process step: Evaluation
Cognitive level: Application

148. A patient with acute myocardial infarction is experiencing frequent premature ventricular contractions (PVCs). The probable cause of the PVCs can be attributed to all of the following *except:*
A. Decreased carbon dioxide level
B. Decreased potassium level
C. Ischemic myocardium
D. Sympathetic response to injury

CORRECT ANSWER—A. A hypoxic or ischemic myocardium, decreased potassium level, hypercapnia, digoxin toxicity, bradycardia, and stimulation of the sympathetic nervous system can elicit PVCs. Premature ventricular contractions are ectopic impulses that originate in the ventricles. Because PVCs usually are conducted in a retrograde manner, the QRS complex appears wide and bizarre. An increased potassium level correlates with bradycardia, idioventricular arrhythmias, and asystole and is indicated on the ECG by tall, tented T waves, flattened P waves, and widened QRS complexes. In the patient with an acute myocardial infarction, the decreased carbon dioxide level most often is related to tachypnea.
Nursing process step: Evaluation
Cognitive level: Knowledge

149. A multiple-gated acquisition (MUGA) scan provides data on:
A. Cardiac index
B. Ejection fraction
C. Cardiac output
D. Systemic vascular resistance

CORRECT ANSWER—B. The most commonly used radionuclide technique for assessing ventricular performance is gated cardiac blood pool imaging with MUGA scan. The MUGA scan measures ejection fraction and helps the clinician evaluate left ventricular wall motion.
Nursing process step: Evaluation
Cognitive level: Knowledge

150. The initial medical treatment for ventricular
fibrillation is:
A. Defibrillation
B. Cardioversion
C. Pacing
D. I.V. bolus of lidocaine

CORRECT ANSWER—A. Defibrillation produces
momentary asystole in an attempt to completely
depolarize the myocardium and allow the natural pacemaker to resume normal activity. Early
defibrillation using successive shocks is more important than adjunctive drug therapies. Cardioversion or synchronized countershock is an appropriate intervention if the patient has a pulse,
which is never the case with ventricular fibrillation. Lidocaine is a second-line drug that would
be used if defibrillation fails. Pacing is used for
patients with heart blocks or symptomatic
bradyarrhythmias but as a last resort with asystole.
Nursing process step: Implementation
Cognitive level: Knowledge

151. A previously normotensive patient is admitted
to the intensive care unit with a blood pressure
of 200/120 mm Hg. Which condition could precipitate such an event?
A. Clinical depression requiring treatment with a
monoamine oxidase (MAO) inhibitor
B. Anxiety requiring treatment with alprazolam
C. Paranoid schizophrenia
D. Manic depression requiring treatment with
lithium

CORRECT ANSWER—A. Hypertensive emergencies can occur in patients who have primary (essential) or secondary hypertension, as well as in
those who have been normotensive in the past. A
hypertensive emergency in a previously
normotensive patient suggests acute glomerulonephritis, a drug reaction to an MAO inhibitor,
or toxemia associated with pregnancy. Alprazolam or lithium therapy would not induce a hypertensive emergency. Paranoid schizophrenia is
not associated with a hyperdynamic state.
Nursing process step: Assessment
Cognitive level: Application

152. The goal of treating a hypertensive emergency is to:
A. Reduce the blood pressure by half the diastolic value
B. Treat the underlying cause of the emergency
C. Reduce the systolic and diastolic values quickly but safely
D. Always treat the systolic value first

CORRECT ANSWER—C. The goal of treatment in a hypertensive emergency is to lower the systolic and diastolic blood pressures as quickly and safely as possible to avoid hypertensive encephalopathy, cerebrovascular accident, left heart failure, and pulmonary edema. The actual level to which the pressures should be lowered depends on the clinical situation. Hypertensive emergencies are marked by acute life-threatening increases in diastolic blood pressure over 120 mm Hg. Although the diastolic blood pressure must be reduced, how much of a decrease depends on the patient's clinical and hemodynamic response to treatment. Systolic blood pressure is not the only concern; diastolic and mean arterial blood pressures should also be considered when treating a patient in a hypertensive emergency. Treating the underlying cause of the emergency is not an immediate priority.
Nursing process step: Planning
Cognitive level: Analysis

153. Which of the following hemodynamic parameters would the nurse document and monitor during a hypertensive emergency?
A. Invasive arterial blood pressure
B. Cuff blood pressure
C. Central venous pressure
D. All of the above

CORRECT ANSWER—D. Depending on the type of treatment the patient receives during a hypertensive emergency, several hemodynamic parameters may be useful in monitoring the response to treatment. Invasive arterial blood pressure or cuff blood pressure measurements may be monitored. Central venous pressure, mean right atrial pressure, or pulmonary artery pressure can help determine the patient's fluid volume status during diuretic therapy. Systemic vascular resistance, pulmonary vascular resistance, and cardiac output may be helpful in monitoring the patient's progress if potent vasodilators are administered.
Nursing process step: Implementation
Cognitive level: Comprehension

154. Increased central venous pressure (CVP) can be an initial clinical sign of:
  A. Pulmonary congestion
  B. Right-sided heart failure
  C. Left-sided heart failure
  D. Cardiogenic shock

CORRECT ANSWER—**B.** Because CVP reflects right ventricular end-diastolic pressure, it increases when right-sided heart failure is present. In patients with left-sided heart failure, CVP initially may be low because of decreased venous return to the right side of the heart. If left ventricular failure progresses and causes a backup of blood to the pulmonary circulation and the right side of the heart, CVP will increase. Pulmonary congestion and pulmonary hypertension trigger increases in pulmonary systolic and diastolic pressures. Cardiogenic shock is first indicated by low cardiac output and decreased CVP; eventually, as global heart failure occurs, CVP increases.
Nursing process step: Evaluation
Cognitive level: Evaluation

155. To help the physician diagnose pheochromocytoma, which laboratory test might be ordered?
  A. Blood urea nitrogen and creatinine levels
  B. 24-hour urine test for vanillylmandelic acid (VMA)
  C. Plasma renin activity
  D. Renal angiography

CORRECT ANSWER—**B.** Pheochromocytoma is a catecholamine-secreting tumor of the adrenal medulla. The laboratory diagnosis involves measuring plasma catecholamine, epinephrine, and norepinephrine levels and taking 24-hour urine measurements of catecholamine metabolites, including VMA and homovanillylmandelic acid. Angiography can be used to localize the tumor, but it is not considered necessary for the initial diagnosis. Blood urea nitrogen and creatinine levels allow the nurse to monitor renal involvement, which usually does not occur with this type of tumor. Renin is an enzyme secreted by the kidneys in response to decreased glomerular filtration rate. The plasma renin level, combined with the plasma aldosterone level, aids in the differential diagnosis of primary versus secondary hyperaldosteronism.
Nursing process step: Assessment
Cognitive level: Application

156. During the admission assessment, a patient with unstable angina complains of chest pain after meals. The nurse should plan to provide:
A. Clear liquid meals
B. Three small meals daily
C. Low-cholesterol, high-fat, low-sodium diet
D. Six small meals daily

CORRECT ANSWER—D. Small, frequent meals often are preferable for cardiac patients, especially those with angina triggered by meals, because metabolic demands increase after eating. The nurse could also suggest that the patient take a sublingual nitroglycerin tablet before meals. Studies have shown that hot or cold fluids do not negatively affect heart patients. However, the patient should be instructed to avoid caffeine, although data in this area are not conclusive. The patient does not require clear liquid meals. Six small meals a day incorporating a low-cholesterol, low-fat, low-sodium diet will provide sufficient calories for this patient.
Nursing process step: Planning
Cognitive level: Application

157. Which position is most beneficial for a cardiac patient?
A. Trendelenburg's position
B. Semi-Fowler's position
C. Supine position
D. Reverse Trendelenburg's position

CORRECT ANSWER—B. Semi-Fowler's position involves placing the patient supine in the bed and slightly elevating both the feet and head without gatching the bed. This position promotes the return of blood from the lower extremities and avoids adding to pulmonary congestion. Trendelenburg's position can be detrimental to a cardiac patient because it increases venous return to the heart, increases the workload of the heart, and causes pulmonary congestion. The supine position also can cause pulmonary congestion. Reverse Trendelenburg's position may cause pitting edema in the extremities and, because venous return to the heart might decrease in this position, the compensatory mechanism of tachycardia will increase myocardial oxygen consumption.
Nursing process step: Implementation
Cognitive level: Application

158. A first-degree atrioventricular (AV) block is most likely to be seen with which type of myocardial infarction?

A. Lateral wall
B. Inferior wall
C. Anteroseptal wall
D. Posterior wall

CORRECT ANSWER—**B.** An inferior wall myocardial infarction is most often related to occlusion of the right coronary artery (RCA). The RCA supplies blood to the AV node in approximately 90% of the population; consequently, blocks occurring at the AV junction are more common with inferior wall myocardial infarctions. These infarctions are associated with varying degrees of AV block. Heart blocks affecting the inferior wall usually are transient. Prolonged PR intervals occur in approximately 13% of patients with acute myocardial infarctions, mostly those involving the inferior wall. Approximately 75% of these patients go on to develop second-degree AV block, Mobitz type I; about half of these patients go on to develop a second- or third-degree or complete heart block.
Nursing process step: Assessment
Cognitive level: Evaluation

159. Two of the primary treatment goals for a patient in acute heart failure are:

A. Normal cardiac index and adequate tissue perfusion
B. Normal wedge pressure and normal right atrial pressure
C. Normal heart rate and normal respiratory rate
D. Clear lungs and normal heart sounds

CORRECT ANSWER—**A.** The first goal of treatment in acute heart failure is to meet metabolic tissue demands by decreasing demands on the heart, decreasing the work of the heart, and improving cardiac performance and output. Measures that normalize heart rate and fluid status can decrease the demands on the heart, leading to a normal cardiac index and adequate tissue perfusion. Normal respiratory rate and clear lungs are signs of normalized fluid status and heart function. Normal heart sounds may or may not be assessed in patients with heart failure; these sounds are indicative of many cardiac diseases and depend on the patient's underlying condition. In patients whose heart failure is directly related to coronary artery disease, another goal is to limit ischemia and infarct size. Normal hemodynamic parameters may not be attainable for a patient with acute heart failure; instead, individual baseline values need to be established.
Nursing process step: Evaluation
Cognitive level: Evaluation

160. A patient with a diagnosis of unstable angina returns from the cardiac catheterization laboratory. No significant coronary artery disease was found, and a definitive diagnosis of Prinzmetal's angina was made. Prinzmetal's angina is thought to be caused by:
  A. Mitral regurgitation
  B. Chronic anemia
  C. Coronary artery spasm
  D. Hypoxemia

CORRECT ANSWER—C. The clinical syndrome of Prinzmetal's angina, also called variant angina, results from coronary artery spasm. The resulting ECG changes include transient ST-segment elevation. A definitive diagnosis is made in the cardiac catheterization laboratory by inducing coronary artery spasm. Treatment is directed at reducing the constriction, usually with nitrates and calcium channel blockers. A patient with hypoxemia or chronic anemia may develop anginal pain caused by decreased oxygen supply to the cardiac muscle. Symptoms of mitral regurgitation include fatigue, weakness, heart failure, atrial fibrillation, and, possibly, hypotension.
Nursing process step: Assessment
Cognitive level: Knowledge

Questions 161 to 163 refer to the following information:
A 17-year-old male patient arrives at the trauma unit with a stab wound to the chest. He is tachycardic and hypotensive, with a narrow pulse pressure. During the physical examination, the nurse notes distended neck veins, central cyanosis, apprehension, and restlessness. Breath sounds are clear bilaterally; heart tones are distant.

161. Based on the physical assessment, the nurse suspects the patient's symptoms most likely are caused by:
  A. Cardiac rupture
  B. Acute pulmonary edema
  C. Tension pneumothorax
  D. Cardiac tamponade

CORRECT ANSWER—D. The patient displays the classic signs of cardiac tamponade. Neck veins are distended because of the inability of the heart to pump the venous volume through the cardiac chambers. Hypotension and cyanosis result from reduced cardiac output. Heart tones are muffled because of the pericardial effusion causing the tamponade. Patients with cardiac rupture usually die immediately; however, some patients with atrial rupture survive and may display symptoms similar to those of cardiac tamponade. The presence of clear, bilateral breath sounds rules out tension pneumothorax and pulmonary edema.
Nursing process step: Assessment
Cognitive level: Analysis

162. The patient initially responds favorably to fluid resuscitation, with an improvement in vital signs. Shortly thereafter, the nurse observes that the patient's abdomen has become rigid and tender and his neck veins have distended further. The nurse should prepare the patient for emergency:

A. Thoracotomy
B. Pericardiocentesis
C. Laparotomy
D. Cardiac catheterization

CORRECT ANSWER—**B.** Patients with cardiac tamponade typically respond well initially to fluid replacement but demonstrate signs of increased filling pressures shortly thereafter; the distended neck veins reflect this phenomenon. The rigid abdomen could signify either venous engorgement of the liver secondary to tamponade or emergence of symptoms from a separate abdominal injury. Emergency pericardiocentesis is both diagnostic and therapeutic in a patient with tamponade and impending cardiac failure; there may be no time to prepare for a thoracotomy. However, thoracotomy is the definitive treatment after an accurate diagnosis is made. Laparotomy would be performed if an abdominal injury was identified. Cardiac catheterization is not indicated.
Nursing process step: Planning
Cognitive level: Analysis

163. The patient is taken to the operating room for emergency thoracotomy. A laceration of the right ventricle is found. Postoperative nursing priorities related to this injury wound include:

A. Providing early nutrition and encouraging ambulation
B. Observing for infection, bleeding, and arrhythmias
C. Monitoring for infection, oliguria, and pneumonia
D. Implementing early ventilator weaning and extubation

CORRECT ANSWER—**B.** All the responses are correct, but only option B describes complications directly related to the patient's stab wound. Infection may result if the weapon used during the attack was contaminated, bleeding can occur from the laceration site or from the surgical repair, and arrhythmias may occur if the stab wound damaged conductive tissue in the right ventricle.
Nursing process step: Planning
Cognitive level: Analysis

164. The nurse would monitor for GI distention and return of bowel sounds most closely in a postoperative patient who has undergone:

A. Femoral-popliteal bypass grafting
B. Femoral-tibial bypass grafting
C. Aorto-bifemoral bypass grafting
D. Axillary-femoral bypass grafting

CORRECT ANSWER—**C.** Of the surgeries listed, only the aorto-bifemoral bypass requires laparotomy and manipulation of the intestines. Patients undergoing this procedure are at high risk for postoperative ileus.
Nursing process step: Assessment
Cognitive level: Comprehension

165. When evaluating a patient with an automatic implantable cardioverter defibrillator (AICD), the nurse should:
A. Determine how many times the device has discharged
B. Verify the patient's level of angina
C. Review the daily pulse diary with the patient
D. Auscultate for extra heart sounds produced by the device

CORRECT ANSWER—**A.** The nurse's evaluation of a patient with an AICD should include information about the number of times the device has discharged, symptoms before device discharge, blood levels of any antiarrhythmic medications, electrolyte levels if the device has been discharging, and educational and psychosocial evaluation of the patient. Angina is an important symptom to evaluate, but is not related to the AICD. Patients are not asked to maintain a daily pulse diary after AICD implantation, but they are advised to keep a history of symptoms experienced before the device discharges. AICDs do not affect heart sounds.
Nursing process step: Evaluation
Cognitive level: Evaluation

166. The most appropriate diet for a patient newly diagnosed with myocardial infarction is:
A. Low-sodium and low-cholesterol
B. General, as tolerated
C. Nothing-by-mouth (NPO)
D. Clear-liquid

CORRECT ANSWER—**D.** Metabolic demands increase after food is ingested; therefore, many physicians prefer to have patients receive clear liquids on the first day after admission for acute myocardial infarction. The patient also may be experiencing nausea and vomiting, in which case clear liquids are preferable. The patient can advance the diet as tolerated, but smaller, more frequent meals are recommended.
Nursing process step: Implementation
Cognitive level: Application

167. Which nursing intervention will have the greatest impact on the condition of a patient with acute heart failure?
A. Monitoring intake and output
B. Limiting the number of visitors
C. Encouraging coughing and deep breathing
D. Assessing the patient's knowledge of the disease

CORRECT ANSWER—**A.** Successful management of a patient with heart failure includes limiting physical activity, providing oxygen, and optimizing fluid balance. In heart failure, compensatory mechanisms cause the retention of fluid and sodium. In addition to limiting the patient's sodium intake, the physician often prescribes diuretics to eliminate both sodium and fluid. Intake and output must be closely monitored along with daily weight. The nurse should limit the number of visitors only if the patient's condition worsens in response to the increased activity from visitors. Encouraging coughing and deep breathing to avoid atelectasis and assessing the patient's knowledge of the disease are important nursing interventions. However, the patient's fluid status has the greatest impact on his failing heart.
Nursing process step: Implementation
Cognitive level: Application

168. Upon the initial assessment of a patient with unstable angina, which finding would warrant the nurse's immediate attention?
  A. Denial of the disease process
  B. Complaint of hunger
  C. Apparent anxiety
  D. Complaint of back discomfort

CORRECT ANSWER—D. During the initial assessment of this patient, pursuing the complaint of back discomfort takes priority. The nurse should first establish the type of discomfort the patient is experiencing by eliciting qualitative data from the patient. Back discomfort may or may not turn out to be anginal pain. A patient who denies the disease process needs to be reeducated about the disease to avoid disease-related injury. A complaint of hunger does not take precedence over evaluating and treating back discomfort. Anxiety is normal in such cases, but severe anxiety can exacerbate angina. After assessing the patient's back pain, the nurse should investigate the cause of the anxiety.
Nursing process step: Implementation
Cognitive level: Analysis

169. Sympathetic blocking agents may be used during a hypertensive emergency. These drugs work by:
  A. Stimulating the sympathetic nervous system
  B. Vasoconstricting the peripheral arteriolar bed
  C. Decreasing the activity of the sympathetic nervous system
  D. None of the above

CORRECT ANSWER—C. Although the exact mechanisms of action for each sympatholytic agent used during hypertensive emergencies are not completely known, the basic action of each of these drugs is to decrease outflow from the sympathetic nervous system. Stimulation of the sympathetic nervous system releases catecholamines and causes vasoconstriction of the arteriolar bed—both of which could exacerbate a hypertensive emergency.
Nursing process step: Intervention
Cognitive level: Comprehension

170. The nurse is caring for a patient who has been receiving high doses of a nitroprusside I.V. infusion for 4 days to control a hypertensive emergency. The nurse notices mental status changes and begins to suspect:

A. Thiocyanate and cyanide intoxication
B. Acute renal failure
C. Acute heart failure
D. Alveolar ventilation shunting

CORRECT ANSWER—A. Symptoms of thiocyanate and cyanide intoxication include mental status changes, blurred vision, nausea, tetanus, and other vague symptoms. Although thiocyanate and cyanide intoxication are uncommon, they usually occur when high doses of nitroprusside are given or when nitroprusside is administered for a prolonged period. Alveolar ventilation shunting can occur with the administration of nitroprusside, resulting in decreased PaO_2 and mental status changes. However, problems resulting from alveolar ventilation shunting tend to appear early in the course of therapy, and this patient has been receiving nitroprusside for 4 days. Acute renal failure and acute heart failure are not associated with the administration of high doses of nitroprusside. Nevertheless, either of these events could cause changes in mental status—from hypoxemia in acute heart failure or from the buildup of waste products in acute renal failure.
Nursing process step: Evaluation
Cognitive level: Analysis

171. The nurse would expect which of the following pulmonary problems to develop in a patient in cardiogenic shock?

A. Decreased pulmonary vascular resistance
B. Pulmonary vasodilation
C. Decreased PaO_2
D. Decreased pulmonary artery pressure

CORRECT ANSWER—C. Pulmonary changes associated with poor alveolar-capillary gas exchange occur in patients in cardiogenic shock. These changes result from pulmonary vasoconstriction, increased pulmonary vascular resistance, increased left atrial pressure, and hypoxia of the lung tissues caused by decreased blood flow. As a result, PaO_2 drops to 70 mm Hg or lower. Pulmonary artery pressure is increased, not decreased, in cardiogenic shock.
Nursing process step: Planning
Cognitive level: Analysis

172. Which type of blood pressure measurement is the most accurate way of monitoring a patient in cardiogenic shock?
A. Intra-arterial pressure
B. Automated cuff pressure
C. Palpable blood pressure
D. Auscultatory blood pressure

CORRECT ANSWER—**A.** Measuring arterial blood pressure with a cuff may yield inaccurate results in shock states, especially if the patient is treated with vasopressor agents. Intra-arterial pressures often are higher than cuff pressures and are not always the same in each artery. Even though intra-arterial monitoring is not perfect, it is the best method for assessing blood pressure in patients in cardiogenic shock. Palpable blood pressure and auscultatory blood pressure readings are not as reliable as intra-arterial blood pressure in these patients.
Nursing process step: Assessment
Cognitive level: Application

173. Which dietary restriction would best apply to a patient with acute heart failure?
A. Restricted sodium
B. Low cholesterol
C. Low fat
D. Reduced caloric intake

CORRECT ANSWER—**A.** A compensatory mechanism in heart failure is the retention of sodium and water, along with the inability of the kidneys to excrete sodium. A normal sodium intake of 5 to 8 g/day cannot be tolerated by most patients with heart failure. Sodium intake should be restricted to about 2 g/day. A low-cholesterol, low-fat diet would be recommended for a patient with a history of heart failure; the nurse should educate the patient about these dietary changes before discharge. A reduced caloric intake would not be recommended for all patients with acute heart failure; it would be based on the patient's individual condition.
Nursing process step: Implementation
Cognitive level: Application

174. Asystole sometimes can be mistaken for which type of arrhythmia?
  A. Idioventricular rhythm
  B. Pulseless ventricular tachycardia
  C. Fine ventricular fibrillation
  D. Complete heart block

CORRECT ANSWER—C. In some cases, ventricular fibrillation masquerades as asystole; however, the more common cause of a false report of asystole is operator error. Asystole must be differentiated from fine ventricular fibrillation, which appears as a slightly wavy baseline on the ECG, to ensure appropriate medical intervention. Coarse ventricular fibrillation, which is more easily terminated than fine ventricular fibrillation, is marked by large waves on the ECG. Idioventricular rhythms produce a heart rate of about 32 beats/minute and identifiable QRS complexes. Pulseless ventricular tachycardia is indicated by a rapid succession of QRS complexes. In complete heart block, P waves and QRS complexes are present, but there is no relationship between the two.
Nursing process step: Assessment
Cognitive level: Analysis

175. The nurse caring for a patient with sick sinus syndrome would expect to administer which drug first?
  A. Isoproterenol
  B. Atropine
  C. Dopamine
  D. Norepinephrine

CORRECT ANSWER—B. Sick sinus syndrome is a degenerative process of the sinoatrial node that can produce sinus bradycardia, slow atrial fibrillation, or alternating periods of bradycardia and tachycardia. Atropine is the drug of choice for a patient with sick sinus syndrome who is experiencing symptomatic bradycardia, or a heart rate less than 60 beats/minute. Isoproterenol is indicated for the immediate but temporary control of hemodynamically significant bradycardia that does not respond to atropine. Dopamine is indicated for hypotension in patients who are not hypovolemic. Norepinephrine is indicated for hypotension associated with shock states.
Nursing process step: Implementation
Cognitive level: Application

176. The preferred treatment for a hypertensive
urgency is:
  A. Oral antihypertensive agents
  B. I.V. antihypertensive agents
  C. Antianxiety agents
  D. Loop diuretics

CORRECT ANSWER—**B.** A hypertensive urgency
is a situation in which blood pressure should be
controlled within 24 hours. Differentiating a hypertensive urgency from a hypertensive emergency sometimes is not possible; therefore, I.V.
medications are preferred because their onset of
action is faster than that of oral agents. Antianxiety medications and loop diuretics also can be
administered intravenously; these agents may
help decrease blood pressure if anxiety and fluid
overload contribute to hypertension.
Nursing process step: Intervention
Cognitive level: Application

177. What is the most appropriate method of oxygen
delivery for a patient in cardiogenic shock?
  A. Face mask
  B. Face tent with high humidity
  C. Venturi mask to maintain PaO_2 between 60
  and 80 mm Hg
  D. Any method that maintains PaO_2 between 70
  and 100 mm Hg

CORRECT ANSWER—**D.** Adequate oxygenation
must be maintained in a patient in cardiogenic
shock. This involves giving the patient oxygen as
needed to maintain a PaO_2 level between 70 and
100 mm Hg. Different methods of oxygen therapy deliver different levels of inspired oxygen
concentration. The patient's response to oxygen
therapy will determine the type of device to be
used. Oxygen delivery devices include nasal cannula, face mask, partial rebreather mask, nonrebreather mask, Venturi mask, transtracheal oxygen, and CPAP (constant positive airway
pressure) mask. Aerosolized oxygen from a nebulizer can be delivered by face mask, hood, or
tent to provide needed humidity.
Nursing process step: Implementation
Cognitive level: Application

178. Because of high pressures in the left side of the
heart, which two valves are most often affected
by disease?
  A. Aortic and mitral
  B. Aortic and pulmonic
  C. Pulmonic and tricuspid
  D. Pulmonic and mitral

CORRECT ANSWER—**A.** The valves most commonly affected by disease are the aortic and mitral valves. Although the tricuspid and pulmonic
valves are affected less often, they can become
significantly diseased, which may result in
death. Pulmonic valve disorders commonly result from congenital malformations.
Nursing process step: Assessment
Cognitive level: Knowledge

179. The murmur associated with aortic stenosis is classified as a systolic murmur. It can best be heard by placing the diaphragm of the stethoscope over the:
  A. Apex of the heart
  B. Fifth intercostal space, midclavicular line
  C. Fourth intercostal space, left sternal border
  D. Aortic area

CORRECT ANSWER—D. The systolic murmur associated with aortic stenosis is a harsh, crescendo-decrescendo murmur found over the aortic area, which is at the right sternal border and second intercostal space. The patient may also have a split S_2 sound, and an increased point of maximum impulse. The apex of the heart is located approximately at the fifth intercostal space and at the left midclavicular line.
Nursing process step: Assessment
Cognitive level: Comprehension

180. Which test would best detect signs of rejection in a patient who has received a heart transplant?
  A. Endomyocardial biopsy
  B. Blood culture
  C. White blood cell count
  D. Electrophysiologic studies

CORRECT ANSWER—A. Endomyocardial biopsy principally is used to monitor patients for rejection after heart transplant. It also can be used to detect myocarditis, as well as cardiac toxicity in patients receiving chemotherapy. In addition, endomyocardial biopsy can help differentiate restrictive cardiomyopathy from constrictive pericarditis. Positive blood cultures in a heart transplant patient are a sign of infection. However, the patient's white blood cell count probably would not be increased because of the immunosuppressants given to prevent rejection. Electrophysiologic studies are used to evaluate the electrical activity of the heart, not to detect signs of rejection.
Nursing process step: Evaluation
Cognitive level: Analysis

181. The nurse would observe which finding during the later stages of hypovolemic shock?
  A. Decreased lactate level
  B. Hypoglycemia
  C. Confusion and agitation
  D. Decreased hemoglobin level

CORRECT ANSWER—C. Compensatory mechanisms fail when blood volume decreases by 25% and cerebral perfusion is reduced, resulting in confusion, agitation, and stupor. Reduced tissue perfusion leads to lactic acidosis and, consequently, increased lactate level. An intense adrenergic discharge occurs, resulting in hyperglycemia. Hemoglobin level may actually increase secondary to hemoconcentration in a dehydrated patient, unless the hypovolemia is due to hemorrhage.
Nursing process step: Assessment
Cognitive level: Evaluation

182. The critical care nurse knows that the leading cause of chest trauma is:
  A. Industrial crush accidents
  B. Falls from great heights
  C. High-speed automobile crashes
  D. Stab injuries

CORRECT ANSWER—**C.** Critical care nurses have a social responsibility to educate the public about avoidable causes of chest trauma. The majority of injuries to the chest result from rapid deceleration during a high-speed automobile crash. The use of seat belts can help prevent serious injury. The other responses all cause chest trauma, but not at the high rate associated with car accidents.
Nursing process step: Implementation
Cognitive level: Application

183. The nurse would expect to auscultate a bruit over all of the following structures *except:*
  A. Partially occluded carotid artery
  B. Completely occluded carotid artery
  C. Abdominal aortic aneurysm
  D. Femoral artery with 80% stenosis

CORRECT ANSWER—**B.** A bruit is the consequence of turbulent flow through a stenosed artery or the communication of an artery and a vein, such as in an arteriovenous fistula placed for renal dialysis. Because no blood flows through a completely occluded artery, bruits are not heard. However, bruits commonly are heard over the abdominal aorta when stenosis or an aneurysm exists.
Nursing process step: Assessment
Cognitive level: Comprehension

184. An appropriate intervention for a patient who develops second-degree atrioventricular (AV) block, Mobitz type II, is:
  A. Temporary pacemaker insertion
  B. Isoproterenol therapy
  C. No intervention if the patient is asymptomatic
  D. Electrical cardioversion

CORRECT ANSWER—**A.** Almost always, a second-degree AV block, Mobitz type II, originates below the level of the bundle of His. Because the transmission of the atrial impulse never reaches the ventricles, a bilateral blockage of the bundle branches exists. The prophylactic insertion of a ventricular pacing wire is the treatment of choice because second-degree AV block can easily degenerate into complete heart block. Electronic pacing provides better control than isoproterenol therapy and does not increase myocardial oxygen consumption. Electrical cardioversion is used to treat atrial fibrillation, atrial flutter, and unstable supraventricular tachycardia, as well as ventricular tachycardia in patients with a pulse who are unstable and do not respond to pharmacologic intervention. The risk of rapid clinical deterioration still exists in an asymptomatic patient, and pacemaker insertion is necessary for such a patient.
Nursing process step: Planning
Cognitive level: Application

185. The nursing evaluation of a patient being treated for a hypertensive crisis would indicate that:
A. Blood pressure is within prescribed limits
B. Hemodynamic parameters reflect normal blood volume
C. ECG reveals normal sinus rhythm
D. All of the above

CORRECT ANSWER—D. The nurse caring for a patient being treated for a hypertensive crisis would evaluate the effectiveness of treatment based on blood pressure, hemodynamic parameters, electrolyte levels, and cardiac rhythm.
Nursing process step: Evaluation
Cognitive level: Evaluation

186. Patient and family teaching for a patient who develops shock after an acute myocardial infarction should focus on:
A. Cardiac rehabilitation
B. Drug action and side effects
C. Current treatment plan
D. Reading materials related to the patient's condition

CORRECT ANSWER—C. Patient and family teaching must take into account the individual's readiness to learn. Patients who develop shock after an acute myocardial infarction need concise information related to their immediate care, not information related to future events, such as cardiac rehabilitation. The nurse should explain the treatment plan and the reasons for treatment in a manner that will decrease the patient's anxiety. The nurse should also explain why the patient is receiving a particular medication; however, information on mechanisms of action and side effects is unnecessary at this point. Reading materials are not appropriate for a patient in shock; although they may provide a diversion for family members, they are inappropriate until the patient's condition is stabilized.
Nursing process step: Implementation
Cognitive level: Application

187. The nurse working in an intensive care unit would prepare for which of the following for a symptomatic patient with acute cardiac tamponade?
A. Pericardial window procedure
B. Pericardiocentesis
C. Pericardiotomy
D. Mediastinal chest tube insertion

CORRECT ANSWER—B. In a patient with effusion greater than 200 ml or one who becomes symptomatic with the effusion, immediate evacuation of the accumulated fluid may be necessary. Both the pericardial window procedure and pericardiotomy are performed in the operating room, mostly for repeat effusions. A mediastinal chest tube drains the mediastinal cavity only. Thus, pericardiocentesis is the treatment of choice for draining fluid from the pericardial space.
Nursing process step: Implementation
Cognitive level: Application

188. The nurse would administer I.V. fluids to a patient experiencing:
   A. Widened pulse pressure
   B. Pulsus paradoxus
   C. Decreased systemic vascular resistance
   D. Decreased heart rate

CORRECT ANSWER—B. Pulsus paradoxus can occur in an intravascularly depleted patient because the reduced venous return is affected by changes in intrathoracic pressure during respiration. A possible cause of widened pulse pressure is hypervolemia resulting from increased stroke volume. Systemic vascular resistance is expected to increase as a compensatory mechanism in hypovolemia, thereby maintaining blood pressure. Compensatory tachycardia, not a decreased heart rate, usually occurs with hypovolemia.
Nursing process step: Implementation
Cognitive level: Analysis

189. The nurse would monitor which value to assess the response to treatment of a patient with a ventricular septal defect?
   A. Systemic vascular resistance
   B. Central venous pressure
   C. Pulmonary capillary wedge pressure
   D. Pulmonary vascular resistance

CORRECT ANSWER—D. In a patient with a ventricular septal defect, blood is shunted from the left ventricle to the right ventricle because of higher pressures on the left side of the heart. As pressures build on the right side, pulmonary blood flow increases, which can lead to right-sided heart failure and permanent pulmonary vascular injury. To appropriately manage such patients, the nurse must closely monitor pulmonary vascular resistance. Systemic vascular resistance reflects the impedance that the left ventricle must overcome to eject its volume. Central venous pressure indirectly reflects venous return to the right side of the heart. Normally, pulmonary capillary wedge pressure reflects pressure in the left ventricle just before contraction. However, in a patient with a ventricular septal defect, pulmonary capillary wedge pressure is not an accurate measure of left ventricular pressure because an opening exists in the septum separating the ventricles.
Nursing process step: Implementation
Cognitive level: Evaluation

190. Which crystalloid solution would be most appropriate for a hypotensive patient who has had flulike symptoms, including severe nausea, vomiting, and diarrhea, for 1 week?
A. Dextrose 5% in 0.9% sodium chloride solution with 40 mEq/liter of potassium chloride at a rate of 150 ml/hour
B. Dextrose 10% in .45% sodium chloride solution with 20 mEq/liter of potassium chloride at a rate of 50 ml/hour
C. Dextrose 5% in water with 2 g/liter of magnesium sulfate at a rate of 50 ml/hour
D. Total parenteral nutrition, including a 20% lipid solution

CORRECT ANSWER—A. A patient who has lost upper and lower GI fluids also has lost a large amount of electrolytes, especially sodium, chloride, and potassium. A solution of dextrose 5% in 0.9% sodium chloride solution with 40 mEq/liter of potassium chloride will replace extracellular and intracellular fluid losses as well as potassium, which is lost through the GI tract. The nurse should administer this solution at a high rate and assess the patient's cardiopulmonary response to the rate of infusion. The solutions in options B and C are administered at too slow a rate; they also will not provide the necessary electrolytes or replenish intracellular and extracellular fluids. Total parenteral nutrition should be reserved for patients who cannot receive enteral nutrition for an extended period and those who are obviously catabolic from starvation. Lipid solutions are not crystalloids.
Nursing process step: Implementation
Cognitive level: Analysis

191. The nurse must remain alert for the following condition, which typically is asymptomatic in the early stages after trauma:
A. Cardiac contusion
B. Cardiac laceration
C. Aortic dissection
D. Cardiac failure

CORRECT ANSWER—A. Cardiac contusion is a commonly missed or delayed diagnosis in patients who do not display obvious chest trauma. Symptoms are caused by inflammatory changes and often occur late. Cardiac laceration and aortic dissection result from more obvious chest trauma and generally are recognized early. Cardiac failure, cardiogenic shock, and cardiac arrest are reported complications of cardiac contusion.
Nursing process step: Assessment
Cognitive level: Evaluation

192. The treatment plan for a patient who has undergone mechanical aortic valve replacement would include all of the following *except:*
A. Anticoagulant therapy
B. Prophylactic antibiotic therapy before dental procedures
C. Cardiac rehabilitation
D. Prophylactic antiarrhythmic therapy

CORRECT ANSWER—D. Treatment for a patient who has undergone a mechanical valve replacement is slightly different than for a patient who has received a porcine valve replacement (bioprosthesis). Patients who have received a mechanical device, such as the Starr-Edwards or Björk-Shiley valve, require lifelong anticoagulant therapy; this is not necessary for patients with bioprostheses. Because of the risk of developing infective endocarditis, the patient should receive prophylactic antibiotic therapy before any surgical or dental procedure. Cardiac rehabilitation is indicated for any patient who undergoes cardiac surgery.
Nursing process step: Planning
Cognitive level: Application

193. Early postoperative care of a patient who has undergone abdominal aneurysm resection includes:
A. Providing adequate oral and I.V. fluids to prevent dehydration
B. Recommending that the patient stop smoking
C. Providing a soft, low-cholesterol diet
D. Administering adequate analgesia

CORRECT ANSWER—D. The large abdominal incision necessary for abdominal aneurysm resection is painful and can interfere with postoperative respiratory care and early ambulation. Providing analgesia via the I.V., I.M., or epidural route is essential. Oral food and fluids are contraindicated in the early postoperative period because of the patient's ileus. I.V. fluids, however, are essential for overcoming postoperative shifting of fluid from the intravascular space to the interstitial space, which can result in hypotension. Smoking cessation is important but not an early priority.
Nursing process step: Implementation
Cognitive level: Application

194. Which medication is the nurse most likely to administer to a patient with a cardiac contusion?
A. Heparin
B. Warfarin
C. Ibuprofen
D. Nitroglycerin

CORRECT ANSWER—C. Much of the pain experienced by a patient with a cardiac contusion is secondary to inflammatory changes in the chest and pericardium; therefore, ibuprofen is appropriate. Nitroglycerin would be indicated if the patient had evidence of myocardial ischemia, but vasodilators are otherwise of little value in patients with cardiac contusion. Anticoagulants generally are contraindicated in patients with chest trauma because of the risk of hemorrhage from associated injuries.
Nursing process step: Implementation
Cognitive level: Analysis

195. The nurse concludes that a patient who has undergone peripheral percutaneous transluminal angioplasty (PTA) has significantly improved distal blood flow when the ankle/brachial index (ABI) goes from:
A. 0.3 to 0.8 after the procedure
B. 0.9 to 0.4 after the procedure
C. 0.5 to 0.6 after the procedure
D. 0.6 to 0.5 after the procedure

CORRECT ANSWER—A. The ABI is a comparison of the blood pressure in the brachial artery with that in the ankle (pedal or posterior tibial pulse). The ankle pressure exceeds the brachial pressure in healthy individuals; a normal ABI is equal to or greater than 1.0. Patients with intermittent claudication have an ABI of 0.4 to 0.8; those with resting pain or severe ischemia have an ABI of less than 0.4. Although there are no set standards for what constitutes an improved ABI after PTA, a change of 0.5 to 0.6 most likely would be of little clinical benefit.
Nursing process step: Evaluation
Cognitive level: Comprehension

196. When discussing the home-care regimen for a patient with cardiomyopathy, the nurse should stress the importance of:
A. Monitoring the patient's daily weight and notifying the physician of any weight gain over 2 pounds
B. Encouraging good nutrition and following a low-cholesterol diet
C. Providing sufficient fluids to satisfy the thirst mechanism and prevent dehydration
D. Understanding that some depression is inevitable and that exercise can be used to alleviate it

CORRECT ANSWER—A. A weight gain of more than 2 pounds equals more than 1 liter of excess fluid, which could precipitate pulmonary edema in a patient with cardiomyopathy. When discharged, the patient will be prescribed diuretics and given fluid restrictions; a low-sodium diet also is indicated. Limiting cholesterol intake is not required unless the patient also has coronary artery disease or hyperlipidemia. Depression is common in patients with chronic disease and should be treated as needed with psychological or pharmacologic therapy. A patient with cardiomyopathy is unlikely to have the energy to exercise to alleviate depression.
Nursing process step: Implementation
Cognitive level: Analysis

197. The nurse should teach a patient with an automatic implantable cardioverter defibrillator (AICD) about the:
A. Need for follow-up appointments with the physician
B. Symptoms to report to the physician
C. Sensitivity of the device to magnetic fields
D. All of the above

CORRECT ANSWER—D. After implantation of an AICD, the patient must see the physician about every 2 months. Any unusual symptoms must be reported along with the number of shocks delivered by the device. Magnetic fields can inhibit the device and should be avoided.
Nursing process step: Intervention
Cognitive level: Knowledge

198. A 58-year-old male patient is diagnosed with right-sided heart failure and is admitted to the medical unit for observation. The nurse would expect to assess for which of the following signs and symptoms in this patient?

A. Dyspnea on exertion and bibasilar crackles

B. Dependent edema and hepatic engorgement

C. Distended neck veins and a systolic murmur

D. Angina-like pain when patient is in the supine position and fever

CORRECT ANSWER—B. Right-sided heart failure commonly is caused by left-sided heart failure; however, it also can occur independently of left-sided heart failure, for example, as a result of primary pulmonary hypertension. Symptoms of right-sided heart failure include distended neck veins, dependent edema, and hepatic engorgement. Symptoms of left-sided heart failure include orthopnea, dyspnea on exertion, crackles, low PaO_2, S_3 heart sound, and a systolic murmur. Angina-like pain when patient is in the supine position and a fever may indicate that pericarditis is developing.

Nursing process step: Assessment

Cognitive level: Comprehension

RESPIRATORY SYSTEM

Respiratory System

1. A patient who suffered a gunshot wound to the right chest is being treated in the intensive care unit for a sucking chest wound. His respiratory rate is 36 breaths/minute and oxygen saturation is 85%. The nurse would plan to evaluate symptoms in this patient because the:

A. Opening in the chest wall is smaller than the diameter of the airways

B. Opening in the chest wall is larger than the diameter of the airways

C. Opening in the chest wall is smaller than the diameter of the trachea

D. Opening in the chest wall is larger than the diameter of the trachea

CORRECT ANSWER—D. An open sucking chest wound results when the opening in the chest wall is larger than the diameter of the trachea. When this occurs, air enters the pleural space through the chest wall opening, causing the lung to collapse. If the opening is smaller than the diameter of the trachea, subjective symptoms are minimal. The overall airway diameter is not the important factor; the ratio of the trachea diameter to the wound size is what determines the patient's symptoms.

Nursing process step: Planning
Cognitive level: Comprehension

2. The nurse would implement aspiration precautions for each of the following patients *except:*

A. A 15-year-old male with multiple facial fractures

B. An 85-year-old male admitted for surgery to correct paralytic ileus

C. A 55-year-old male who underwent arthroscopic surgery 8 hours ago

D. A 45-year-old female who had a generalized tonic-clonic seizure 1 hour ago

CORRECT ANSWER—C. Patients at high risk for aspiration include those with a decreased level of consciousness (such as patients who have suffered seizures), those receiving tube feedings, those with neuromuscular disorders, those who recently received general anesthesia, and elderly patients. The 15-year-old male patient with multiple facial fractures will require tube feedings. The 85-year-old male patient is at risk because of his age and the general anesthesia used during surgery. The 45-year-old female patient has a variable level of consciousness as a result of the seizure; therefore, she also is at risk for aspiration. The 55-year-old male patient who underwent arthroscopic surgery would have received regional anesthesia; therefore, he would not be at risk for aspiration.

Nursing process step: Implementation
Cognitive level: Analysis

3. A 38-year-old patient with sarcoidosis is admitted because of recurrent pneumothorax. A chest tube is inserted, and the lung is reexpanded. Given the patient's history, the health care team decides to sclerose the lung. The nurse understands that sclerotherapy is advantageous for this patient because the:

A. Sclerosing agent will seal the hole in the lung
B. Pleura will become fibrotic when the sclerosing agent is added, making it unable to expand and accept air
C. Sclerosing agent will seal the pleura to the lung and remove the potential space
D. Lung will be unable to collapse as the external layer will be fibrosed

CORRECT ANSWER—C. Sarcoidosis is a multisystemic granulomatous disorder that typically causes lymphadenopathy, pulmonary infiltration, and skeletal, liver, eye, or skin lesions. The lungs are almost always involved; pulmonary clinical manifestations may include pleural effusions, spontaneous pneumothoraces, and hemoptysis. After a pneumothorax has occurred, sclerosing seals the pleura to the lung, removing the potential space and hindering pneumothorax development. Unfortunately, sclerotherapy may need to be repeated if pockets of unsclerosed tissue remain after the initial sclerosing. **Nursing process step:** Implementation **Cognitive level:** Comprehension

---

Questions 4 to 6 refer to the following information:
After being evaluated in the emergency department (ED), a 28-year-old female patient is admitted to the intensive care unit with an acute exacerbation of asthma. She states that she has been using inhaled albuterol every hour for the past day without relief. While in the ED, she received nebulized albuterol treatments every 20 minutes, subcutaneous epinephrine, I.V. methylprednisolone, and I.V. aminophylline. Arterial blood gas readings are pH, 7.45; partial pressure of carbon dioxide in arterial blood ($PaCO_2$), 28 mm Hg; partial pressure of oxygen in arterial blood (PaO_2), 80 mm Hg; HCO_3^-, 24 mm Hg; and fraction of inspired oxygen (FIO_2), .60 via a nonrebreather mask. Her respirations are 40 breaths/minute, and she exhibits a paradoxical breathing pattern.

4. Based on the clinical findings, the nurse would expect to initiate treatment for:
   A. Hypersensitivity reaction
   B. Status asthmaticus
   C. Adult respiratory distress syndrome (ARDS)
   D. Pneumonia

CORRECT ANSWER—**B.** Because the patient is experiencing an exacerbation of asthma, the nurse can assume that asthma is a preexisting condition. Asthma is a chronic reactive disorder of the airways that produces episodic, reversible airway obstruction via bronchospasm, increased mucus secretion, and mucosal edema. The patient has not responded to conventional therapy for asthma, which includes bronchodilators, steroids, and aminophylline. Asthma refractory to conventional therapy is called status asthmaticus. Hypersensitivity reactions are initiated by an inappropriate immune response, such as an allergic reaction. Neither pneumonia nor ARDS is caused by an exacerbation of asthma. Pneumonia is an acute infection of the lung's functional tissue resulting in inflammation of the alveoli. ARDS may be caused by several other conditions, such as aspiration of stomach contents, that increase capillary permeability in the lung circulation and result in pulmonary edema.
Nursing process step: Planning
Cognitive level: Analysis

5. The arterial blood gas levels indicate that the patient has:
   A. Respiratory alkalosis with hypoxemia
   B. Respiratory acidosis with compensation
   C. Respiratory alkalosis without compensation
   D. Respiratory acidosis without hypoxemia

CORRECT ANSWER—**A.** The $PaCO_2$ is decreased because of the patient's increased respiratory rate. A PaO_2 of 80 mm Hg on room air is normal. However, the FIO_2 of .60 indicates a blockage of oxygen at the arterial-alveoli interface. This obstruction prevents inspired air from passing through the respiratory membrane and diffusing into the erythrocytes, leading to hypoxemia. This condition is referred to as an arterial-alveoli gradient (A-a gradient) or shunt. Respiratory acidosis with compensation would be reflected by elevated $PaCO_2$ and bicarbonate levels. Respiratory alkalosis without compensation would be reflected by decreased $PaCO_2$ level without any change in bicarbonate level. Respiratory acidosis without hypoxemia would be reflected by an elevated $PaCO_2$ level (caused by inadequate ventilation to maintain CO_2 level within normal limits), and a PaO_2 level of 80 mm Hg on room air indicates that no hypoxemia is present.
Nursing process step: Assessment
Cognitive level: Analysis

6. The patient may experience which major adverse effect as a result of the medications she received in the emergency department?
A. Nausea
B. Nervousness
C. Tachycardia
D. Hypertension

CORRECT ANSWER—**C.** Bronchodilators, aminophylline, and epinephrine all cause tachycardia. Consequently, the patient should be closely observed for this adverse effect. These drugs must be used cautiously in certain patients, such as young children and elderly patients with heart disease or cardiac impairment, in whom tachycardia could be especially detrimental. Patients receiving aminophylline I.V. infusions should have their serum blood levels of theophylline monitored; toxicity has been reported at theophylline levels greater than 20 mcg/ml. Patients receiving subcutaneous epinephrine may be monitored with a continuous ECG to check for rate and rhythm disturbances, especially if patient is receiving more than one injection. Nervousness and nausea are minor adverse effects of these drugs. Hypotension, not hypertension, typically occurs as a result of tachycardia or decreased venous return caused by hyperinflation of the lungs.
Nursing process step: Assessment
Cognitive level: Comprehension

7. A patient with a C3 to C4 spinal injury and tracheostomy is evaluated for swallowing ability. The nurse knows that the correct procedure for such evaluation involves:
A. Having the patient swallow, deflating the cuff, suctioning, then reinflating the cuff
B. Inflating the cuff, suctioning, having the patient swallow, then deflating the cuff
C. Deflating the cuff, having the patient swallow, reinflating the cuff, then suctioning
D. Deflating the cuff, suctioning, having the patient swallow, then reinflating the cuff

CORRECT ANSWER—**C.** Evaluating swallowing ability is important for determining how a patient with a spinal cord injury will obtain caloric intake. To determine whether the patient can properly direct food or fluid, the patient's cuff should be deflated, the patient should swallow dyed food or fluid, the cuff should be reinflated, and the patient should be suctioned to check for aspiration of the color-marked materials.
Nursing process step: Implementation
Cognitive level: Comprehension

Questions 8 to 10 refer to the following information:

A 65-year-old female patient weighing 60 kg and with a history of chronic obstructive pulmonary disease (COPD) is placed on the following ventilator settings for weaning: FIO_2, .40; tidal volume, 600 cc; intermittent mandatory ventilation (IMV), 8 breaths/minute; positive end-expiratory pressure (PEEP), 5 cm H_2O and pressure support, 10 cm H_2O. Twenty minutes after the ventilator changes have been made, the nurse assesses the patient and notices diaphoresis and labored respirations. The patient's vital signs are heart rate, 160 beats/minute; blood pressure, 160/90 mm Hg; and temperature, 99° F (37.2° C).

8. Which of the following is the most likely cause of the patient's clinical condition?
A. Low FIO_2
B. High tidal volume
C. Low tidal volume
D. IMV setting

CORRECT ANSWER—D. IMV frequently is used for weaning patients from mechanical ventilation and usually works well. The disadvantage of IMV is that it increases the work of breathing. A patient with chronic lung disease typically cannot handle the increased work of breathing and will begin to show signs of respiratory distress shortly after being placed on IMV. Pressure support is a ventilatory parameter that can be adjusted to decrease the work of breathing; it may need to be increased in this situation instead of returning the patient to assist-control mode. Because this patient weighs 60 kg and tidal volume is calculated at 10 to 15 cc per kilogram of body weight (usually 10 cc/kg to prevent overdistention of the alveoli), a tidal volume of 600 cc is appropriate. An FIO_2 of .40 is more than adequate for a patient with chronic disease. If the FIO_2 is too high, the hypoxic drive is suppressed and the patient will not attempt to breathe spontaneously.
Nursing process step: Evaluation
Cognitive level: Analysis

9. The nurse discusses the patient's condition with the physician and the respiratory therapist. A decision is made to:

A. Increase the PEEP to 10 cm H_2O
B. Increase the tidal volume to 700 cc
C. Increase the pressure support to 14 cm
D. Switch to inverse ratio ventilation

CORRECT ANSWER—C. Pressure-support ventilation is a mode of mechanical ventilation commonly used in conjunction with IMV to decrease the work of breathing. It eliminates the resistance of the ventilator circuit and allows the patient to increase endurance during weaning. PEEP and inverse ratio ventilation are used to improve PaO_2, usually in patients with adult respiratory distress syndrome. The patient's tidal volume should be adequate; the calculation for tidal volume is 10 cc per kilogram of body weight, and this patient is receiving 600 cc ($10 \text{ cc} \times 60 \text{ kg}$).
Nursing process step: Implementation
Cognitive level: Application

10. The nurse is aware that intermittent mandatory ventilation (IMV) can:

A. Increase respiratory muscle strength
B. Decrease respiratory muscle strength
C. Increase respiratory muscle endurance
D. Decrease respiratory muscle endurance

CORRECT ANSWER—A. IMV is useful for weaning patients with chronic obstructive pulmonary disease from mechanical ventilation because it allows the respiratory muscles to become stronger. This occurs through the same mechanism involved in weight lifting: repetitive motion against resistance increases the size of muscle fibers. However, care must be taken to prevent respiratory muscle fatigue. Increasing the patient's muscle strength can increase the patient's pulmonary endurance. Pressure-support ventilation used in conjunction with IMV will improve respiratory muscle endurance.
Nursing process step: Assessment
Cognitive level: Comprehension

11. The nurse caring for a patient with adult respiratory distress syndrome (ARDS) should assess for which of the following changes in pulmonary function?

A. Decreased compliance and decreased functional residual capacity
B. Increased compliance and increased functional residual capacity
C. Decreased minute ventilation and increased tidal volume
D. Increased minute ventilation and decreased tidal volume

CORRECT ANSWER—A. Two hallmarks of ARDS are decreased lung compliance and decreased functional residual capacity. Decreased lung compliance occurs secondary to the development of diffuse hypercellular, edematous lung tissue. Decreased lung compliance and decreased functional residual capacity also result from the increased fluid and debris present in the alveoli. Minute ventilation is calculated as the respiratory rate multiplied by the tidal volume. An increase in tidal volume does not cause a decrease in minute ventilation, and a decrease in tidal volume does not cause an increase in minute ventilation.
Nursing process step: Planning
Cognitive level: Knowledge

12. A 16-year-old male is brought to the emergency department after a football practice in which he was tackled aggressively and suffered injuries to the neck and upper chest. He is dyspneic and complains of hoarseness and dysphagia. Based on these findings, the nurse would suspect that the patient has which type of injury?
A. Oropharyngeal injury
B. Tracheobronchial tear
C. Laryngeal injury
D. Esophageal injury

CORRECT ANSWER—**C.** Hoarseness and dysphagia can result from laryngeal or cervical injury. Esophageal injuries are associated with acute substernal chest pain, fever, and shock. Tracheobronchial injuries are marked by hemoptysis, mediastinal emphysema, recurrent pneumothorax, and massive air leakage. Tracheobronchial tears cause air to accumulate in the thoracic cavity; if left untreated, these injuries can lead to lobular atelectasis, hemoptysis, and persistent air leak syndrome. Oropharyngeal injuries are associated with broken or displaced teeth, tongue injury, and obstructive pharyngeal injury.
Nursing process step: Assessment
Cognitive level: Application

13. A patient with advanced acquired immunodeficiency syndrome (AIDS) is diagnosed with active tuberculosis. Which of the following regimens would the nurse expect the physician to prescribe?
A. Isoniazid and rifampin
B. Ethambutol, pyrazinamide, and isoniazid
C. Isoniazid, rifampin, ethambutol, and pyrazinamide
D. Ethambutol, ciprofloxacin, pyrazinamide, and streptomycin

CORRECT ANSWER—**C.** A patient with advanced AIDS is less able to fight tuberculosis because of decreased cellular immunity. Usually, a 21-day course of treatment is required to identify the specific sensitivity of the tuberculous organism to antibacterial medications. However, multi-drug-resistant tuberculosis is prevalent among patients with AIDS. To avoid inadequate treatment and prevent development of resistant tuberculosis, the patient is prescribed a four-drug regimen until specific sensitivities are established; the medication regimen is then adjusted. This patient would receive isoniazid (a tuberculostatic), rifampin (which is tuberculocidal), pyrazinamide (which is highly specific for *Mycobacterium tuberculosis*), and ethambutol *or* streptomycin. Ethambutol and streptomycin are not given together to this patient. Ciprofloxacin usually is not a first-line drug used to treat resistant tuberculosis.
Nursing process step: Planning
Cognitive level: Application

Questions 14 to 17 refer to the following information:
A patient with pneumonia is on a mechanical ventilator and requires suctioning every 2 hours. He is producing a large amount of thick, tenacious, yellow secretions. In the afternoon, the nurse notices that the amount of secretions has abruptly decreased.

14. The patient's peak inspiratory pressure (PIP) increases from 26 to 36 mm Hg. All other vital signs are normal. What process probably is occurring?
   A. Pneumonia is resolving
   B. Pulmonary emboli are forming
   C. Pneumothorax is occurring
   D. Mucus plugs are forming

CORRECT ANSWER—**D.** The nurse must monitor for any trend in the secretions produced by the patient. An abrupt decrease in the amount of secretions is a sign that secretions are being retained; the higher PIP used to ventilate the patient reflects the increased airway resistance caused by retained secretions. PIP typically increases abruptly, not gradually. If the pneumonia were resolving, PIP would be low. Pneumothorax and pulmonary emboli typically cause respiratory distress, which is not the case for this patient.
Nursing process step: Assessment
Cognitive level: Analysis

15. Aggressive chest physiotherapy is instituted but is not successful in removing the secretions. Which type of drug would the nurse expect the physician to prescribe next?
   A. Anticholinergic
   B. Mucolytic
   C. Antibiotic
   D. Diuretic

CORRECT ANSWER—**B.** Mucolytics thin the mucus by lysing white blood cells. An anticholinergic or diuretic would thicken secretions; an antibiotic would not help the patient expectorate secretions.
Nursing process step: Planning
Cognitive level: Comprehension

16. The physician prescribes 1 ml of a 10% solution of acetylcysteine via a nebulizer. What other type of drug should be given with this medication?
   A. Bronchodilator
   B. Mucolytic
   C. Mydriatic
   D. Anti-inflammatory agent

CORRECT ANSWER—**A.** Acetylcysteine is used as adjunctive therapy to treat patients with abnormal or viscid mucous secretions. Acetylcysteine can cause adverse reactions, such as bronchospasm, although their incidence is higher with the 20% solution. However, because of the potential for bronchospasm, acetylcysteine should always be administered with a bronchodilator. Mucolytics can be used to prepare patients for bronchoscopy and other bronchial studies. Mydriatic agents, which dilate pupils, and anti-inflammatory agents are not indicated.
Nursing process step: Implementation
Cognitive level: Analysis

17. The use of which drug would increase the patient's risk of developing nosocomial pneumonia?
   A. Aminophylline
   B. Labetalol hydrochloride
   C. Cimetidine
   D. Spironolactone

CORRECT ANSWER—C. Cimetidine and other histamine$_2$ blockers make the pH of the gastric flora more basic. The normally low pH in the stomach usually kills bacteria that would otherwise travel from the GI tract into the lungs. Because cimetidine changes the pH of the stomach, more bacteria can grow in the GI tract and migrate to the respiratory tract; this process is facilitated by the lack of glottic closure in a patient with an artificial airway. Aminophylline, labetalol, and spironolactone are not associated with such adverse effects as leukopenia, which could increase the risk of nosocomial infection or pneumonia.
Nursing process step: Assessment
Cognitive level: Comprehension

18. A 65-year-old male patient is admitted for respiratory distress that he claims has been steadily increasing over the past 24 hours. His medical history reveals an intake of six beers a day and smoking of three packs of cigarettes a day. He was diagnosed with chronic obstructive pulmonary disease (COPD) 3 years ago. The patient is dyspneic and cyanotic, and complains of chest pain. Breath sounds are diminished on the right side and distant on the left side. Given these findings, the nurse would suspect that the patient is experiencing:
   A. Exacerbation of COPD
   B. Spontaneous pneumothorax
   C. Myocardial infarction
   D. Pleural infection

CORRECT ANSWER—B. Spontaneous pneumothorax is a common complication in patients with COPD or lung cancer and in cigarette smokers ages 20 to 40. Typical findings include dyspnea, chest pain, cyanosis, and absent or distant breath sounds on the affected side. Pleural rubs are common in patients with pleural infections, whereas breath sounds usually are coarse in patients with pulmonary problems resulting from myocardial infarction.
Nursing process step: Assessment
Cognitive level: Evaluation

19. Which physiologic component affects the work of breathing?
   A. Functional residual capacity
   B. Compliance
   C. Negative inspiratory force
   D. Reserve volume

CORRECT ANSWER—B. Three physiologic components affect the work of breathing: compliance, airway resistance, and lung- and thoracic-wall expandability. Negative inspiratory force is a weaning parameter. Functional residual capacity and reserve volume are volumes of air in the lungs at different times. ·
Nursing process step: Assessment
Cognitive level: Knowledge

20. A 72-year-old female with chronic bronchitis has been placed on a mechanical ventilator since developing pneumonia and acute respiratory failure. Her ventilator settings are FiO_2, .40; tidal volume, 600 cc; and assist control, 10 breaths/minute. She has a 7-cm endotracheal tube in her airway. She has been receiving antibiotics for the past 10 days, and her chest X-ray film is clear. The size of the endotracheal tube can increase the work of breathing by increasing the airway's:
A. Negative inspiratory force
B. Minute ventilation
C. Resistance
D. Maximum inspiratory pressure

CORRECT ANSWER—C. The size of an endotracheal tube directly affects airway resistance—the smaller the tube, the greater the resistance. For each one-half centimeter decrease in tube size, airway resistance is increased twofold. Negative inspiratory force measures how effectively a patient can move a volume of air to maintain adequate ventilation. Minute ventilation and maximum inspiratory pressure indicate the level of lung compliance, which also affects the work of breathing.
Nursing process step: Assessment
Cognitive level: Analysis

21. A patient is admitted to the intensive care unit with an acute exacerbation of asthma. Auscultation reveals nearly absent breath sounds. Thirty minutes after administering albuterol via nebulizer, the nurse auscultates diffuse inspiratory and expiratory wheezes throughout all lung fields. This finding most likely represents:
A. Increased airflow
B. No change in airflow
C. Decreased airflow
D. No correlation with airflow

CORRECT ANSWER—A. Changes in breath sounds provide a general indication of response to treatment. Nearly absent breath sounds or no chest sounds indicate severe airflow obstruction. A noisy chest is a sign that air is flowing through the air passages, even though they are still partially obstructed.
Nursing process step: Assessment
Cognitive level: Evaluation

22. A patient with pneumonia is admitted to the intensive care unit with the following signs and symptoms: abrupt, shaking chills; temperature, 101° F (38.3° C); tympanic respirations, 34 breaths/minute; dyspnea and sharp pain during inspiration; and production of rust-colored sputum. Which organism is the most likely cause of the pneumonia in this patient?
A. *Mycoplasma*
B. *Pneumococcus*
C. *Haemophilus influenzae*
D. *Klebsiella*

CORRECT ANSWER—B. Pleuritic chest pain, chills, and rust-colored sputum are the most common signs of pneumococcal pneumonia. Infection with *Mycoplasma* typically results in fever, myalgia, headache, minimally productive cough, and nonpleuritic chest pain. *Haemophilus influenzae* causes chills, fever, cough, and purulent sputum. Infection with *Klebsiella* manifests suddenly and is characterized by blood-tinged sputum and tachycardia.
Nursing process step: Assessment
Cognitive level: Analysis

23. A left-sided tension pneumothorax is best described as an accumulation of air in the:
A. Left pleural space, resulting in collapse of the left lung
B. Right pleural space, resulting in collapse of the left lung
C. Left pleural space, resulting in collapse of the left lung and compression of the right thoracic structures
D. Left pleural space, resulting in collapse of the right lung and compression of the right thoracic structures

CORRECT ANSWER—C. Tension pneumothoraces result in collapse of the lung on the injured side, increased intrathoracic pressure on the injured side, and compression of the thoracic structures on the uninjured (opposite) side. Thus, a left-sided tension pneumothorax would involve an accumulation of air in the left pleural space that results in collapse of the left lung and compression of the right thoracic structures.
Nursing process step: Assessment
Cognitive level: Comprehension

24. A simple, closed pneumothorax can be caused by:
A. Bullet lodged in the pleural space
B. Mechanical ventilation
C. Knife wound
D. Thoracotomy

CORRECT ANSWER—B. Simple, closed pneumothoraces occur in the absence of an external wound; there is no communication between the pleural space and atmospheric air. This type of pneumothorax can occur in the intensive care unit as a result of mechanical ventilation, central I.V. line placement (if the pleural space is pierced but there is no communication with external atmospheric pressures), or cardiopulmonary resuscitation (during which the rib pierces the pleural cavity).
Nursing process step: Assessment
Cognitive level: Comprehension

25. Injury to the lungs, aortic arch, and vertebral column is associated with fractures of which structures?
A. Ribs 1 and 2
B. Ribs 3 to 5
C. Ribs 7 to 9
D. Clavicles

CORRECT ANSWER—A. Fractures of the first two ribs are associated with high-impact trauma and injury to the lungs, aorta, and vertebral column. Fractures of ribs 3 to 9 most commonly are associated with blunt trauma and underlying lung injury. Lower-rib injuries also are associated with liver tears and other abdominal injuries. Clavicular injury usually does not result in injury to the lungs, aortic arch, or vertebral column.
Nursing process step: Assessment
Cognitive level: Knowledge

Questions 26 and 27 refer to the following information:
A 35-year-old female patient is admitted to the intensive care unit 6 hours after being involved in a multiple-vehicle accident. The patient has a steering wheel imprint on her chest and significant pain and discomfort with breathing. On arrival at the emergency department, she had infiltrates and bloody sputum. Her current chest X-ray film shows progressive alveolar capillary injury and patchy infiltrates. She continues to have bloody secretions (as evidence by suctioning).

26. The nurse suspects that the patient's primary lung problem involves:
A. Infection
B. Adult respiratory distress syndrome (ARDS)
C. Pulmonary contusions
D. Hemothorax

CORRECT ANSWER—C. A pulmonary (lung) contusion results from the chest wall hitting an object, such as a steering wheel, or from the blunt force of an explosion. Hemorrhage and edema occur within the area of the contusion and gradually involve surrounding tissue. A lung contusion commonly is associated with pulmonary hematoma or laceration. ARDS typically presents as a diffuse process. An infection usually does not cause bloody sputum. A hemothorax would be seen on the chest X-ray film; it generally is not associated with patchy infiltrates.
Nursing process step: Assessment
Cognitive level: Analysis

27. Given the assessment findings, the nurse would expect the patient's lung compliance to be:
A. Increased
B. Decreased
C. Within normal limits
D. Better later than earlier

CORRECT ANSWER—B. Compliance decreases as the lungs become more difficult to ventilate. Consequently, as the patient's pulmonary condition worsens, lung compliance will decrease.
Nursing process step: Evaluation
Cognitive level: Evaluation

28. Where on the ventilator can the nurse determine the level of auto–positive end-expiratory pressure (PEEP) the patient may be inadvertently receiving?
A. Peak airway pressure setting
B. Plateau pressure setting
C. Spontaneous minute ventilation reading
D. Pressure support reading

CORRECT ANSWER—A. During end expiration, the inspiratory port of the ventilator is occluded. If auto-PEEP occurs, it will register where the peak inspiratory pressure is read. In order for auto-PEEP to be determined, the inspiratory port must be occluded. Depending on the ventilator used, each of the other parameters is found on a separate dial and can be read independently of each other. Also, none of the other options indicate the level of auto-PEEP the patient is receiving.
Nursing process step: Evaluation
Cognitive level: Comprehension

29. Which ventilator change would the nurse antici-pate to decrease a patient's auto–positive end-ex-piratory pressure (PEEP)?
A. Increase the respiratory rate
B. Increase the tidal volume
C. Decrease the oxygen flow rate
D. Change the setting from assist-control ventila-tion to synchronized intermittent mechanical ventilation

CORRECT ANSWER—D. The primary goal in de-creasing auto-PEEP is to increase the patient's ex-halation time. Ventilator changes that accom-plish this goal include decreasing the respiratory rate or tidal volume, increasing the oxygen flow rate, and changing the setting from assist-control ventilation to synchronized intermittent mechan-ical ventilation.
Nursing process step: Implementation
Cognitive level: Comprehension

30. Aspiration of which fluid is associated with the greatest potential for pulmonary injury?
A. Clear liquid with a pH of 2.0
B. Tube feedings
C. Fresh water
D. Salt water

CORRECT ANSWER—A. The pH of aspirated ma-terial largely determines the extent of lung inju-ry. As the pH falls below 2.5, the severity of lung injury increases. Although aspiration of neutral pH fluids, such as tube feedings, causes hypoxia, pulmonary edema, and changes in surfactant, ne-crosis is rare; the sequelae usually are transient and more easily reversed. The nature and extent of pulmonary damage also is determined by the volume aspirated. Near-drowning victims aspi-rate less than 25 milliliters of fluid per kilogram of body weight; the principal changes that occur are inflammation and fluid and electrolyte imbal-ances, which may lead to hypercapnia, hypoxe-mia, and acidosis, and, rarely, permanent lung in-jury.
Nursing process step: Assessment
Cognitive level: Knowledge

31. Inspiratory and expiratory stridor may be found in a patient:
A. Who is experiencing an exacerbation of goiter
B. Who is experiencing an acute asthmatic attack
C. Who has aspirated a piece of meat
D. Who has severe laryngotracheitis

CORRECT ANSWER—C. Inspiratory and expirato-ry stridor is a low-pitched crowing sound heard in patients who have a foreign body obstructing the trachea or mainstem bronchi. Acute asthmat-ic attacks are characterized by wheezing, where-as goiter attacks and severe laryngotracheitis are associated with inspiratory stridor only.
Nursing process step: Assessment
Cognitive level: Knowledge

Questions 32 and 33 refer to the following information:
Three days after undergoing surgical repair for fractures of the first four ribs, a 25-year-old male patient has a left chest tube in place that exhibits consistent air leakage, bloody suction material, and mediastinal subcutaneous emphysema.

32. The nurse suspects these findings are caused by:
   A. Infectious pleural effusions
   B. Tracheobronchial tear
   C. Diffuse pulmonary hemorrhage
   D. Pulmonary embolism

CORRECT ANSWER—B. Injury to the tracheobronchial tree can cause incomplete separation of the lumens from the surrounding fascia. In many cases, extension of pneumothorax does not become evident until 3 to 4 days after the injury. Diffuse pulmonary hemorrhage, infectious pleural effusions, and pulmonary embolism are unlikely causes of subcutaneous emphysema or pleural leaks.
Nursing process step: Assessment
Cognitive level: Analysis

33. The nurse caring for this patient would expect to prepare for:
   A. Insertion of a second chest tube
   B. Change in antibiotic therapy
   C. Ventilation/perfusion (V/Q) scan
   D. Bronchoscopy

CORRECT ANSWER—D. The definitive diagnostic test for tracheobronchial tearing is bronchoscopy, which permits direct inspection and visualization of the trachea and bronchi through a flexible fiber-optic or rigid bronchoscope. The other options are not appropriate for diagnosing or treating tracheobronchial tears.
Nursing process step: Planning
Cognitive level: Comprehension

34. A patient with flail chest is placed on a mechanical ventilator for internal stabilization. What is the usual length of time a patient is intubated to ensure rib healing?
   A. 1 to 5 days
   B. 5 to 10 days
   C. 15 to 25 days
   D. 25 to 30 days

CORRECT ANSWER—C. Healing of rib and lung parenchyma injuries usually takes 2 to 3 weeks. The patient will remain in the intensive care unit until the ribs have healed to the point that they can create negative inspiratory pressure gradients. Time also is required for weaning the patient from the ventilator and developing the patient's pulmonary stamina.
Nursing process step: Implementation
Cognitive level: Knowledge

35. Which pulmonary artery pressure readings reflect the need for diuresis in a patient with severe pulmonary contusions?
   A. Pulmonary artery systolic pressure/pulmonary artery diastolic (PAS/PAD) pressures, 22/12 mm Hg; pulmonary capillary wedge pressure (PCWP), 10 mm Hg
   B. PAS/PAD, 50/25 mm Hg; PCWP, 18 mm Hg
   C. PAS/PAD, 35/16 mm Hg; PCWP, 12 mm Hg
   D. PAS/PAD, 15/8 mm Hg; PCWP, 6 mm Hg

CORRECT ANSWER—B. Normal pulmonary artery catheter pressures include PAS of 15 to 30 mm Hg and PAD of 4 to 12 mm Hg. PCWP, a measure of the preload of the left ventricle, should be between 4 and 12 mm Hg. Increased pulmonary artery pressure readings are associated with increased pulmonary vascular pressures related to disease and hypervolemia. A patient with pulmonary contusions has preexisting capillary damage and is at increased risk for third-space fluid shifts. Diuresis helps prevent pulmonary edema and respiratory compromise.
Nursing process step: Implementation
Cognitive level: Evaluation

36. Positive end-expiratory pressure (PEEP) decreases systemic blood pressure by:

A. Enhancing venous return to the right atrium

B. Increasing forward flow through the systemic circulation

C. Decreasing stroke volume of the left ventricle

D. Compressing intrathoracic vessels and increasing preload

CORRECT ANSWER—C. PEEP compresses intrathoracic vessels, which impedes venous return to the right atrium and ventricle and decreases preload of the left ventricle. The decreased stroke volume of the left ventricle causes a decrease in cardiac output and systemic blood pressure. Compression of the intrathoracic vessels hinders outflow. Patients requiring PEEP therapy who do not have normal blood volume will need increased blood volume to increase the volume in the intravascular space as well as vasopressors to maintain adequate blood pressure.

Nursing process step: Implementation

Cognitive level: Comprehension

37. What is the most prominent finding on a chest X-ray film of a patient with adult respiratory distress syndrome (ARDS)?

A. Infiltrates

B. Bilateral infiltrates

C. Kerley's B lines

D. Enlarged cardiac silhouette

CORRECT ANSWER—B. Bilateral infiltrates are the classic diagnostic finding on a chest X-ray film of a patient with ARDS. Kerley's B lines and an enlarged cardiac silhouette are consistent with cardiogenic pulmonary edema, not ARDS (which is also known as noncardiogenic pulmonary edema).

Nursing process step: Evaluation

Cognitive level: Evaluation

38. A 35-year-old male with a history of alcoholic pancreatitis is transferred to the intensive care unit after developing acute respiratory distress 3 days after admission to the hospital. He is on a 100% nonrebreather mask, breathing at 40 breaths/minute. His chest X-ray film appears normal. His arterial blood gas results include pH, 7.48; $PaCO_2$, 33 mm Hg; PaO_2, 69 mm Hg; and HCO_3^-, 24 mEq/liter. The nurse would implement measures to treat which primary acid-base disturbance?

A. Metabolic acidosis

B. Metabolic alkalosis

C. Respiratory acidosis

D. Respiratory alkalosis

CORRECT ANSWER—D. The primary acid-base disturbance is alkalosis, indicated by a pH of greater than 7.45. The decreased $PaCO_2$ is a sign of respiratory alkalosis. The HCO_3^- is normal, although a change in this parameter would indicate a metabolic problem. Metabolic acidosis is evidenced by decreased pH and HCO_3^-; metabolic alkalosis is evidenced by increased pH and HCO_3^-.

Nursing process step: Implementation

Cognitive level: Analysis

39. A patient with a diaphragmatic injury is likely to report all of the following *except:*
A. Nausea and vomiting
B. Chest pain
C. Shoulder pain
D. Shortness of breath

CORRECT ANSWER—B. A patient with a diaphragmatic injury may be asymptomatic or may complain of abdominal pain, nausea and vomiting, postprandial discomfort, shortness of breath, and shoulder pain. Chest pain commonly is not associated with a diaphragmatic injury.
Nursing process step: Assessment
Cognitive level: Analysis

Questions 40 and 41 refer to the following information:
A female patient is admitted to the intensive care unit with pulmonary contusions after a motor vehicle accident. Her arterial blood gas levels in the emergency department at 7 p.m. were: pH, 7.25; $PaCO_2$, 58 mm Hg; PaO_2, 70 mm Hg; and HCO_3^-, 20 mEq/liter. Her pulse oximetry reading is 85%.

---

40. The patient is given two ampules of sodium bicarbonate. Her pulse oximetry reading at 8 p.m. is 92%. What does this change reflect?
A. Increase in oxygen-carrying capacity of the blood
B. Increase in oxyhemoglobin binding
C. Decrease in oxygen tension
D. Decrease in venous oxygen tension

CORRECT ANSWER—B. Pulse oximetry, which determines arterial oxygen saturation (SaO_2), is based on the ability of the saturation probe to detect oxygen-hemoglobin binding. The more hemoglobin that is bound to oxygen molecules, the higher the saturation reading. Saturation readings can be altered by acidosis, carbon dioxide concentration, increased temperature, and 2,3-diphosphoglycerate (2,3-DPG) level. If the patient is acidotic, hyperthermic, or hypercapnic or has an increased 2,3-DPG level, the oxyhemoglobin bonds are more easily broken and oxygen is released to the tissues; this is known as a "shift to the right." The pulse oximetry reading will decrease, reflecting the desaturation of the hemoglobin. If the patient is alkalotic or hypothermic or has a low carbon dioxide concentration or a decreased 2,3-DPG level, the bonds between hemoglobin and oxygen are stronger and the saturation reading is increased (this is known as a "shift to the left"). When a patient is given sodium bicarbonate, the serum becomes more alkaline; this increases the affinity of the hemoglobin for oxygen and increases the saturation reading. Oxygen-carrying capacity is determined by the hemoglobin content of the blood, which is unchanged in this patient. Oxygen tension is proportional to oxygen saturation and would increase in this case.
Nursing process step: Evaluation
Cognitive level: Analysis

41. After administering multiple doses of sodium bicarbonate to the patient, the nurse obtains samples for two arterial blood gas (ABG) analyses, neither of which were received by the laboratory. Rather than subject the patient to another blood sample collection for ABG analysis at 9 p.m., the physician takes a venous sample of blood to the laboratory for pH analysis. The patient's pulse oximetry reading indicates arterial oxygen saturation of 94%. Venous pH is 7.49. What does this suggest about the patient's tissue oxygenation?
A. Tissue oxygenation is greater at 9 p.m. than 7 p.m.
B. Tissue oxygenation is greater at 7 p.m. than 9 p.m.
C. No significant change in oxygenation has occurred in the tissues
D. No conclusions can be drawn; venous pH is not an appropriate index for evaluating oxygen saturation

CORRECT ANSWER—B. At 7 p.m., the patient had a pH of 7.25 and a PaO_2 of 70 mm Hg. In acidosis, oxygen is readily transferred from hemoglobin to the tissues. At 9 p.m., the patient has a pH of 7.49; although the PaO_2 at this time is unknown, the bonds between oxygen and hemoglobin are stronger in an alkalotic environment. Because no changes were made to the patient's oxygen therapy, the stronger bonds between oxygen and hemoglobin would decrease the release of oxygen to the tissues. Consequently, the patient's tissue oxygenation would be greater at 7 p.m. than at 9 p.m. Venous pH is an acceptable index for evaluating oxygen saturation.
Nursing process step: Evaluation
Cognitive level: Analysis

42. A patient with fractured ribs is experiencing decreased ventilation because of refractory pain. Actions to correct this situation would include:
A. Strapping the chest with adhesive bandages and providing I.V. pain medications
B. Placing a restrictive band around the upper thorax and providing oral pain medications
C. Providing a cough pillow and performing an intercostal nerve block
D. Providing a cough pillow and performing a spinal nerve block

CORRECT ANSWER—C. Multiple-rib fractures are associated with significant pain that hinders a patient's respiratory effort. Atelectasis, pneumonia, and respiratory failure may result. Strapping or binding the chest would further impede expansion. Local administration of long-acting anesthetic agents to block the associated intercostal nerves is appropriate, especially if the pain is refractory to lidocaine or other local anesthetics. A cough pillow provides the patient with physical and psychological support during coughing and deep-breathing exercises.
Nursing process step: Implementation
Cognitive level: Analysis

43. The nurse notices that an asthmatic patient's pulsus paradoxus has changed from 60 mm Hg to 30 mm Hg, which indicates:
A. Increased blood pressure
B. Decreased hyperinflation
C. Increased hyperinflation
D. Decreased blood pressure

CORRECT ANSWER—B. A decreasing pulsus paradoxus is associated with decreases in airflow obstruction (decreased hyperinflation) and work of breathing. Decreased airflow obstruction would cause the blood pressure to increase, not decrease. However, pulsus paradoxus does not correlate with blood pressure measurements, but rather with the level of pulmonary airflow obstruction.
Nursing process step: Assessment
Cognitive level: Evaluation

44. The nurse is assessing a patient being treated for exacerbation of asthma. Which findings provide the best warning of an impending fatal asthma attack?

A. Previous intubation, rapid onset of symptoms, and no response to bronchodilator therapy

B. Cyanosis, rapid onset of symptoms, and peak expiratory flow rate above 300 cc after bronchodilator therapy is initiated

C. Altered level of consciousness, development of symptoms over 3 days, and inability to speak after bronchodilator therapy is initiated

D. Sinus tachycardia, worsening of symptoms at night, and peak expiratory flow rate less than 150 cc

CORRECT ANSWER—A. Unless status asthmaticus is promptly and correctly treated and the patient responds to therapy, fatal respiratory failure will occur. The following findings are associated with a fatal asthma attack: rapid onset and deterioration of symptoms, wide diurnal variation in airflow obstruction, little or no response to bronchodilator therapy after 1 hour of treatment, altered level of consciousness, central cyanosis, PaO_2 below 50 mm Hg with a $PaCO_2$ above 45 mm Hg, previous or recurrent episodes of status asthmaticus or pulsus paradoxus, and previous intubation.

Nursing process step: Evaluation
Cognitive level: Evaluation

45. All of the following measures increase pulmonary compliance *except:*

A. Continuous positive airway pressure

B. Decreased inspiratory flow rate

C. Deep-breathing and coughing exercises

D. Chest physiotherapy

CORRECT ANSWER—B. Compliance is a measure of the ease with which the lungs and chest wall expand. A decreased inspiratory flow rate can reduce airway pressure by lengthening the time in which a breath is delivered, but it probably will not directly affect compliance. Continuous positive airway pressure increases compliance by maintaining a constant flow of air into the pulmonary tissue and making inhalation easier. Chest physiotherapy and deep-breathing and coughing exercises facilitate secretion removal and alveolar expansion.

Nursing process step: Implementation
Cognitive level: Application

46. A nurse suspects that a patient has just aspirated a foreign object. The correct order of care for this patient would be to:

A. Place the patient in semi-Fowler's position, administer oxygen, and suction the patient

B. Administer oxygen, place the patient in high-Fowler's position, and suction the patient

C. Suction the patient, administer oxygen, and place the patient in low-Fowler's position

D. Place the patient in a lateral decubitus position, suction the patient, and administer oxygen

CORRECT ANSWER—D. The gravity-dependent areas of the lung are at greatest risk when a patient aspirates. Placing the patient in a lateral decubitus position localizes the injury. Suctioning facilitates removal of the aspirated materials, and oxygen can help prevent any hypoxia or hypoxemia resulting from the injury. Placing the patient in the semi- or low-Fowler's position does not help localize the area of injury.

Nursing process step: Planning
Cognitive level: Application

47. A patient with fractures of the ribs or sternum is most likely to have:
   A. Dyspnea and localized pain
   B. Angina
   C. Dyspnea and backache
   D. Pain on deep inspiration and touch

CORRECT ANSWER—D. A patient with rib or sternal fractures is likely to have pain that worsens with chest-wall movement, deep inspiration, or touch. Dyspnea and localized pain are associated with flail chest; angina is associated with cardiac contusion. Dyspnea and backache are associated with rupture of the aorta and the major vessels.
Nursing process step: Assessment
Cognitive level: Comprehension

48. The second stage of adult respiratory distress syndrome (ARDS) is characterized by:
   A. Progressive respiratory failure
   B. Progressive shunting
   C. Persistent hyperventilation
   D. Persistent hypercapnia

CORRECT ANSWER—C. ARDS occurs in four stages. The first stage, which encompasses the initial injury and resuscitation, is characterized by lactic acidosis leading to compensatory respiratory alkalosis caused by hyperventilation. Stage two, in which the patient appears stable but arterial blood gas values continue to worsen, is characterized by persistent hyperventilation. Stage three is marked by progressive respiratory failure. Stage four, the terminal phase, is characterized by progressive hypoxemia, hypercapnia, lactic acidosis, and alveolar shunting.
Nursing process step: Assessment
Cognitive level: Evaluation

49. The nurse would plan to treat which primary problem in a patient with adult respiratory distress syndrome (ARDS)?
   A. Oxygenation
   B. Ventilation
   C. Perfusion
   D. Effusion

CORRECT ANSWER—A. Inadequate oxygenation is the primary problem in ARDS, which causes severe refractory hypoxemia. ARDS results from an acute lung injury, which causes bilateral pulmonary infiltrates and significantly reduces lung compliance. The pathologic cause of ARDS is diffuse alveolar damage, which leads to the mismatch between ventilation and perfusion that causes the severe hypoxemia. Effusions may occur if ARDS is caused by infection, but they are a secondary complication, not the primary problem, in a patient with ARDS.
Nursing process step: Planning
Cognitive level: Comprehension

Questions 50 and 51 refer to the following information:
A 65-year-old female patient with bronchitis has been in the intensive care unit for 4 weeks and is on mechanical ventilation. The physician orders that weaning parameters be obtained.

---

50. The nurse would obtain which parameters?
A. Tidal volume, negative inspiratory force, and reserve volume
B. Vital capacity, negative inspiratory force, and functional residual capacity
C. Tidal volume, reserve volume, and functional residual capacity
D. Vital capacity, negative inspiratory force, and minute ventilation

CORRECT ANSWER—D. Weaning parameters include vital capacity, negative inspiratory force, minute ventilation, and respiratory rate. Reserve volume is the air remaining in the lungs at the end of a forced expiration; functional residual capacity is the air left in the lungs at the end of a normal exhalation. Reserve volume and functional residual capacity are not weaning parameters.
Nursing process step: Implementation
Cognitive level: Knowledge

51. While evaluating weaning parameters, the nurse must remember that the parameters may be skewed because they:
A. Require patient cooperation
B. Are continuous
C. Are done on the ventilator
D. Are difficult to obtain

CORRECT ANSWER—A. Weaning parameters require the patient to be able or willing to follow instructions, such as taking a deep breath. Weaning parameters often appear poor because the patient would not or could not do what was asked. Weaning parameters are not continuous and are not difficult to obtain. Although weaning parameters are done on the ventilator, this should not skew the results.
Nursing process step: Evaluation
Cognitive level: Analysis

52. A patient with significant drainage following chest tube placement for a trauma-induced hemothorax is being considered for autotransfusion. Contraindications for autotransfusion include all of the following *except:*
A. Decreased urine output and creatinine level of 5.0 mg/dl
B. Injury occurring within 2 hours of initiation of therapy
C. Abdominal perforation with ruptured diaphragm
D. History of Hodgkin's disease 2 years before the injury

CORRECT ANSWER—B. Autotransfusion is contraindicated in any patient with a known malignancy because of the risk of introducing malignant cells into the circulation; in inadequate renal or hepatic function because of the inability to sufficiently clear the by-products of hemolysis, which occurs with reinfusion; in wounds more than 3 hours old because of the risk of contamination; and in significant contamination caused by bowel, stomach, or esophageal wounds.
Nursing process step: Implementation
Cognitive level: Comprehension

53. A 62-year-old female patient with chronic obstructive pulmonary disease is placed on the following ventilator settings: FIO_2, .35; tidal volume, 700 cc; intermittent mandatory ventilation, 8 breaths/minute; and pressure support, 10. Her arterial blood gas readings at these settings are pH, 7.42; $PaCO_2$, 58 mm Hg; PaO_2, 121 mm Hg; and HCO_3^-, 35 mEq/liter. The nurse should be concerned about the patient's PaO_2 reading because it:
   A. Is dangerously low
   B. May blunt her hypoxic drive
   C. May cause oxygen toxicity
   D. May cause bronchospasm

54. Which value reflects compensation in a patient with chronically elevated $PaCO_2$ level?
   A. pH
   B. $PaCO_2$
   C. PaO_2
   D. HCO_3^-

55. Which parameter is the best way to evaluate a patient's response to a bronchodilator?
   A. Forced vital capacity
   B. Oxygen saturation
   C. Forced expiratory volume
   D. Peak expiratory flow

CORRECT ANSWER—B. A patient with chronic lung disease has lost the carbon dioxide (CO_2) drive for breathing, and the body accepts a higher CO_2 level. It is essential not to blunt the hypoxic drive, which helps stimulate respiration. A high FIO_2 can cause oxygen toxicity and would decrease the stimulus for breathing in this patient. A high PaO_2 will not cause oxygen toxicity or bronchospasm. A PaO_2 of 90 mm Hg is more than enough to provide adequate oxygenation for cellular metabolism; a patient would actually be safe with a PaO_2 as low as 65 mm Hg.
Nursing process step: Evaluation
Cognitive level: Analysis

CORRECT ANSWER—D. HCO_3^- increases as the body compensates metabolically for the chronically elevated $PaCO_2$. However, the response is not immediate; it takes several days for the kidneys to retain HCO_3^-.
Nursing process step: Assessment
Cognitive level: Evaluation

CORRECT ANSWER—D. A peak expiratory flow meter is a portable device that provides rapid assessment of the severity of disease and the patient's response to treatment. Measuring peak expiratory flow does not require a full-forced expiration, so this parameter is less likely than other measures (such as forced vital capacity or forced expiratory volume) to cause coughing and bronchospasm. Also, most asthmatic patients monitor peak expiratory flows at home and are familiar with the maneuver. A change in oxygen saturation is a late sign of bronchospasm or its resolution.
Nursing process step: Planning
Cognitive level: Comprehension

56. A 22-year-old male patient who underwent a bone marrow transplant is admitted to the intensive care unit with increased shortness of breath, cough, and hypoxemia. He is diagnosed with cytomegalovirus (CMV) pneumonia. Which drug most commonly is prescribed for this condition?
 A. I.V. co-trimoxazole
 B. I.V. ganciclovir and immunoglobulin
 C. I.V. pentamidine and corticosteroids
 D. I.V. tobramycin

CORRECT ANSWER—B. Ganciclovir can be used alone or in combination with I.V. immunoglobulin to treat CMV pneumonia. Most CMV infections result from reactivation of the CMV virus in seropositive patients. The medications listed in the other options are ineffective against viruses. Prophylactic use of immunoglobulin infusion, ganciclovir, or high-dose acyclovir can reduce the incidence and severity of CMV pneumonia.
Nursing process step: Implementation
Cognitive level: Comprehension

57. Assessment of a patient with a chest tube includes:
 A. Noting bubbling within the drainage chamber
 B. Assessing drainage every 24 hours
 C. Auscultating breath sounds every 4 hours and as needed
 D. Percussing for subcutaneous emphysema every 8 hours

CORRECT ANSWER—C. The nurse should frequently auscultate breath sounds in a patient with a chest tube to ensure that the tube is patent, expansion is achieved and maintained, and the patient's pulmonary status is not declining; such assessments should occur at least every 4 hours and as needed. Chest tube drainage should be assessed at least once every shift for stable patients and more frequently for those who have just had the chest tube placed or who have had significant drainage. Subcutaneous emphysema is best evaluated by palpation or auscultation. Bubbling should not occur within the drainage chamber of the chest tube.
Nursing process step: Assessment
Cognitive level: Application

58. A patient with a significant spontaneous pneumothorax would have which sign or symptom?
 A. Sudden bilateral chest pain
 B. Increased fremitus
 C. Uneven chest expansion
 D. Decreased work of breathing

CORRECT ANSWER—C. Signs and symptoms of spontaneous pneumothorax include difficulty breathing even without exercise, sudden unilateral chest pain, shortness of breath, increased work of breathing, uneven chest-wall movement, decreased or absent fremitus, and distant or absent breath sounds.
Nursing process step: Assessment
Cognitive level: Evaluation

59. The respiratory tract normally is protected from ingested liquid or solid materials by all of the following structures *except*:
A. Epiglottis
B. Vocal cords
C. Tongue
D. Pharyngeal palate

CORRECT ANSWER—C. The epiglottis, vocal cords, pharyngeal palate, pharyngeal constrictor muscles, and cervical esophagus are coordinated to prevent aspiration of liquid or solid materials. The tongue propels food and fluid back toward the pharynx and esophagus, but it does not protect the trachea from aspiration.
Nursing process step: Assessment
Cognitive level: Knowledge

Questions 60 and 61 refer to the following information:
An 80-kg, 52-year-old female patient with adult respiratory distress syndrome has been on a mechanical ventilator for 8 days. Her current ventilator settings are as follows: synchronized intermittent mandatory ventilation (SIMV), 14 breaths/minute; tidal volume, 800 cc; FIO_2, .60; and positive end-expiratory pressure (PEEP), 8 cm H_2O. During the past 24 hours, her peak airway pressures have been 30 to 40 cm H_2O, and she has been hemodynamically stable, with a blood pressure of 110/50 mm Hg and a heart rate of 86 beats/minute.

Over the next 2 hours, the patient's airway pressures increase to 50 cm H_2O and her blood pressure drops to 90/50 mm Hg, with a heart rate of 100 beats/minute. Occlusion of the expiratory circuit during end expiration reveals an airway pressure of 15 cm H_2O. When the patient is taken off the ventilator for suctioning, her blood pressure returns to the baseline level.

60. The nurse suspects that the fluctuations in the patient's condition are caused by:
A. Expiratory delay
B. Inspiratory pause
C. Too-low tidal volume
D. Auto-PEEP

CORRECT ANSWER—D. Auto-PEEP results from an accumulation of pressures within the alveoli. Auto-PEEP may cause decreased expiratory time, which results in incomplete exhalation of alveolar air. Auto-PEEP is associated with changes similar to those that occur when PEEP is increased, including possible decreased venous return, decreased cardiac output, tachycardia, and barotrauma. Expiratory delay and inspiratory pause do not increase end-expiratory pressures. Because this patient weighs 80 kg and tidal volume is calculated at 10 to 15 cc per kilogram of body weight, a tidal volume of 800 cc is appropriate. If the tidal volume were too low, the patient may exhibit signs of atelectasis, such as dyspnea and hypoxia.
Nursing process step: Evaluation
Cognitive level: Evaluation

61. The patient's condition suddenly deteriorates. She is tachycardic, hypotensive, diaphoretic, and hypoxic. An arterial blood gas analysis is performed, and a chest roentgenograph is taken. Airway pressure increases to 60 cm H_2O, and the patient is difficult to ventilate manually when taken off the ventilator. Breath sounds are diminished on the right side, although chest expansion is equal. The nurse plans to intervene based on the potential causes of these findings, which include:

A. Pneumothorax and right-sided mainstem intubation

B. Pneumothorax, kinked endotracheal tube, and mucus plug

C. Pneumothorax, endotracheal cuff leak, and mucus plug

D. Endotracheal cuff leak, mucus plug, and migration of the endotracheal tube into the carina

CORRECT ANSWER—B. Pneumothorax, mucus plug, kinked endotracheal tube, and an endotracheal tube too close to the carina can cause the symptoms experienced by this patient. An endotracheal cuff leak does not increase airway pressure. Right-sided mainstem intubation causes diminished breath sounds on the left side.
Nursing process step: Planning
Cognitive level: Evaluation

62. Nursing care of a patient who has aspirated solid food chunks includes all of the following *except:*

A. Administering supplemental oxygen

B. Maintaining normal blood volume

C. Preparing the patient for pulmonary angiography

D. Turning the patient on his side and suctioning immediately

CORRECT ANSWER—C. Because aspiration causes diffusion defects and edema of the affected airways, oxygen therapy often is required. Turning the patient on his side and suctioning immediately helps limit the injury by removing aspirated material from the lungs. Maintaining normal blood volume and perfusion aids oxygen delivery and carbon dioxide removal. Pulmonary angiography is not helpful in diagnosing or treating aspiration; this test is used to detect blood flow abnormalities in the pulmonary circulation. Direct bronchoscopy can be used to remove foreign material, but there is a risk of pushing the foreign bodies further into the pulmonary system.
Nursing process step: Implementation
Cognitive level: Application

63. The nurse maintains an adequate water level in the water-seal chamber of a chest tube drainage system because the water seal:
A. Controls the suction level of the chest tube system
B. Controls the rate of drainage from the pleural cavity
C. Prevents air and pleural fluid from reentering the pleural cavity
D. Determines the amount of drainage from the pleural cavity

CORRECT ANSWER—C. The water-seal chamber maintains a seal with the pleural cavity and prevents air or fluid from being pulled back into the pleural space. The rate of drainage is determined by the amount of suction applied and the rate of bubbling in the suction-control chamber. The amount of drainage is determined by the quantity of fluid within the pleural cavity and the patency of the chest tube and drainage systems. The suction level is the result of the amount of water placed in the suction-control chamber, not the water-seal chamber.
Nursing process step: Implementation
Cognitive level: Comprehension

Questions 64 and 65 refer to the following information:
After administering a nebulized bronchodilator to an asthmatic patient, the nurse notices a sustained decrease (from 93% to 86%) in oxygen saturation on the pulse oximetry readings.

64. The nurse realizes this decrease resulted from:
A. Increased airway resistance
B. Increased pulmonary vasoconstriction
C. Increased perfusion to less ventilated alveoli
D. Increased ventilation to less perfused pulmonary capillaries

CORRECT ANSWER—D. Bronchodilators can worsen hypoxemia while decreasing airway resistance. During an asthma attack, the bronchial walls hypertrophy and clearance of secretions decreases, causing a bronchiolar obstruction. This obstruction reduces alveolar ventilation, and blood is diverted away from poorly ventilated alveoli as a result of pulmonary vasoconstriction caused by hypoxemia. When bronchodilators are administered, the alveoli near poorly perfused capillaries are opened. A ventilation-perfusion mismatch occurs, and hypoxemia results.
Nursing process step: Assessment
Cognitive level: Analysis

65. Which treatment is appropriate in this situation?
  A. Providing vigorous chest physiotherapy
  B. Increasing FIO_2
  C. Continuing to administer the bronchodilator
  D. Stopping bronchodilator therapy

CORRECT ANSWER—B. An increased FIO_2 will deliver a higher concentration of oxygen to the alveoli; the oxygen will diffuse into the pulmonary capillaries and prevent further vasoconstriction. Continued administration of bronchodilators without increasing FIO_2 will not treat the hypoxemia, which is secondary to the ventilation-perfusion mismatch. Vigorous chest physiotherapy will not improve the hypoxemia and may exacerbate status asthmaticus by increasing reactivity of the airways and causing further bronchoconstriction. Stopping bronchodilator therapy also would not improve the patient's clinical condition. Continuing bronchodilator therapy with a subsequent increase in FIO_2 will improve both ventilation and perfusion and thus improve oxygenation.
Nursing process step: Implementation
Cognitive level: Application

66. A patient with multiple rib fractures asks to be "taped up," like he has seen in the movies. The nurse correctly explains that binding the thoracic cavity with tape is no longer recommended because:
  A. Taping makes assessment of rib fractures more difficult
  B. Taping leads to increased atelectasis and pneumonia
  C. Taping increases pain associated with rib fractures
  D. Taping can compromise cardiac function by compressing the thoracic cavity

CORRECT ANSWER—B. Binding the chest with tape or restrictive bands increases the patient's risk of atelectasis and pneumonia. An inability to assess rib fractures and compromised cardiac function are not the primary reasons why taping is no longer recommended. Because of its stabilizing effect, taping would decrease, not increase, pain associated with rib fractures.
Nursing process step: Implementation
Cognitive level: Synthesis

Questions 67 to 69 refer to the following information:
A 25-year-old male patient is admitted to the intensive care unit after an industrial accident in which he fell 26 feet and suffered multiple fractures of his fourth and sixth ribs on the right side. He also sustained a minor head injury. The patient has been receiving I.V. morphine sulfate for pain.

67. Twenty-four hours after the accident, the patient's chest X-ray film shows a complete whiteout of the lower lobe of the right lung. The nurse knows this finding indicates which type of injury?
A. Multiple rib fractures
B. Detached sternum
C. Inhalation injury
D. Flail chest

CORRECT ANSWER—**D.** Flail chest is characterized by multiple fractures of multiple ribs in which one section of the chest wall moves freely. Multiple rib fractures refer to single fractures of multiple ribs. A detached sternum occurs when the cartilage holding the sternum in a fixed position breaks, allowing the sternum to move independently of the chest wall. An inhalation injury is characterized by dyspnea that occurs suddenly or gradually after inhalation of chemicals or hot gases.
Nursing process step: Assessment
Cognitive level: Knowledge

68. The nurse should plan appropriate measures to treat which primary problem associated with this type of injury?
A. Hypoventilation caused by pain and sedation
B. Hypoventilation caused by head injury and sedation
C. Hyperventilation caused by head injury
D. Asynchronous respirations

CORRECT ANSWER—**A.** Flail chest causes hypoventilation because of pain. The patient typically receives analgesics for the pain; however, these medications place the patient at risk for oversedation, which also causes hypoventilation. The patient suffered only a minor head injury, which should not affect his breathing. Nevertheless, the nurse should continue to monitor his neurologic status and evaluate for any change. Flail chest causes the patient to have paradoxical chest movement with each respiration, and absent breath sounds may be detected over the affected side. Asynchronous respirations are a sign of diaphragmatic fatigue.
Nursing process step: Planning
Cognitive level: Application

69. While obtaining vital signs, the nurse notices that a portion of the patient's chest wall moves inward on inspiration and outward on expiration. The nurse realizes this paradoxical movement is caused by:
A. Increased negative pressure on inspiration
B. Increased pain on inspiration
C. Decreased tidal volume on inspiration
D. Decreased inflow on inspiration

CORRECT ANSWER—**A.** The negative pressure generated on inspiration causes the flail part of the chest to be drawn inward on inspiration. Conversely, a flail chest moves outward on expiration, when there is less negative pressure in the thorax. This paradoxical movement causes severe pain, but the pain does not cause the paradoxical movement. Because of the increase in negative pressure, the affected lung contracts on inspiration and bulges on expiration, leading to hypoxia. The decreased tidal volume and inflow to the affected lung are caused by flail chest; they do not cause flail chest.
Nursing process step: Implementation
Cognitive level: Analysis

70. Vocal fremitus typically is increased in a patient with:
   A. Pneumothorax
   B. Hemothorax
   C. Pulmonary hemorrhage
   D. Subcutaneous emphysema

CORRECT ANSWER—**C.** Vocal fremitus increases with increased lung density, as seen in patients with pulmonary hemorrhage. Fremitus decreases in conditions in which air (as in pneumothorax and subcutaneous emphysema) or blood (as in hemothorax) occupy the pleural space.
Nursing process step: Assessment
Cognitive level: Evaluation

71. Nursing care of a patient undergoing intubation includes all of the following *except:*
   A. Auscultating central breath sounds
   B. Applying pressure to the cricoid cartilage when directed by the physician
   C. Administering an anesthetic and muscle relaxant as ordered
   D. Ensuring that the endotracheal or nasotracheal tube is properly secured

CORRECT ANSWER—**A.** Applying pressure to the cricoid cartilage, administering sedatives and neuromuscular blockers, ensuring tube safety, and assisting the physician are all expected roles of the bedside nurse. When auscultating for bilateral breath sounds, the nurse should listen to the peripheral, not central, chest; this is a more accurate means of determining that the tube has entered the trachea and not the esophagus. Bilateral measurement allows the nurse to assess for tube placement above the carina, as opposed to a single mainstem intubation.
Nursing process step: Implementation
Cognitive level: Application

Questions 72 to 76 refer to the following information:
A 25-year-old male patient is admitted to the critical care unit after a motorcycle accident. His injuries include multiple leg fractures, ruptured spleen, and perforated bowel. He received 8 units of blood during surgery to remove his spleen and set his fractures.

72. The nurse would plan to evaluate for which syndrome in this high-risk patient?

A. Syndrome of inappropriate antidiuretic hormone (SIADH)

B. Marfan syndrome

C. Adult respiratory distress syndrome (ARDS)

D. Stevens-Johnson syndrome

CORRECT ANSWER—C. The patient has multiple risk factors for ARDS, including multiple blood transfusions, multiple fractures, and increased risk of sepsis. SIADH most commonly is associated with malignant diseases, central nervous system disorders, nonmalignant pulmonary hypertension, and administration of such drugs as chlorpropamide, vincristine, cyclophosphamide, and barbiturates. Marfan syndrome is a generalized disorder of the connective tissue; it has skeletal, ocular, and cardiovascular manifestations. Stevens-Johnson syndrome is a reaction of the skin and mucous membranes in response to infections (such as herpes simplex), vaccinations, drugs, cancer, or infectious mononucleosis.
Nursing process step: Planning
Cognitive level: Analysis

73. The patient is placed on a mechanical ventilator at the following settings: FIO_2, .50; tidal volume, 700 cc; and assist control with a rate of 10 breaths/minute. Arterial blood gas levels include pH, 7.32; $PaCO_2$, 32 mm Hg; PaO_2, 51 mm Hg; and HCO_3^-, 19 mEq/liter. What is the patient's primary acid-base disturbance?

A. Respiratory acidosis

B. Respiratory alkalosis

C. Metabolic acidosis

D. Metabolic alkalosis

CORRECT ANSWER—C. A pH of 7.32 indicates acidosis, and an HCO_3^- of 19 mEq/liter indicates a metabolic problem. Because the $PaCO_2$ level is not increased, the acid-base disturbance does not have a respiratory component. Both metabolic and respiratory alkalosis can be immediately ruled out by the patient's pH (pH less than 7.42 reflects acidosis; pH greater than 7.42 indicates alkalosis).
Nursing process step: Assessment
Cognitive level: Analysis

74. Based on the patient's injuries, what is the most likely cause of the acid-base disturbance?

A. Sepsis

B. Pancreatitis

C. Gastritis

D. Colitis

CORRECT ANSWER—A. A perforated bowel may allow fecal matter to escape into the abdominal cavity, thereby increasing the risk of sepsis and metabolic acidosis. Pancreatitis can cause metabolic acidosis, but it does not occur immediately after trauma has occurred. Gastritis and colitis also are not immediate consequences of trauma, although they may occur as long-term adverse effects of treatment and hospitalization.
Nursing process step: Evaluation
Cognitive level: Evaluation

75. Which ventilator change would the nurse make in this situation?
A. Increasing tidal volume
B. Increasing FIO_2
C. Increasing respiratory rate
D. Switching to intermittent mandatory ventilation (IMV)

CORRECT ANSWER—B. The patient's PaO_2 is dangerously low, so the nurse would increase FIO_2. Increased FIO_2 will increase diffusion of oxygen across the alveolar-capillary membrane because of the increase in the partial pressure of oxygen within the alveoli. Increasing the tidal volume, increasing the respiratory rate, or switching to IMV will not improve PaO_2; these maneuvers do not improve the ability of oxygen to diffuse across the alveolar-capillary membrane.
Nursing process step: Implementation
Cognitive level: Application

76. A pH of 7.32, as evidenced by the most recent arterial blood gas analysis, would cause which change in the oxyhemoglobin dissociation curve?
A. Shift to the right
B. Shift to the left
C. No change
D. pH does not correlate with oxyhemoglobin dissociation curve

CORRECT ANSWER—A. Acidosis is one physiologic change that can cause the oxyhemoglobin dissociation curve to shift to the right. When a shift to the right occurs, hemoglobin more readily gives up oxygen to the tissues. Consequently, although less oxygen is in the blood, the oxygen can enter the tissues and can prevent hypoxia. Other physiologic changes that cause a shift to the right on the oxyhemoglobin dissociation curve include hyperthermia, hypercapnia, and increased 2,3-diphosphoglycerate (2,3-DPG) level. Conversely, a shift to the left can be caused by alkalosis, hypothermia, hypocapnia, and decreased 2,3-DPG level. A shift to the left causes hemoglobin to bind more tightly to oxygen; therefore, not as much oxygen is released to the tissues. Any one or a combination of these conditions can cause a shift in the oxyhemoglobin dissociation curve.
Nursing process step: Assessment
Cognitive level: Knowledge

77. While examining a patient with multiple penetrating injuries to the thoracoabdominal area, the nurse notes bowel sounds in the patient's chest. This finding indicates:
A. Esophageal rupture
B. Gastric outlet obstruction
C. Diaphragmatic injury
D. Intestinal perforation

CORRECT ANSWER—C. A patient with a diaphragmatic injury may have bowel sounds in the chest area. This may result from herniation of the intestinal tract through the diaphragmatic rupture or from radiation of bowel sounds through the diaphragm. Esophageal rupture produces subcutaneous crepitus in the chest wall, respiratory distress, epigastric pain, and hematemesis. Gastric outlet obstruction results in eructation, epigastric fullness and discomfort, anorexia, nausea, and vomiting. Intestinal perforation causes intense abdominal pain, abdominal rigidity, and fever.
Nursing process step: Assessment
Cognitive level: Evaluation

78. A 45-year-old female asthmatic patient has required mechanical ventilation for the past 5 days. She is receiving albuterol via nebulizer, I.V. methylprednisolone, and a continuous I.V. infusion of midazolam and vecuronium. Because of the concurrent use of these drugs, the nurse must closely monitor for:
A. Narcotic withdrawal syndrome
B. Muscle weakness
C. Hypothermia
D. Electrolyte imbalances

CORRECT ANSWER—B. The concurrent I.V. infusion of vecuronium (a neuromuscular blocker) and methylprednisolone (a corticosteroid) can cause severe myopathy that may last for weeks to months after the infusion is stopped; therefore, the nurse must monitor for muscle weakness. Continuous infusion of these drugs should be limited to 48 hours if possible. The nurse should frequently assess muscle function using a peripheral nerve stimulator, and the patient should be allowed partial return of muscle function by decreasing or stopping the infusion periodically. Vecuronium and methylprednisolone are not narcotics, so assessing for narcotic withdrawal syndrome is not indicated. The nurse should monitor for electrolyte imbalances secondary to dehydration, which is associated with acute asthma. However, neither electrolyte imbalances nor hypothermia are associated with the concurrent administration of a nondepolarizing muscle relaxant and a corticosteroid.
Nursing process step: Evaluation
Cognitive level: Analysis

79. Which drug will increase serum levels of theophylline?
A. Phenobarbital
B. Cimetidine
C. Phenytoin
D. Rifampin

CORRECT ANSWER—B. Theophylline interacts with numerous medications. Cimetidine, oral contraceptives, and quinolone antibiotics all decrease the hepatic clearance of theophylline and increase serum level of the drug. Phenobarbital, phenytoin, and rifampin will decrease the theophylline level. The nurse must watch for signs of toxicity and monitor serum theophylline level whenever a patient also is being receiving cimetidine.
Nursing process step: Implementation
Cognitive level: Comprehension

Questions 80 to 82 refer to the following information:
A 65-year-old male patient with chronic obstructive pulmonary disease has a tracheostomy and a gastrostomy tube in place. He is being weaned from the mechanical ventilator and is receiving intermittent tube feedings.

80. While suctioning the patient, the nurse notices milky, white secretions instead of the previously thin, clear secretions. What is the probable cause?
A. Malpositioned tracheostomy tube
B. Bowel obstruction
C. Aspiration of tube feedings
D. Gastroesophageal reflux

CORRECT ANSWER—C. A patient with an artificial airway loses the glottic closure that normally prevents aspiration. Other risk factors for aspiration include advanced age, decreased mental status, hypoxemia, supine position, and tube (especially gastric) feedings. A nurse who suctions milky secretions from any patient receiving tube feedings should suspect aspiration, especially if the aspirate is characteristically different from previous aspirates. Although a malpositioned tracheostomy tube, bowel obstruction, or gastroesophageal reflux can promote aspiration, they are less likely to be the cause in this situation.
Nursing process step: Assessment
Cognitive level: Analysis

81. Which of the following would help the nurse assess and validate the patient's condition?
A. Arterial blood gas studies
B. A chest X-ray film
C. Measurement of the glucose level in the patient's sputum
D. A sputum culture

CORRECT ANSWER—C. Normal mucus does not contain glucose. The presence of glucose in the sputum would indicate that the tube feeding has been aspirated. Changes in chest X-ray films would not be evident for about 24 hours after aspiration has occurred. The other diagnostic studies are not specific to this problem.
Nursing process step: Assessment
Cognitive level: Evaluation

82. Which intervention would be most effective for decreasing the risk of aspiration in this patient?
A. Elevating the head of the bed
B. Decreasing the rate of tube feedings
C. Suctioning the patient frequently
D. Turning the patient every 2 hours

CORRECT ANSWER—A. Elevating the head of the bed to at least 45 degrees can prevent aspiration. Although slowing the infusion rate may help, it can prevent the patient from receiving the total amount of the infusion. Suctioning the patient frequently increases the risk of aspiration. Turning the patient every 2 hours will not decrease this risk.
Nursing process step: Implementation
Cognitive level: Application

83. Nursing care for a patient with a chest tube includes:
A. Turning the patient every 2 hours and using antiembolism stockings to prevent deep vein thrombosis
B. Using incentive spirometry every 2 hours while the patient is on bed rest
C. Obtaining daily chest X-ray films to evaluate tube placement and pulmonary status
D. All of the above

CORRECT ANSWER—D. A patient with a chest tube is at risk for deep vein thrombosis, atelectasis, infection, and decreased activity tolerance. Turning and use of incentive spirometry facilitates adequate cardiovascular and pulmonary function. Daily chest X-ray films are recommended for evaluating tube placement and assessing the pulmonary system for complications associated with chest tube placement and prolonged bed rest.
Nursing process step: Implementation
Cognitive level: Application

84. A 47-year-old male patient with unresolved hemothorax is febrile, with chills and sweating. He has a nonproductive cough and chest pain. His chest tube drainage is turbid. A possible explanation for these findings is:
A. Lobar pneumonia
B. Empyema
C. *Pneumocystis carinii* pneumonia
D. Infected chest tube wound site

CORRECT ANSWER—B. Any condition that produces fluid accumulation or sequestration of fluid with infective properties can lead to empyema, an accumulation of pus in a body cavity, especially the pleural space, as a result of bacterial infection. An infected chest tube site, lobar pneumonia, and *Pneumocystis carinii* pneumonia can lead to the fever, chills, and sweating associated with infection. In this case, turbid drainage indicates that empyema has developed. Pneumonia typically causes productive cough and an infected chest tube wound, but not turbid drainage.
Nursing process step: Evaluation
Cognitive level: Analysis

85. An asthmatic patient who requires mechanical ventilation suddenly is in acute distress. He is hypotensive, has an increased peak airway pressure, and is difficult to ventilate with the resuscitator bag. What is the most likely cause of the patient's acute respiratory distress?

A. Mucus plug

B. Pulmonary infection

C. Pneumothorax

D. Malpositioned endotracheal tube

CORRECT ANSWER—C. Because of the high airway pressures generated by the trapping of air and decreased lung compliance, an asthmatic patient is at increased risk for pneumothorax. A mucus plug initially will increase airway pressures and decrease oxygen saturation levels, but it does not usually cause hypotension unless the hypoxemia is severe and leads to cardiovascular compromise. Pulmonary infection may cause increased secretions, which can increase peak airway pressures; however, this does not occur in acute situations. A malpositioned endotracheal tube can cause diminished or absent lung sounds on the contralateral side, little if any chest excursion on the contralateral side, expiratory wheezing, and, occasionally, uncontrollable coughing.

Nursing process step: Implementation

Cognitive level: Analysis

86. A patient has a pulmonary artery catheter in place. His pulmonary artery pressures are as follows: systolic, 35 mm Hg; diastolic, 12 mm Hg; and mean, 26 mm Hg. The pulmonary capillary wedge pressure is 10 mm Hg. His ventilator settings are FIO_2, .75; assist-control mode, 12 breaths/minute; and tidal volume, 850 cc. The positive end-expiratory pressure (PEEP) recently was increased to 10 cm H_2O to improve oxygenation. When assessing the next set of pulmonary pressure readings, the nurse notices that all of the pressures are elevated. The nurse suspects this is due to:

A. Increased interstitial fluid levels from the addition of PEEP

B. Increased intrathoracic pressures transmitted to the pulmonary circulation

C. Increased intra-alveolar fluid levels

D. Increased interstitial pressures transmitted to the alveoli

CORRECT ANSWER—B. The addition of PEEP to positive-pressure ventilation increases intrathoracic pressures because the volume of air left in the lungs at the end of expiration increases instead of returning to baseline volume. This pressure is transmitted to the pulmonary vessels and is reflected in higher pulmonary artery pressures. The addition of PEEP does not increase interstitial fluid levels or pressures, but it does reduce intra-alveolar fluid levels.

Nursing process step: Assessment

Cognitive level: Analysis

Questions 87 to 91 refer to the following information:

A 69-year-old male patient with a history of emphysema is admitted to the intensive care unit complaining of acute shortness of breath. His vital signs are temperature, 101° F (38.3° C); pulse, 142 beats/minute; and respirations, 22 breaths/minute. His chest X-ray film shows infiltrate in the lower lobe of the right lung. He is placed on oxygen therapy, at a rate of 4 liters of oxygen via nasal cannula, and has the following arterial blood gas levels: pH, 7.46; $PaCO_2$, 32 mm Hg; PaO_2, 63 mm Hg; and HCO_3^-, 25 mEq/liter.

87. What is the primary acid-base disturbance in this patient?
A. Respiratory alkalosis
B. Respiratory acidosis
C. Metabolic alkalosis
D. Metabolic acidosis

CORRECT ANSWER—A. The elevated pH indicates that alkalosis is the primary acid-base disturbance, and the decreased $PaCO_2$ with a normal HCO_3^- suggests that the problem is respiratory in origin. Acidosis is not an option because the pH is elevated; because the HCO_3^- level is within normal limits (24 to 28 mEq/liter), the metabolic system is not involved.
Nursing process step: Assessment
Cognitive level: Evaluation

88. The nurse institutes measures to control the patient's temperature because an elevated temperature can:
A. Increase CO_2 production
B. Decrease CO_2 production
C. Increase HCO_3^- production
D. Decrease HCO_3^- production

CORRECT ANSWER—A. Carbon dioxide is a byproduct of metabolism. Because elevated temperature increases metabolism, the nurse would expect $PaCO_2$ to increase, not decrease. The patient has enough leeway in his arterial blood gas level for an increase in $PaCO_2$ because his reading currently is below normal. Nevertheless, the nurse must monitor for any increase in $PaCO_2$, which could lead to respiratory acidosis. An increase in temperature would not affect the HCO_3^- level.
Nursing process step: Implementation
Cognitive level: Analysis

89. An increased metabolic rate in this patient will lead to:
A. Increased work of breathing
B. Increased functional residual capacity
C. Increased peak expiratory flow rate
D. Increased vital capacity

CORRECT ANSWER—**A.** An increase in metabolic rate leads to increased production of CO_2. The body's natural response is to increase the respiratory rate to excrete the excess CO_2. An increased respiratory rate increases the energy and oxygen requirements of the respiratory muscles. Functional residual capacity is the air remaining in the lungs at the end of a normal exhalation; it is not affected by metabolism. Peak expiratory flow rate (the rate at which air moves through the airways) and vital capacity (the amount of air inhaled during a deep breath) are not affected by metabolism.
Nursing process step: Assessment
Cognitive level: Evaluation

90. The nurse obtains another set of vital signs and notes that the patient's respiratory rate has decreased to 12 breaths/minute and he appears more lethargic. The nurse would institute measures for which developing condition?
A. Congestive heart failure
B. Increased intracranial pressure
C. Acute respiratory failure
D. Cerebrovascular accident

CORRECT ANSWER—**C.** This patient has a history of chronic obstructive pulmonary disease and an infiltrate on his chest X-ray film; he also is febrile. The increased work of breathing caused by the increased metabolism has pushed this borderline patient into acute respiratory failure. The lethargy is caused by hypoxia and hypercapnia, not a neurologic condition, such as increased intracranial pressure or cerebrovascular accident. Congestive heart failure would have been apparent on the chest X-ray film.
Nursing process step: Implementation
Cognitive level: Evaluation

91. The patient's next arterial blood gas analysis reveals the following: pH, 7.32; $PaCO_2$, 62 mm Hg; PaO_2, 50 mm Hg; and HCO_3^-, 24 mEq/liter. The nurse would expect the next intervention to involve:
A. Placing a 100% nonrebreather mask on the patient
B. Intubating the patient and placing him on a mechanical ventilator
C. Starting I.V. aminophylline and steroids
D. Administering an acetaminophen suppository and placing the patient on a hypothermia blanket

CORRECT ANSWER—**B.** This patient must be intubated and mechanically ventilated to improve oxygenation while maintaining and controlling ventilation. Although the oxygen level is dangerously low, using a 100% nonrebreather mask is likely to blunt the patient's hypoxic drive. Drug therapy would follow after oxygenation has been stabilized and the respiratory acidosis is corrected by controlling ventilation. Although fever can contribute to an increased level of carbon dioxide and correcting the patient's hyperthermia is an appropriate intervention, maintaining the airway and breathing takes priority.
Nursing process step: Planning
Cognitive level: Application

92. When teaching an asthmatic patient about inhaled corticosteroids, the nurse would instruct the patient to:
   A. Take the drug before using a bronchodilator
   B. Rinse the mouth after administering the drug
   C. Use the drug only when short of breath
   D. Call the physician if changes in vision occur

CORRECT ANSWER—B. The two major adverse effects of inhaled corticosteroids are oral candidiasis (thrush) and change in voice, which are caused by deposits of the drug in the mouth and vocal cords. These adverse effects can be decreased if the patient uses a spacing device, which greatly increases the deposition of inhaled medication directly to the lungs, and rinses the mouth after using the drug. A bronchodilator, if prescribed, should be taken before an inhaled corticosteroid so the corticosteroid can be deposited in the smaller airways after bronchodilation has occurred. Inhaled corticosteroids are used to prevent inflammation and must be taken consistently; most bronchodilators are now prescribed on an as-needed basis. Ingested corticosteroids can cause glaucoma or cataracts, which would affect a patient's vision; however, inhaled corticosteroids usually are not associated with these adverse effects.
Nursing process step: Planning
Cognitive level: Application

Questions 93 to 95 refer to the following information:
An 82-year-old female patient with insulin-dependent diabetes is admitted to the intensive care unit from a nursing home after experiencing weight loss, night sweats, shortness of breath, and hemoptysis during the past 2 weeks. Her chest X-ray film reveals an infiltrate on the upper lobe of the right lung.

93. Based on these findings, the nurse would antici-
pate implementing interventions to treat:
  A. Pneumonia
  B. Tuberculosis
  C. Lung cancer
  D. Pleural effusion

CORRECT ANSWER—B. Signs and symptoms of
tuberculosis include weight loss, night sweats,
anorexia, shortness of breath, and hemoptysis.
The patient's age and chronic illness place her at
increased risk for tuberculosis. The incidence of
tuberculosis is three times higher in persons over
age 65. In addition, the incidence of tuberculosis
in nursing homes is increasing. Pneumonia may
be associated with infiltrates and shortness of
breath, but not with the other symptoms listed.
Lung cancer may be evident on the X-ray film as
a mass or tumor; it typically is not associated
with night sweats, and the other symptoms listed above may occur. Pleural effusion usually occurs in the base of the lung, and typically does
not present with the symptoms this patient is experiencing.
Nursing process step: Planning
Cognitive level: Application

94. The patient is started on isoniazid and rifampin.
What additional medication typically is given to
minimize the adverse effects caused by isonia-
zid?
  A. Pyridoxine hydrochloride
  B. Ethambutol hydrochloride
  C. Magnesium sulfate
  D. Cyanocobalamin

CORRECT ANSWER—A. Pyridoxine (vitamin B_6)
commonly is administered to minimize peripheral neuropathy associated with isoniazid. Ethambutol hydrochloride is an antitubercular agent,
which probably would not be added because the
patient has just been started on concomitant isoniazid and rifampin therapy. Magnesium sulfate
and cyanocobalamin are not indicated for a patient receiving isoniazid or rifampin; however, if
the patient was malnourished, cyanocobalamin
(vitamin B_{12}) may be prescribed.
Nursing process step: Implementation
Cognitive level: Comprehension

95. The nurse would plan to monitor the results of
which test during the patient's isoniazid therapy?
  A. Uric acid test
  B. Liver function studies
  C. Creatinine clearance test
  D. Visual acuity test

CORRECT ANSWER—B. Elderly patients receiving isoniazid are at increased risk for hepatitis;
therefore, baseline and monthly liver function
studies should be done. If symptoms of hepatitis
occur and the aspartate aminotransferase (AST)
level rises five times above normal, isoniazid
therapy should be stopped. Isoniazid does not
cause nephrotoxic injury; therefore, neither a creatinine clearance test nor a uric acid test is indicated. A visual acuity test is not necessary
because isoniazid does not affect vision.
Nursing process step: Planning
Cognitive level: Application

96. The nurse should warn a patient about the dangers of continuously using an inhaled bronchodilator during an asthma attack, explaining that:
A. Life-threatening arrhythmias can occur
B. Asthma can become resistant to treatment
C. Shortness of breath can worsen
D. Heart failure can occur

CORRECT ANSWER—**A.** Arrhythmias can result from the stimulant effects of beta$_2$-adrenergic blockers, including bronchodilators. If a patient uses the inhaler continuously without response, the underlying etiology of the asthma attack most likely is inflammation, not bronchospasm. The problem is not unresponsiveness to the bronchodilator, but the need for a medication to treat the underlying etiology. Lack of appropriate treatment, not continued use of the bronchodilator, will worsen shortness of breath. Tachycardia, not heart failure, is associated with excess use of bronchodilators.
Nursing process step: Implementation
Cognitive level: Synthesis

97. A 25-year-old male struck by a car is found face-down and unconscious in a drainage ditch. He has bruises across the chest, multiple facial injuries, and a fractured left arm. He is transported to the emergency department, where the nurse notes rhonchi and wheezing on the right side. Left-sided breath sounds are unremarkable, and his arterial blood gas levels indicate a PaO$_2$ of 90 mm Hg and a PaCO$_2$ of 43 mm Hg. Given these assessment findings, the nurse suspects the patient has which condition?
A. Pulmonary contusion
B. Aspiration
C. Pneumothorax
D. Hemothorax

CORRECT ANSWER—**B.** A patient at risk for aspiration is likely to have suffered a loss of consciousness or an injury to the physical structures that normally prevent aspiration. Surgical anesthesia, alcohol intoxication, narcotic overdose, traumatic injury (especially a head injury), and cerebrovascular accident produce the decreased level of consciousness that predisposes a patient to aspiration. Trauma patients are at increased risk for aspiration, especially if they have eaten recently, because undigested food can cause the patient to vomit. Rhonchi and wheezing are consistent with aspiration. Hemothorax and pneumothorax would be accompanied by diminished or absent breath sounds in this patient. Pulmonary contusion can occur from a blunt injury to the lung tissue; however, edema and hemorrhage of the functional lung tissue would be more consistent with pulmonary contusion. The patient with pulmonary contusion would have compromised arterial blood gas (ABG) levels as well as signs and symptoms of adult respiratory distress syndrome (ARDS) and cardiac tamponade; the patient with aspiration may have compromised ABG levels as well as signs and symptoms of ARDS, but would not exhibit signs of cardiac tamponade.
Nursing process step: Assessment
Cognitive level: Synthesis

Questions 98 and 99 refer to the following information:

A 25-year-old male patient is found facedown in a deep puddle of rainwater after apparently suffering a generalized seizure. He is brought to the emergency department by paramedics, who provided ventilatory assistance via a bag-valve-mask system (Ambu bag). The patient's vital signs include heart rate, 160 beats/minute; respirations, 15 breaths/minute; and blood pressure, 140/60 mm Hg. His arterial blood gas analysis reveals pH, 7.29; PaO_2, 55 mm Hg; $PaCO_2$, 58 mm Hg; and HCO_3^-, 24 mEq/liter.

98. The patient's arterial blood gas (ABG) analysis reflect which acid-base imbalance?
   A. Uncompensated respiratory alkalosis
   B. Partially compensated metabolic acidosis
   C. Uncompensated respiratory acidosis
   D. Compensated respiratory acidosis

CORRECT ANSWER—C. In a patient with a compensated acid-base imbalance, the body system that is primarily not affected will compensate in an effort to bring the pH toward the normal range (7.35 to 7.45). If the disturbance is respiratory in nature, the kidneys will respond. If the cause is nonrespiratory (metabolic) in origin, the kidneys are primarily affected and the respiratory system is stimulated. Although the kidneys are slower to compensate than the pulmonary system, the response is strong when it occurs. In this case, the patient's primary disturbance is respiratory acidosis (normal $PaCO_2$ is 35 to 45 mm Hg), but his kidneys have not begun to compensate. Kidneys respond to respiratory acidosis by excreting more acid in the urine and reabsorbing the bicarbonate ion. This patient's bicarbonate level (HCO_3^-) is still within normal limits (22 to 26 mm Hg), and his pH is still below normal. If compensation had occurred, ABG analysis would have revealed a pH near normal (for example, 7.40).
Nursing process step: Assessment
Cognitive level: Evaluation

99. The paramedics report that the patient was apneic at the scene, and near-drowning is suspected. The nurse would plan to assess for all of the following laboratory findings *except*:

A. Hypervolemia
B. Leukocytosis
C. Increased hemoglobin level
D. Hemodilution

CORRECT ANSWER—C. A patient who aspirates a significant quantity of fresh water typically has signs of hypervolemia, hemodilution, and hemolysis minutes after the water is absorbed into the circulation. Hemodilution causes the hemoglobin level to decrease, not increase. A patient who aspirates salt water typically shows signs of fluid shifting from the surrounding tissue into the alveolar sacs. In response to aspiration and potential infection, the body may produce an increased number of white blood cells to combat the threat of infection, as evidenced by leukocytosis.
Nursing process step: Planning
Cognitive level: Analysis

100. In a patient with significant pulmonary contusions, the nurse would expect to implement which pulmonary therapy?

A. Chest physiotherapy and postural drainage
B. Bronchodilator therapy
C. Chest tube insertion
D. Mucolytic therapy

CORRECT ANSWER—A. Pulmonary contusions often lead to atelectasis. Frequent postural drainage and chest physiotherapy to the affected segments help clear these areas. Within 48 to 72 hours after pulmonary contusions occur, the bloody mucus should become darker and thinner; eventually it will return to a normal appearance. Bronchodilators are used for bronchodilation; mucolytics are helpful for removing thickened secretions. Chest tubes are indicated for pneumothorax or hemothorax.
Nursing process step: Implementation
Cognitive level: Analysis

Questions 101 to 104 refer to the following information:
A 48-year-old male patient was involved in a motor vehicle accident and was admitted to intensive care unit 48 hours ago with the following injuries: right-sided flail chest, subdural hematoma, and multiple fractures of the pelvis and right femur. His condition continues to worsen, and he is diagnosed with adult respiratory distress syndrome (ARDS). His last arterial blood gas readings included pH, 7.24; $PaCO_2$, 65 mm Hg; PaO_2, 51 mm Hg; and HCO_3^-, 19 mEq/liter. His ventilator settings include FIO_2, 1.00; tidal volume, 800 cc; assist control, 12 breaths/minute; and positive end-expiratory pressure (PEEP), 15 cm H_2O. Vital signs include temperature, 101° F (38.3° C); heart rate, 154 beats/minute; blood pressure, 90/70 mm Hg; and respirations, 28 breaths/minute. His intracranial pressure, monitored via a subarachnoid screw, is elevated and continues to increase. His pulmonary artery pressures include systolic, 42 mm Hg; diastolic, 19 mm Hg; and mean, 29 mm Hg. His pulmonary capillary wedge pressure is 18 mm Hg. The patient has a cardiac output of 4 liters/minute and a systemic vascular resistance of 850 dynes/second/cm^{-5}.

---

101. Based on the patient's blood pressure and pulmonary capillary wedge pressure, the nurse would:
A. Increase I.V. fluids
B. Begin a dopamine I.V. infusion
C. Administer blood products
D. Decrease PEEP

CORRECT ANSWER—B. Even though the patient is hypotensive, the nurse should not administer additional fluids or blood products because they will leak into the alveoli from the damaged pulmonary capillaries. The injured alveolar-capillary membrane allows leakage of protein into the alveoli, causing an osmotic gradient that pulls even more fluid into the alveoli. The nurse's goal is to keep the patient as intravascularly dry as possible while maintaining adequate blood pressure and cardiac output; this will minimize the leakage of water from the vascular spaces into the interstitial spaces and alveoli. Vasopressors, such as dopamine, would help accomplish this goal. Decreasing PEEP may improve blood pressure but would worsen oxygenation.
Nursing process step: Implementation
Cognitive level: Application

102. Inverse ratio ventilation allows:
A. Peak inspiratory pressure to increase
B. Peak inspiratory pressure to decrease
C. Negative inspiratory pressure to increase
D. Mean airway pressure to decrease

CORRECT ANSWER—B. Inverse ratio ventilation allows peak inspiratory pressure to decrease, causing less barotrauma while increasing mean airway pressure; this leads to more stable airways and better gas exchange. Negative inspiratory pressure is not affected.
Nursing process step: Implementation
Cognitive level: Comprehension

103. The patient's fractured pelvis and femur suggest that the precipitating cause of ARDS is:
A. Sepsis
B. Fat emboli
C. Excessive blood loss
D. Bone marrow loss

CORRECT ANSWER—B. A fat embolus is likely to be the precipitating cause of ARDS when fractures of the pelvis and femur are present. Long-bone and pelvic fractures allow fat globules to escape into the systemic circulation; this fat travels into the pulmonary circulation and causes an embolism. The patient shows no signs of sepsis, such as elevated cardiac output or elevated systemic vascular resistance; however, he should be monitored for this potential complication. Excessive bone marrow loss has not been associated with ARDS. Excessive blood loss requiring multiple blood transfusions is a potential cause of ARDS, but this patient did not require transfusions.
Nursing process step: Assessment
Cognitive level: Analysis

104. While evaluating the patient after instituting inverse ratio ventilation, the nurse notices a crackling feeling when touching the patient's thorax and puffiness of his neck and eyelids. The nurse suspects the patient is developing:
A. Subcutaneous emphysema
B. Increased fluid retention
C. Anaphylaxis
D. Mazinsky's syndrome

CORRECT ANSWER—A. Subcutaneous emphysema is evidenced by a crackling sensation under the skin and pockets of air that form along areas where skin is loosely attached to the underlying muscle. Increased fluid retention would cause swelling in dependent areas, not crackling on palpation. Anaphylaxis would cause acute respiratory and circulatory collapse along with swelling and edema; also, no crackling sensation under the skin would be present. Mazinsky's syndrome does not exist.
Nursing process step: Evaluation
Cognitive level: Application

105. The nurse assessing a patient for tracheal displacement should know that the trachea will deviate toward the:
A. Contralateral side in a simple pneumothorax
B. Affected side in a hemothorax
C. Affected side in a tension pneumothorax
D. Contralateral side in a hemothorax

CORRECT ANSWER—D. The trachea will shift according to the pressure gradients within the thoracic cavity. In tension pneumothorax and hemothorax, accumulation of air or fluid causes a shift away from the injured side. If there is no significant air or fluid accumulation, the trachea will not shift. Tracheal deviation toward the contralateral side in simple pneumothorax is seen when the thoracic contents shift in response to the release of normal thoracic pressure gradients on the injured side.
Nursing process step: Assessment
Cognitive level: Analysis

106. Which patient would benefit most from chest physiotherapy?
A. Patient who has undergone coronary artery bypass graft (CABG) surgery and has lobar (segmental) atelectasis
B. Patient with bronchiectasis who produces ½ cup (about 120 ml) of sputum per day
C. Patient with emphysema and a nonproductive cough
D. Patient who has undergone thoracotomy and has crackles over the chest tube insertion site

CORRECT ANSWER—B. Chest physiotherapy is indicated for patients expectorating 30 ml or more of sputum per day. It is not helpful as a treatment for atelectasis or as a prophylaxis for atelectasis after CABG surgery. Crackles over a thoracotomy site usually are caused by fluid or bubbling sounds transmitted from the chest tube. Chest physiotherapy does not help patients with a nonproductive cough, it helps only those with a productive cough. Nonproductive cough is caused primarily by postnasal drip.
Nursing process step: Implementation
Cognitive level: Application

107. The nurse would expect which nursing intervention to be most effective in improving the pulmonary status of each of the three remaining patients in the previous question?
A. Encouraging deep breathing and coughing
B. Placing the patient in the supine position
C. Suctioning the patient routinely
D. Encouraging the patient to splint the incision site

CORRECT ANSWER—**A.** Deep breathing improves the ventilation-perfusion ratio and prevents atelectasis; coughing helps maintain a patent airway. The three patients in this situation should be encouraged to get out of bed; if they are on bed rest, they should be turned at least every 2 hours. Suctioning should be done only if secretions are audible or auscultated as rhonchi. Splinting the incision can be helpful when coughing, but constant splinting will prevent good lung expansion and can cause atelectasis.
Nursing process step: Evaluation
Cognitive level: Application

108. In which position would the nurse place a patient with a chest tube to best facilitate respiration?
A. Lateral decubitus position
B. Low-Fowler's position
C. Semi-Fowler's position
D. Supine position

CORRECT ANSWER—**C.** Placing the patient in semi-Fowler's position facilitates diaphragmatic expansion and exercise of the intercostal muscles. Placing the patient in the low-Fowler's, supine, or lateral decubitus position would not aid chest expansion or respiratory effort.
Nursing process step: Implementation
Cognitive level: Application

109. A 43-year-old patient with pneumothorax has a chest tube in place and is exhibiting signs of dyspnea, tachypnea, cyanosis, and tachycardia. Evaluation of the chest tube drainage system reveals that the tubing is kinked under the patient. The nurse would intervene based on the strong suspicion that the patient's symptoms result from:
A. Excessive suction pressure within the pleural cavity
B. Reaccumulation of fluid within the pleural space
C. Overexpansion of the lung
D. Tension pneumothorax

CORRECT ANSWER—**D.** Inadvertent clamping or disruption of the chest tube drainage system causes pressure to accumulate within the pleural space. If the chest tube drainage system cannot communicate with the area of increased pressure, the patient will exhibit signs and symptoms of tension pneumothorax. If the chest tube is placed for hemothorax, inadvertent clamping of the tube could cause signs and symptoms consistent with reaccumulation of fluid. Excessive suction pressure within the pleural space may draw the drainage ports up against the tissue, thereby decreasing overall drainage. It is not possible to overexpand the lung via a chest tube drainage system.
Nursing process step: Implementation
Cognitive level: Analysis

Questions 110 to 112 refer to the following information:

A 32-year-old male patient with status asthmaticus is admitted to the intensive care unit. Physical examination reveals paradoxical respirations, 34 breaths/minute; sinus tachycardia, 140 beats/minute; and blood pressure, 90/50 mm Hg. The patient has a gray, ashen appearance, is diaphoretic, and cannot speak. No audible sounds are heard on chest auscultation. Arterial blood gas levels on a 50% nonrebreather mask include pH, 7.25; $PaCO_2$, 80 mm Hg; PaO_2, 45 mm Hg; and HCO_3^-, 26 mEq/liter.

110. The patient's arterial blood gas levels indicate:

A. Respiratory acidosis with metabolic compensation

B. Respiratory acidosis with severe hypoxemia

C. Combined respiratory and metabolic acidosis

D. Respiratory alkalosis with severe hypoxemia

CORRECT ANSWER—B. The findings indicate uncompensated respiratory acidosis with hypoxemia. The pH and elevated CO_2 level reflect acidosis, but the HCO_3^- is within normal limits. The increased CO_2 level and normal HCO_3^- level indicate that respiratory, not metabolic, acidosis exists. Severe hypoxemia is occurring despite the increased FIO_2. Metabolic compensation would be evidenced by an abnormal HCO_3^- level. Respiratory acidosis is evidenced by a low CO_2 level. In the earlier stage of an asthma attack, the patient may have respiratory alkalosis, but as the patient tires and the work of breathing increases, CO_2 is retained. In approximately 24 hours, the kidneys will begin to compensate by retaining bicarbonate. Metabolic acidosis is reflected by decreased pH and decreased HCO_3^- level. The worst-case scenario for this patient would be respiratory and metabolic acidosis as well as hypoxemia; this would lead to death.

Nursing process step: Assessment

Cognitive level: Analysis

111. Which intervention should the nurse implement next?

    A. Providing continuous albuterol via a nebulizer

    B. Increasing the oxygen level to 100% via a non-rebreather mask

    C. Preparing for intubation

    D. Administering subcutaneous epinephrine

CORRECT ANSWER—C. The assessment findings suggest excessive work of breathing and an inability of the lungs to maintain adequate oxygenation and ventilation. Intubation with subsequent mechanical ventilation will decrease the work of breathing; neuromuscular paralysis also may be required. Albuterol therapy is not administered continuously. No audible breath sounds on auscultation indicate that the patient is not exchanging any air at the cellular level; therefore, increasing FIO_2 would be inappropriate unless ventilation is improved. Epinephrine would not be administered because it would increase adverse effects, including tachycardia and increased oxygen consumption.

Nursing process step: Planning
Cognitive level: Application

112. After the patient has been on the mechanical ventilator for a few hours, the nurse notices that peak airway pressures have increased from 30 to 50 cm H_2O. The patient is not in respiratory distress, but his blood pressure has decreased from 130/70 mm Hg to 100/50 mm Hg. What process most likely is occurring?

    A. Tension pneumothorax

    B. Onset of auto–positive end-expiratory pressure (PEEP)

    C. Increased bronchoconstriction

    D. Adult respiratory distress syndrome (ARDS)

CORRECT ANSWER—B. Because of incomplete emptying of alveoli during expiration, the patient may be experiencing auto-PEEP, a condition in which PEEP activates without the nurse's setting the PEEP dial on the mechanical ventilator. The clinical manifestations of auto-PEEP are the same as those for PEEP. Tension pneumothorax would cause respiratory distress. Bronchoconstriction would not decrease blood pressure. ARDS commonly does not result from status asthmaticus, and can produce refractory hypoxemia that leads to respiratory distress.

Nursing process step: Assessment
Cognitive level: Analysis

113. Chest tube drainage is facilitated by all of the following *except:*

A. Short-segment squeezing of the tube to remove clots

B. Positioning the chest tube drainage system at the level of the patient's chest

C. Turning the patient every 2 to 4 hours

D. Having the patient use an incentive spirometer

CORRECT ANSWER—B. The chest tube drainage system should be kept below the level of the patient's chest to facilitate gravity drainage. Sequential short-segment squeezing of the chest tube promotes movement of clots or debris through the tube into the drainage system. Short-segment squeezing does not create the prolonged occlusion and increased pressure gradient associated with the classic practice of "stripping a chest tube." Turning the patient every 2 to 4 hours and encouraging safe mobilization will decrease fluid sequestration and facilitate drainage. Use of incentive spirometry helps decrease atelectasis and encourages lung reexpansion.

Nursing process step: Implementation
Cognitive level: Application

114. A patient at risk for aspiration should be positioned:

A. In supine position with legs slightly elevated

B. In Trendelenburg's position with legs elevated on pillows

C. With the head of the bed elevated at least 20 degrees and legs bent to a comfortable position

D. With the head of the bed elevated 5 degrees and the patient's head on a pillow

CORRECT ANSWER—C. Proper positioning during procedures and feedings is essential for preventing aspiration. The patient should be positioned with the head of the bed elevated at least 20 degrees limit gastroesophageal reflux; an elevation of 5 degrees is can increase the risk of gastroesophageal reflux. Positioning the lower extremities to prevent abdominal compression facilitates emptying of the stomach.

Nursing process step: Implementation
Cognitive level: Application

115. Treatment for a patient with severe flail chest and respiratory compromise may include:

A. Chest tube placement at the midclavicular line

B. Chest tube placement at the anterior, third intercostal space

C. Positive-pressure ventilation

D. Sedation and restrictive chest expansion band

CORRECT ANSWER—C. A patient with a severe flail chest (eight or more fractured ribs) and respiratory compromise requires positive-pressure ventilation to coordinate chest-wall movement with lung expansion. Surgical repair also may be necessary if the fractures are severe. Chest tubes are indicated for pneumothorax, hemothorax, and hemopneumothorax. Restricting chest expansion with a chest expansion band could result in pulmonary infection or atelectasis.

Nursing process step: Implementation
Cognitive level: Application

116. A patient with maxillofacial fractures is brought to the emergency department in respiratory arrest. Which type of airway is most likely to be used in this situation?
- A. Oropharyngeal airway
- B. Nasotracheal airway
- C. Endotracheal airway
- D. Tracheostomy

CORRECT ANSWER—C. Endotracheal intubation is preferred for most trauma patients; it provides a controlled airway for mechanical ventilation and an open airway if cardiopulmonary resuscitation is needed. An oropharyngeal airway is inadequate for a patient in respiratory arrest; it does not provide a direct, open airway to the trachea. Nasotracheal intubation is contraindicated in patients with facial injuries; it would make intubation more difficult and further damage the facial area. Tracheostomy is of limited use in an emergency because of the amount of time required to perform the procedure and the potential for bleeding. It is reserved for patients who have a compromised airway secondary to tracheal edema or laryngeal obstruction.
Nursing process step: Planning
Cognitive level: Application

Questions 117 to 119 refer to the following information:
An 80-kg, 72-year-old female patient is admitted to the intensive care unit after falling down stairs 3 days ago. Her neighbors did not find her until this morning. She has bilateral hip fractures and fractures of the last four ribs on the left side. She has a chest tube in place for left-sided pneumothorax and is placed on a mechanical ventilator because of her decreased level of consciousness. The ventilator settings are synchronized intermittent mandatory ventilation (SIMV), 20 breaths/minute; tidal volume, 700 cc; FIO_2, .70; and positive end-expiratory pressure (PEEP), 5 cm H_2O. Her arterial blood gas (ABG) values are pH, 7.25; $PaCO_2$, 55 mm Hg; PaO_2, 65 mm Hg; and HCO_3^-, 16 mEq/liter.

117. Based on the patient's arterial blood gas values, the nurse would plan to treat which of the following acid-base imbalances?
  A. Metabolic alkalosis with hypoxemia
  B. Respiratory acidosis with hypoxemia
  C. Mixed respiratory and metabolic acidosis
  D. Mixed respiratory and metabolic alkalosis

CORRECT ANSWER—C. Metabolic and respiratory acidosis result from decreased bicarbonate and increased carbon dioxide concentrations, respectively. Normal pH is 7.35 to 7.45, with a $PaCO_2$ of 35 to 45 mm Hg and a serum bicarbonate (HCO_3^-) level between 22 and 26 mEq/liter. For each 10 mm Hg increase or decrease in $PaCO_2$, pH can be expected to fall or rise 0.08. Alkalosis is evidenced by pH above 7.45 and requires a decreased $PaCO_2$ level or increased HCO_3^- level. Respiratory acidosis with hypoxemia would not include an HCO_3^- value of 16 mEq/liter; rather, the HCO_3^- level would be in the normal or above-normal range, which is indicative of the body's ability to compensate for the respiratory acidosis.
Nursing process step: Planning
Cognitive level: Analysis

118. To help correct the patient's acid-base imbalance, the nurse would change the ventilator settings to:
  A. Increase tidal volume
  B. Decrease PEEP
  C. Increase oxygen concentration
  D. Decrease respiratory rate

CORRECT ANSWER—A. The typical tidal volume for a ventilated patient is calculated at a rate of 10 to 15 cc/kg body weight. For a patient weighing 80 kg, the expected tidal volume would be 800 to 1,200 cc. Greater expansion and increased volume delivery facilitates removal of CO_2. Decreasing the respiratory rate and PEEP would promote CO_2 accumulation. Increasing oxygen delivery would not directly affect CO_2 or HCO_3^- concentrations.
Nursing process step: Implementation
Cognitive level: Application

119. Three days later, the patient remains sedated and pharmacologically paralyzed. She has bilateral pneumothorax, pneumonia, and increasing oxygen requirements. The ventilator is currently set on assist control at 18 breaths/minute; tidal volume, 850 cc; FIO_2, .95; and PEEP, 7 cm H_2O. Peak airway pressures range from 32 to 45 cm H_2O. Her arterial blood gas levels are pH, 7.42; $PaCO_2$, 48 mm Hg; PaO_2, 60 mm Hg; and HCO_3^-, 25 mEq/liter. Which nursing intervention is appropriate for increasing the patient's arterial oxygen concentration?

A. Increasing PEEP to 12 mm Hg

B. Increasing the assist-control rate to 24 breaths/minute

C. Changing the SIMV setting to 18 breaths/minute

D. Changing the ventilator mode to inverse ratio ventilation

CORRECT ANSWER—D. The patient needs more time for the oxygen to diffuse across her alveoli into the pulmonary circulation. Inverse ratio ventilation reverses the normal pattern of respiration while maintaining the inspiratory plateau, thereby allowing more time for passive alveolar ventilation. Longer inspiratory times also reduce airway pressure. However, decreased expiratory times can cause auto-PEEP, an accumulation of pressures within the alveoli, which can decrease venous return and cardiac output. Increasing PEEP is not recommended in this situation because it may increase the patient's airway pressure and worsen the pneumothorax without significantly increasing alveolar exposure and oxygenation. Changing the SIMV setting on the ventilator is of no benefit because the patient is paralyzed and breathing only at the preset rate. Increasing the assist-control rate may increase the number of times the alveoli are exposed to oxygen; however, it will not promote oxygen diffusion across the membranes and may decrease the $PaCO_2$ level.

Nursing process step: Implementation
Cognitive level: Application

120. Current research on adult respiratory distress syndrome (ARDS) is investigating the use of all of the following medications *except*:

A. Nonsteroidal anti-inflammatory drugs

B. Histamine₂-blockers

C. Antibiotics

D. Calcium channel blockers

CORRECT ANSWER—D. Calcium channel blockers are not included on the list of investigational drugs used to treat ARDS. Nonsteroidal anti-inflammatory drugs, especially ibuprofen, are being studied as a way to interrupt the inflammatory process in the lung. Histamine₂-blockers are being studied for their suppression of histamine release. Antibiotics currently are being used in the treatment of ARDS, and their use continues to be a focus of research.

Nursing process step: Implementation
Cognitive level: Knowledge

Questions 121 to 124 refer to the following information:
A 44-year-old male patient is admitted to the intensive care unit with a diagnosis of Guillain-Barré syndrome.

121. The primary reason for admitting the patient to the intensive care unit is to monitor for:
A. Respiratory failure
B. Cardiac insufficiency
C. Renal failure
D. Adrenal insufficiency

CORRECT ANSWER—**A.** Patients with Guillain-Barré syndrome are at risk for acute respiratory failure because of ascending paralysis that affects the respiratory muscles. The cardiac muscle is not affected, nor are the renal and adrenal systems.
Nursing process step: Planning
Cognitive level: Comprehension

122. Shortly after the patient is admitted, the nurse notices that his respirations becoming shallow and slower. Which intervention would be appropriate?
A. Obtaining a chest X-ray film
B. Obtaining a blood sample for arterial blood gas (ABG) analysis
C. Obtaining a vital capacity reading
D. Auscultating breath sounds

CORRECT ANSWER—**C.** Vital capacity is measured every 2 to 4 hours in a patient with Guillain-Barré syndrome to determine how far the paralysis has ascended. Decreases in vital capacity indicate a potential for acute respiratory failure. Obtaining a vital capacity reading provides quantitative information, whereas auscultating breath sounds provides only subjective data. Obtaining a blood sample for ABG analysis would be appropriate if the patient's vital capacity was decreased; these values would indicate whether the patient was retaining carbon dioxide. A chest X-ray film would not be useful at this point, but X-ray films will be needed to monitor for signs of significant atelectasis.
Nursing process step: Implementation
Cognitive level: Application

123. The patient is placed on a mechanical ventilator with the following settings: FIO_2, .70; tidal volume, 800 cc; and assist control, 14 breaths/minute. Arterial blood gas readings at these settings are pH, 7.59; $PaCO_2$, 25 mm Hg; PaO_2, 251 mm Hg; and HCO_3^-, 26 mEq/liter. What value would the nurse be most concerned about?
A. PaO_2
B. $PaCO_2$
C. HCO_3^-
D. pH

CORRECT ANSWER—**D.** Overventilation has led to respiratory alkalosis, as evidenced by a pH of 7.59 and a $PaCO_2$ of 25 mm Hg. In this alkalotic state, the patient is at risk for seizures. The PaO_2 of 251 mm Hg indicates that the patient can oxygenate tissues with adequate ventilation and can tolerate weaning of the FIO_2. The bicarbonate (HCO_3^-) level is within normal limits.
Nursing process step: Assessment
Cognitive level: Analysis

124. The physician orders a decrease in the respiratory rate to 10 breaths/minute. What other setting could have been changed to obtain the same results?
A. Tidal volume
B. FIO_2
C. Flow rate
D. Inspiratory/Expiratory ratio

CORRECT ANSWER—**A.** Respiratory rate multiplied by tidal volume equals minute ventilation. A decrease in minute ventilation will increase $PaCO_2$, which is the desired effect in this patient. To decrease minute ventilation, the nurse must decrease either the tidal volume or the respiratory rate because these two factors comprise minute ventilation. Manipulation of any other parameters will not affect minute ventilation.
Nursing process step: Implementation
Cognitive level: Application

125. A 25-year-old male patient is brought to the emergency department with a sucking chest wound. His assessment findings include dyspnea, tachypnea, cyanosis, blood pressure of 110/65 mm Hg, and sinus tachycardia at 160 beats/minute. He is given 100% oxygen via face mask while the health care team evaluates him for surgery. Which intervention is the nurse's top priority?
A. Intubating the patient and placing him on assist-control mechanical ventilation
B. Placing an occlusive dressing taped on three sides over the chest wound
C. Administering 2 liters of 0.9% sodium chloride solution intravenously
D. Preparing to assist with surgical exploration of the wound

CORRECT ANSWER—**B.** A sucking chest wound must be sealed to ensure that pressures within the pleural cavity do not pull air through the wound instead of the trachea when the patient breathes. A three-sided occlusive dressing will seal the wound on inhalation, but allow air to escape during exhalation. If a fully occlusive dressing is used, air will have no means of escaping the pleural cavity and tension pneumothorax may develop. If the wound is sealed appropriately, intubation may be unnecessary, although a chest tube will be required. Cardiovascular support is not a clinical priority because the patient has adequate heart rate and blood pressure. Surgical exploration can wait until the other clinical priorities are met.
Nursing process step: Planning
Cognitive level: Application

126. The nurse would expect a patient with suspected hemopneumothorax to have a chest tube placed in the:
A. Second intercostal space, midclavicular line
B. Eighth intercostal space, midaxillary line
C. Fourth intercostal space, midclavicular line
D. Fifth intercostal space, midaxillary line

CORRECT ANSWER—**D.** To drain both air and fluid with a single chest tube, the tube must be placed at the fourth or fifth intercostal space at the midaxillary line. Chest tubes for draining air alone are placed within the second midclavicular intercostal space. Drainage of fluid alone requires placement in the lower intercostal spaces.
Nursing process step: Planning
Cognitive level: Comprehension

127. The nurse would expect which pulmonary function test result in a patient with pulmonary aspiration?
  A. Increased lung volume
  B. Increased compliance
  C. Increased functional residual capacity
  D. Decreased compliance

CORRECT ANSWER—D. Compliance is a measure of the ease with which the pulmonary system expands. Aspiration causes fluid and blood to accumulate within the alveolar space, thereby decreasing compliance. Aspiration also decreases lung volume and functional residual capacity.
Nursing process step: Planning
Cognitive level: Analysis

128. Nursing care of a patient with pulmonary aspiration includes:
  A. Turning and positioning every 4 hours
  B. Immediately administering broad-spectrum antibiotics
  C. Implementing vigorous pulmonary toilet with postural percussion and drainage
  D. Placing the patient in low-Fowler's position to facilitate coughing and deep breathing

CORRECT ANSWER—C. Vigorous pulmonary toilet is essential to prevent atelectasis, mobilize secretions, decrease the work of breathing, improve ventilation, and promote oxygenation. Antibiotics are not indicated unless an infection is documented and the patient's immune response is inadequate. Turning and positioning should be done at least every 2 hours; coughing and deep-breathing exercises should be performed with patient in high-Fowler's position.
Nursing process step: Implementation
Cognitive level: Comprehension

129. A 25-year-old male patient is admitted to the intensive care unit after a drug overdose that required cardiopulmonary resuscitation in the field. His vital signs are heart rate, 130 beats/minute; blood pressure, 150/58 mm Hg; respirations, 18 breaths/minute; and oxygen saturation, 94%. He is on assist-control mechanical ventilation via a #8 oral endotracheal tube. Arterial blood gas studies are pending. A quick physical examination reveals an emaciated male with a femoral arterial line, subclavian central catheter, and endotracheal tube; no spontaneous movements or breaths; and a firm abdomen. The patient's breath sounds and chest expansion are not equal bilaterally. Based on these findings, the nurse suspects that the primary cause of the patient's symptoms is:
  A. Misplaced endotracheal tube
  B. Pulmonary contusion
  C. Pleural effusion
  D. Open pneumothorax

CORRECT ANSWER—A. Unequal breath sounds and chest expansion can result from pneumothorax, collapsed lung, or misplaced endotracheal tube, as occurs with right mainstem intubation. An open pneumothorax is seen when a penetrating object creates communication between the external atmosphere and the pleural space. A closed pneumothorax sometimes results from cardiopulmonary resuscitation. Pleural effusion and pulmonary contusion are not primary causes of unequal chest expansion.
Nursing process step: Assessment
Cognitive level: Application

130. Emergency treatment of tension pneumothorax involves placement of:

A. 18G to 20G needle in the third to fifth posterior intercostal space

B. 14G to 16G needle in the second to fourth anterior intercostal space

C. 14G to 16G needle in the eighth anterior intercostal space

D. 20G to 22G needle in the second posterior intercostal space

CORRECT ANSWER—B. Emergency decompression of tension pneumothorax is achieved by inserting a 14G to 16G needle in the second to fourth anterior intercostal space. The needle is inserted over the rib and approximately 1 centimeter beyond it. This technique permits air to escape and equalize with the external atmosphere while preparations are made for chest tube placement.

Nursing process step: Implementation

Cognitive level: Comprehension

131. Methylene blue is added to the applesauce being used to evaluate the swallowing ability of a patient with a tracheostomy. A successful swallowing test would be indicated by no blue-tinted secretions:

A. In the oral cavity

B. Around the tracheostomy site

C. With tracheal suctioning

D. With pharyngeal suctioning

CORRECT ANSWER—C. Successful swallowing is determined by the ability of the patient to swallow tinted fluid or food without aspiration into the pulmonary system. Tracheal suctioning resulting in blue-tinted secretions indicates that fluid or food is entering the pulmonary system. The other options do not indicate that methylene blue has entered the pulmonary system.

Nursing process step: Evaluation

Cognitive level: Analysis

132. The nurse assesses a 53-year-old victim of a hit-and-run accident who has just been admitted to the intensive care unit. She notes dyspnea, wheezing, fever, bronchospasm, and frothy, nonpurulent sputum. Based on these findings, the nurse suspects:

A. Tuberculosis

B. Asthma

C. Aspiration pneumonitis

D. Pneumonia

CORRECT ANSWER—C. Classic signs of aspiration pneumonitis — dyspnea, wheezing, fever, bronchospasm, leukocytosis, and frothy, nonpurulent sputum — usually occur within 2 hours of gastric acid aspiration. Tuberculosis is characterized by malaise, fatigue, night sweats, and cough in the early stages and by hemoptysis in the late stages. Pneumonia is indicated by a productive or dry cough, cyanosis, and tachypnea. Acute asthma manifests as dyspnea, increased work of breathing, tachycardia, and bronchospasm.

Nursing process step: Evaluation

Cognitive level: Analysis

133. A 45-year-old construction worker is being treated for aspiration pneumonia in the intensive care unit. His static compliance measurement on Tuesday was 70 ml/cm H_2O; on Wednesday, it was 58 ml/cm H_2O. This means that:
A. The lungs were more difficult to ventilate on Tuesday than Wednesday
B. The lungs were more difficult to ventilate on Wednesday than Tuesday
C. Pulmonary volume was greater on Tuesday than Wednesday
D. Pulmonary volume was less on Tuesday than Wednesday

CORRECT ANSWER—B. Static compliance measures the distensibility of the lung system in a no-flow state. Decreased static compliance indicates a decrease in the ease with which the lungs expand. Even though compliance may decrease, the lungs may be able to achieve expansion and volumes equal to those achieved with better compliance. Static compliance, therefore, should not be used as a measure of pulmonary volume. In this case, however, the work of breathing would be increased.
Nursing process step: Evaluation
Cognitive level: Analysis

134. Successful removal of excessive airway secretions in a ventilated patient is evidenced by all of the following *except:*
A. Peak airway pressures decreasing from 35 cm H_2O to 28 cm H_2O
B. Compliance decreasing from 35 ml/cm H_2O to 25 ml/cm H_2O
C. CO_2 decreasing from 40 mm Hg to 35 mm Hg
D. Mean airway pressure decreasing from 30 cm H_2O to 24 cm H_2O

CORRECT ANSWER—B. Removing airway secretions decreases the effort required to introduce air into the lungs. Peak inspiratory pressures and mean airway pressure decrease as ease of airflow increases. Compliance increases in response to decreased opposition to airflow. $PaCO_2$, a measure of pulmonary ventilation, decreases as ventilation increases.
Nursing process step: Evaluation
Cognitive level: Evaluation

135. A patient involved in a multiple-vehicle accident 4 weeks ago is now in the intensive care unit. The physician performed a tracheostomy 12 days ago because of prolonged respiratory failure. When providing tracheostomy care, the nurse notices the tracheostomy tube pulsating. This is indicative of which type of fistula?
A. Tracheoesophageal fistula
B. Tracheobronchial fistula
C. Tracheoarterial fistula
D. Tracheovenous fistula

CORRECT ANSWER—C. Significant airway disease involving the tracheal tissue can occur in as little as 6 hours after tube placement. It also can result from difficult intubation or a tracheostomy in which the retropharyngeal or tracheal tissue is nicked and later becomes infected. Airway disease also can result from the pressure of an overdistended tracheal cuff or a poorly positioned airway. A tracheoarterial fistula may involve the innominate (brachiocephalic), right carotid, or lowest thyroid artery. A tracheoesophageal fistula is identified by coughing while swallowing, pulmonary secretions contaminated by gastric secretions, increased tracheal secretions, or gastric distention. A tracheobronchial fistula usually causes subcutaneous crepitus and dyspnea, not pulsation of the tracheostomy tube. A tracheovenous fistula may cause nonpulsatile bleeding.
Nursing process step: Assessment
Cognitive level: Evaluation

136. During the morning assessment, the nurse notices a large amount of bright red blood draining from a patient's tracheostomy site into the mechanical ventilator tubing. Her immediate reaction would be to:

A. Inflate the tracheal tube to its maximum capacity

B. Vigorously lavage and suction the patient's airway

C. Increase positive end-expiratory pressure on the ventilator

D. Put pressure on the tracheal stoma

CORRECT ANSWER—**A.** Bright red blood draining from a tracheostomy site, especially when the tracheostomy tube has not been suctioned, may be caused by a tracheoarterial fistula. This hemorrhage can lead to rapid death. Maximizing tracheal pressure using the tracheostomy cuff helps decrease the bleeding. Vigorous suction and lavage can worsen bleeding, and pressure on the stoma will not compress the affected artery. Increasing positive end-expiratory pressure will not help stop the bleeding.

Nursing process step: Implementation
Cognitive level: Application

Questions 137 to 140 refer to the following information:

Two weeks after undergoing coronary artery bypass graft surgery, a 64-year-old male patient with chronic obstructive pulmonary disease (COPD) is readmitted to the intensive care unit (ICU) because of complications. He has atrial arrhythmias, a sternal wound infected by methicillin-resistant *Staphylococcus aureus*, and an acute exacerbation of COPD, which was treated with vancomycin and corticosteroids; he has never fully resolved the exacerbation. On readmission to the ICU, the patient appears confused and difficult to arouse. Assessment findings include temperature, 101° F (38.3° C); blood pressure, 90/50 mm Hg; heart rate, 100 beats/minute with sinus tachycardia and premature atrial contractions; white blood cell count, 17.2 segmented neutrophils/mm^3, 84 band cells/mm^3, and 18 lymphocytes/mm^3; and respirations, 40 breaths/minute using accessory muscles to breathe on 2 liters of oxygen via nasal cannula. The chest X-ray film shows an infiltrate on the right lower lobe of the lung; sputum culture and sensitivity are positive for cocci.

137. What type of isolation would be most appropriate for this patient?

A. Strict

B. Universal

C. Respiratory

D. Wound

CORRECT ANSWER—**A.** Because of the patient's history of resistant pneumonia, strict isolation would best prevent the spread of a nosocomial infection. Universal precautions are mandated for all patients. The two sources of infection, wound and respiratory, would be best addressed via strict isolation.

Nursing process step: Implementation
Cognitive level: Comprehension

138. All of the following medications are helpful in managing an acute exacerbation of chronic obstructive pulmonary disease (COPD) *except:*
  A. Nebulized albuterol
  B. Systemic corticosteroids
  C. Inhaled ipratropium bromide
  D. Inhaled cromolyn sodium

CORRECT ANSWER—D. Cromolyn sodium, an inhalant, is used prophylactically for allergic and exercise-induced asthma. Nebulized albuterol, a bronchodilator, helps open the airways. Systemic corticosteroids decrease inflammation in the airways; they are used for COPD and asthma. Inhaled ipratropium, a bronchodilator, also is used to treat COPD. In addition, patients with COPD often receive antibiotics because of the high risk of infection associated with retained secretions and inadequate immune system response.
Nursing process step: Implementation
Cognitive level: Comprehension

139. The patient's arterial blood gas values are pH, 7.28; PaO_2, 55 mm Hg; $PaCO_2$, 98 mm Hg; HCO_3^-, 30 mm Hg; and oxygen saturation, 86%. Based on these findings, which nursing intervention is most appropriate?
  A. Suctioning the patient
  B. Preparing the patient for intubation
  C. Delivering 100% oxygen via a nonrebreather mask
  D. Placing the patient in semi-Fowler's position

CORRECT ANSWER—B. The patient's increased carbon dioxide level, labored breathing, and decreased mental status indicate he is tiring and will require intubation and mechanical ventilation. Giving a patient with chronic obstructive pulmonary disease 100% oxygen will cause him to retain more carbon dioxide. Suctioning helps clear the airway, but it will not correct the signs of muscle fatigue. Placing the patient in semi-Fowler's position is the least appropriate action to take considering that arterial blood gas values indicate imminent respiratory arrest.
Nursing process step: Implementation
Cognitive level: Application

140. After implementing the previous intervention, the nurse would anticipate an initial change in the patient's:
  A. Mental status
  B. Temperature
  C. Carbon dioxide level
  D. pH

CORRECT ANSWER—C. Because carbon dioxide diffuses rapidly across the alveoli-capillary membrane, the CO_2 level can be corrected more quickly than the other parameters. A decrease in $PaCO_2$ will increase pH and thereby improve mental status because hypercapnia causes mental confusion. The patient's temperature probably is elevated because of infection (as evidenced by the increased white blood cell count) but would not be affected by intubation and mechanical ventilation.
Nursing process step: Evaluation
Cognitive level: Analysis

141. A 66-year-old patient has a chest tube placed for hemothorax. Bubbling in the water-seal chamber could indicate all of the following *except:*

A. Loose suction-control connection

B. Loosening of chest tube connections

C. Leak within the pleural cavity

D. Leak in the chest tube system

CORRECT ANSWER—A. A chest tube placed for hemothorax should not have bubbling in the water-seal chamber unless the system is compromised or pneumothorax has developed. Loosening of the chest tube connections and leaks within the three-bottle system allow air to enter the system, causing bubbling in the water-seal chamber. A loose suction-control connection would decrease the amount of suction applied to the system, but it would not cause bubbling in the water-seal chamber.

Nursing process step: Evaluation

Cognitive level: Comprehension

142. The physician orders cuff deflations every 8 hours for a patient with an endotracheal tube. The nurse knows that the primary concern with frequent deflation and inflation of the cuff is that it increases the risk of:

A. Tracheal rupture

B. Tracheal edema

C. Tracheoesophageal fistula

D. Tracheal aspiration

CORRECT ANSWER—D. Routine cuff deflation is unnecessary when quality low-pressure cuffs are used to secure endotracheal tubes. Because fluids within the oral cavity accumulate above the cuff, aspiration can occur when the cuff is deflated. Conscientious suctioning of the oropharynx decreases the risk of aspiration but will not prevent it. Tracheal rupture, tracheal edema, and tracheoesophageal complications may occur, but they are not the primary concern related to frequent deflation and inflation of the cuff.

Nursing process step: Implementation

Cognitive level: Comprehension

143. Early treatment for a patient with acute gastric acid aspiration includes:

A. Diuresis to maintain central venous pressure (CVP) between 0 and 3 mm Hg

B. Fluid therapy to maintain CVP between 2 and 6 mm Hg

C. Antibiotic therapy to eradicate gram-negative organisms

D. Antibiotic therapy to eradicate gram-positive organisms

CORRECT ANSWER—B. Hypotension from fluid loss into extravascular spaces, also called noncardiogenic pulmonary edema, often results from epithelial damage caused by large-volume gastric acid aspiration. Therefore, fluid therapy would be an appropriate intervention. However, it must be balanced to minimize the hydrostatic component of intrapulmonary capillary leakage. Antibiotics are not recommended until there is evidence of infection, preferably from microscopic examination and culture.

Nursing process step: Implementation

Cognitive level: Application

144. Before the nurse hyperextends a trauma patient's neck for orotracheal intubation, which radiologic result is recommended?
A. Anteroposterior chest X-ray film
B. Right lateral chest X-ray film
C. Cervical spine series
D. Thoracic spine series

CORRECT ANSWER—C. Before a trauma patient is intubated, the cervical spine should be evaluated for injuries that might be exacerbated by intubation. If emergency intubation is required, orotracheal intubation can be performed if the spine is manually immobilized. Anteroposterior and lateral chest X-ray films are helpful for evaluating parenchymal or direct pulmonary tissue injury, but they provide no data on the integrity of the cervical spine. A thoracic spine series is useful for evaluating the thoracic portion of the spine only.
Nursing process step: Planning
Cognitive level: Knowledge

145. Five days after a patient was intubated for a pulmonary contusion, the chest X-ray film shows infiltrates. How soon after the injury would the nurse expect to see evidence of clearing on the chest X-ray film?
A. 48 hours
B. 72 hours
C. 96 hours
D. 120 hours

CORRECT ANSWER—B. Evidence of contusion on chest X-ray films should start to clear within 72 hours after the injury. Persistent infiltrates may be evidence of pneumonia, aspiration, or adult respiratory distress syndrome.
Nursing process step: Evaluation
Cognitive level: Knowledge

146. While a patient is receiving autotransfusion therapy, the nurse prepares to send a blood sample to the laboratory for evaluation. Laboratory values specific to this procedure include:
A. Serum calcium, complete blood count, and urine hemoglobin
B. Serum sodium, partial thromboplastin time, and urine hemoglobin
C. Serum magnesium, partial thromboplastin time, and prothrombin time
D. Serum chloride, platelet count, and urine hemoglobin

CORRECT ANSWER—A. Autologous blood reinfusion causes hemolysis, as evidenced by a decreased hematocrit and increased urine and serum hemoglobin. Hematocrit and hemoglobin are included in a complete blood count. Autologous blood from serosal cavities does not contain fibrinogen but does contain elevated levels of fibrin split products, which would lead to increased prothrombin and partial thromboplastin times; these values should be measured in a patient receiving an autotransfusion. Serum calcium levels should be measured because of the chelating effect of citrate on calcium; citrate often is mixed in the retrieval bag of the autotransfusion unit. Serum sodium, magnesium, and chloride are not values specific to autotransfusion.
Nursing process step: Implementation
Cognitive level: Comprehension

147. A nonventilated 54-year-old male patient is dyspneic and wheezing. Physical assessment reveals accessory muscle use and retraction of the intercostal spaces. The nurse helps the patient to a sitting position, then assesses his breath sounds and finds no improvement. The nurse notes bilateral coarseness and rhonchi and observes that the patient seems to be working harder to breathe. Which intervention is appropriate?
   A. Preparing for chest tube placement
   B. Preparing for suctioning
   C. Administering a sedative
   D. Providing supplemental oxygen

CORRECT ANSWER—B. Retraction of the intercostal spaces indicates obstruction of the inflow of air into the airways. In this situation, the nurse should attempt to remove the obstruction via suctioning. Sedation and oxygen therapy would not correct the underlying problem. Chest tube placement is indicated for hemothorax or pneumothorax, not airway obstruction.
Nursing process step: Implementation
Cognitive level: Application

148. Which diagnostic test is not commonly used to detect early gastric fluid aspiration?
   A. Chest X-ray film
   B. Sputum examination
   C. Bronchoscopy
   D. Pulmonary function study

CORRECT ANSWER—C. Bronchoscopy is used to evaluate patients who have aspirated solid material, which may be removed by a flexible or rigid bronchoscope. Extreme care must be taken not to drive solid or particulate material further into the lung. Bronchoscopy also can be used to remove excess secretions, obtain a biopsy of a tumor, or detect bleeding. Bronchoscopy would not be useful for detecting gastric fluid aspiration. All the other tests listed are used to evaluate a patient's response to aspiration.
Nursing process step: Assessment
Cognitive level: Analysis

149. The nurse is caring for a patient receiving continuous tube feedings. When preparing the patient for chest physiotherapy, the nurse should:
   A. Discontinue the feedings 6 hours before chest physiotherapy
   B. Discontinue the feedings 1 hour before chest physiotherapy
   C. Discontinue the feedings 30 minutes before chest physiotherapy
   D. Continue the feedings at a lower rate during chest physiotherapy

CORRECT ANSWER—B. Discontinuing tube feedings 1 hour before chest physiotherapy is necessary to prevent aspiration. Evaluating intestinal motility, radiologic results, patient comfort, and the amount of residual feeding in the stomach is a standard component of the assessment process. Feedings administered by a tube that enters below the pyloric sphincter need not be discontinued unless the patient experiences reflux into the stomach.
Nursing process step: Implementation
Cognitive level: Application

150. Which position best facilitates coughing?
   A. Supine position
   B. Lateral decubitus position
   C. Low-Fowler's position
   D. High-Fowler's position

CORRECT ANSWER—D. High-Fowler's position, with knees bent and a lightweight pillow placed over the abdomen, increases the expiratory pressures and effort associated with coughing. The low-Fowler's, lateral decubitus, and supine positions do not provide the expiratory assistance afforded by high-Fowler's position.
Nursing process step: Implementation
Cognitive level: Comprehension

151. A 30-year-old office worker who has just undergone emergency surgery for a ruptured appendix is intubated for recovery from anesthesia. On his arrival at the postanesthesia care unit, the nurse notes localized expiratory wheezing, excessive coughing, and bilateral diminished breath sounds. The nurse suspects that the:
   A. Patient has a spontaneous left-sided pneumothorax
   B. Patient has suffered herniation of the cuff over the end of the tube
   C. Tube is positioned at the level of the carina
   D. Tube is displaced into one bronchus

CORRECT ANSWER—C. Low tube placement at the level of the carina results in obstruction or atelectasis of the nonventilated lung. Signs and symptoms of low placement include localized expiratory wheezing, excessive coughing, and bilateral diminished breath sounds. Transferring a ventilated patient within the hospital can displace the tube to the level of the carina or bronchus or back up toward the vocal cords. Displacement of the tube into one bronchus results in uneven or delayed chest expansion, unilateral diminished breath sounds, and localized expiratory wheezing. Herniation of the cuff over the end of the tube causes symptoms associated with obstruction, such as increased airway pressures, difficulty achieving tidal volume, and unequal chest expansion. A left-sided pneumothorax would not cause bilateral diminished breath sounds.
Nursing process step: Assessment
Cognitive level: Comprehension

152. Which finding is common in patients with chronic aspiration?
   A. Bronchial breath sounds in the dependent portions of the lungs
   B. Diffuse bibasilar rales
   C. Rhonchi in the upper lobes of the lungs
   D. Wheezing in the upper airways of both lungs

CORRECT ANSWER—A. Chronic aspiration causes localized consolidation of the dependent portions or bilateral mid-zones of the lungs. Chronic aspiration results from repeated aspiration of small amounts of infected pharyngeal materials that are a source of continuous injury to the lung tissue. Diffuse bibasilar rales indicate fluid in the bases of the lungs and occur in congestive heart failure. Rhonchi in the upper lobes of the lung are caused by air passing through fluid-filled airways, as occurs in upper respiratory tract infection. Wheezing in the upper airways of both lungs occurs when fluid or secretions narrow the airways, causing partial obstruction.
Nursing process step: Assessment
Cognitive level: Evaluation

153. A pulmonary artery catheter is inserted in a patient who has aspirated gastric secretions. Which pulmonary artery systolic pressure (PAS) and pulmonary artery diastolic pressure (PAD) would the nurse expect this patient to have?
  A. PAS, 22 mm Hg; PAD, 12 mm Hg
  B. PAS, 16 mm Hg; PAD, 9 mm Hg
  C. PAS, 42 mm Hg; PAD, 30 mm Hg
  D. PAS, 25 mm Hg; PAD, 18 mm Hg

CORRECT ANSWER—C. Normal PAS is 15 to 30 mm Hg; normal PAD is 4 to 12 mm Hg. Pulmonary artery pressures increase significantly with aspiration of gastric fluid. This results from damage to the alveolar-capillary barrier, which causes alveolar compromise and shunting of blood away from the unventilated areas.
Nursing process step: Assessment
Cognitive level: Evaluation

154. The pathophysiology of traumatic diaphragmatic injury results from:
  A. Increased thoracic pressures
  B. Equalized thoracic and abdominal pressures
  C. Increased intra-abdominal pressures
  D. Asymmetric intrathoracic pressure

CORRECT ANSWER—C. Diaphragmatic injury results from increased intra-abdominal pressures, not equalized thoracic and abdominal pressures, that rupture the muscle. Approximately 5% of diaphragmatic ruptures result from blunt trauma; the remainder are caused by penetrating injury to the chest or abdomen. Increased thoracic pressures cause tension pneumothorax; a mediastinal shift results from asymmetric thoracic volume or pressure.
Nursing process step: Evaluation
Cognitive level: Comprehension

155. When assessing a patient with a lower esophageal perforation, the nurse would check for complications related to:
  A. Left-sided upper pleural effusion
  B. Left-sided upper pneumothorax
  C. Left-sided lower pleural effusion
  D. Right-sided lower pneumothorax

CORRECT ANSWER—C. Esophageal perforations are associated with pleural disease and air leak syndrome. The upper two-thirds of the esophagus are adjacent to the right pleura, while the lower one-third is adjacent to the left pleura. Pleural effusions are common with esophageal injuries and are found on the side proximal to the affected esophagus. Lobar atelectasis, hemoptysis, and persistent air leak syndrome are seen in untreated tracheobronchial injuries. Most pneumothoraces and hemothoraces are related to chest trauma, not specifically to esophageal perforation.
Nursing process step: Assessment
Cognitive level: Analysis

156. A patient complaining of retrosternal chest pain after being involved in a motor vehicle accident is likely to have:
  A. Myocardial infarction
  B. Myocardial contusion
  C. Aortic rupture
  D. Pulmonary contusion

CORRECT ANSWER—C. Aortic rupture is associated with retrosternal chest pain, widened mediastinum, and significant differences in blood pressure between the upper and lower extremities. Chest pain resulting from myocardial infarction usually is defined as crushing; cardiac and pulmonary contusions are not associated with organ-specific pain. A patient with a myocardial contusion may be asymptomatic or complain of angina-like pain; a patient with a pulmonary contusion typically exhibits dyspnea, hypoxemia, and hemoptysis.
Nursing process step: Assessment
Cognitive level: Analysis

NEUROLOGIC SYSTEM

CHAPTER 3

Neurologic System

1. Increased cerebrospinal fluid (CSF) pressure and increased intracranial pressure against the dura can cause:
A. Meningeal irritation
B. Rhinorrhea
C. Otorrhea
D. Papilledema

CORRECT ANSWER—D. Papilledema results from decreased venous outflow, which causes engorgement of the optic disc. Meningeal irritation does not result from increased CSF or intracranial pressure. Rhinorrhea is the leakage of CSF from the nares; otorrhea is the leakage of CSF from the ear. Both conditions may be seen in patients with skull fractures and meningeal laceration.
Nursing process step: Assessment
Cognitive level: Analysis

Questions 2 to 5 refer to the following information:
A 45-year-old executive complains of photophobia, severe headache, and stiff neck. An arteriogram shows an aneurysm of the middle cerebral artery. His vital signs include blood pressure, 120/70 mm Hg; pulse, 88 beats/minute; and respirations, 22 breaths/minute. His initial hemoglobin count is 13.5 g/dl and his initial hematocrit is 39%.

---

2. The patient's symptoms are consistent with:
A. Meningeal irritation resulting from blood in the cerebrospinal fluid (CSF)
B. Secondary bacterial meningitis
C. Encephalitis resulting from blood in the brain parenchyma
D. Idiosyncratic reaction to the dye used in arteriography

CORRECT ANSWER—A. Blood in the CSF mimics the symptoms of meningitis. There is no reason to suspect encephalitis or bacterial meningitis. The symptoms exhibited by this patient typically are seen in subarachnoid hemorrhage, not an allergic reaction.
Nursing process step: Evaluation
Cognitive level: Evaluation

3. This patient should be monitored closely for:
   A. Altered comfort
   B. Further reaction to the dye
   C. Altered level of consciousness
   D. Altered cardiac output

CORRECT ANSWER—C. Vasospasm and rebleeding are common sequelae of subarachnoid hemorrhage. Both of these complications can lead to cerebral ischemia or increased intracranial pressure, which can cause a progressive decrease in the level of consciousness. Although the patient is undoubtedly uncomfortable, a change in level of consciousness is much more significant than an alteration in comfort. The patient's symptoms were not caused by an allergic reaction to the dye. Cardiac output may or may not change significantly.
Nursing process step: Implementation
Cognitive level: Evaluation

4. Treatment for vasospasm resulting from subarachnoid hemorrhage may include:
   A. Administering a calcium channel blocker, such as nimodipine
   B. Reducing circulating blood volume to prevent edema
   C. Administering antihypertensive agents to prevent fluid overload
   D. Administering a beta blocker to reduce spasm

CORRECT ANSWER—A. Nimodipine frequently is prescribed to reduce the vasospasm associated with cerebral hemorrhage. This calcium channel blocker prevents smooth-muscle contraction of the cerebral arteries. Dehydration, beta blockade, and antihypertensive agents can excessively lower mean arterial pressure or cardiac output and predispose the patient to ischemia. Some physicians prefer to combine nimodipine with hypervolemic hemodilution (such as I.V. albumin 5% infused at a rate of 100 ml/hour) to decrease the hematocrit and increase blood flow to the ischemic microcirculation.
Nursing process step: Implementation
Cognitive level: Application

5. The patient is given I.V. dopamine at a rate of 2 mcg/kg/minute and I.V. Plasmanate at a rate of 125 ml/hour. His hematocrit 6 hours later has decreased to 28%. His blood pressure has risen to 145/88 mm Hg, with an increase in pulmonary artery wedge pressure from 10 to 17 mm Hg and cardiac output to 7.5 liters/minute. What do these changes represent?
   A. Additional bleeding from the subarachnoid hemorrhage
   B. Impending herniation and brain stem compression
   C. Increased blood pressure caused by pain and further development of subarachnoid hemorrhage
   D. Desired response to hypervolemic hemodilution to increase perfusion

CORRECT ANSWER—D. The changes in this patient are the expected result of increasing blood pressure and dilution of the blood to aid perfusion in the area beyond which vasospasm has occurred. Rebleeding would not lower the hematocrit as much; the patient's brain stem would herniate first. Herniation would further increase blood pressure, but would not raise the pulmonary artery wedge pressure. Pain would not lower the hematocrit.
Nursing process step: Evaluation
Cognitive level: Synthesis

6. Complications of brain tumors include increased intracranial pressure and:
   A. Hypovolemia
   B. Neurogenic pulmonary edema
   C. Psychotic personality changes
   D. Seizures and focal deficits

CORRECT ANSWER—D. The most common symptoms of a space-occupying lesion (brain tumor) are seizures and focal deficits. Although personality changes may occur, they are not limited to psychosis. Hypovolemia is unlikely unless the patient also has diabetes insipidus. Neurogenic pulmonary edema is more likely to occur with head injuries.
Nursing process step: Evaluation
Cognitive level: Comprehension

7. A space-occupying lesion in the left frontal lobe of the brain can cause:
   A. Receptive aphasia
   B. Expressive aphasia
   C. Seizures with a visual aura
   D. Nystagmus and hyperesthesia

CORRECT ANSWER—B. Broca's motor speech area usually is located in the left frontal lobe of the brain, even in left-handed people. A lesion in this area will cause expressive aphasia. Receptive aphasia is related to problems with Wernicke's motor speech area in the temporal lobe. A visual aura would place the seizure focus in the occipital lobe rather than the frontal lobe. Nystagmus and hyperesthesia are not specifically related to a frontal lesion.
Nursing process step: Assessment
Cognitive level: Evaluation

Questions 8 to 10 refer to the following information:
A male patient has had a reaction to a blood transfusion and currently is in acute renal failure with a blood urea nitrogen (BUN) level of 95 mg/dl and a creatinine level of 8.9 mg/dl. He was confused earlier in the day and received haloperidol 5 mg I.M. His urine output is marginal at 15 to 20 ml/hour. Pulmonary artery pressures are 30 mm Hg and 17 mm Hg. He has become very agitated and had to be restrained to prevent injury. He continually complains of extreme thirst and is confused and disoriented. His pupils are equal and reactive with no motor or sensory deficits, but he has muscle fasciculations in both legs.

8. Which nursing intervention is most appropriate?
   A. Preparing the patient for immediate dialysis and computed tomography scan
   B. Protecting the patient's airway and instituting seizure precautions
   C. Increasing fluid intake to dilute the blood urea nitrogen (BUN) level and to reduce osmolality
   D. Administering additional haloperidol to control patient's agitation and to prevent injury

CORRECT ANSWER—B. The primary nursing intervention is to protect the patient from injury while measures are taken to reduce the BUN level. Although uremic encephalopathy is possible, the BUN level need not be this high to cause encephalopathy. It can occur at much lower levels and may be related to other metabolites or to parathyroid hormone or other abnormalities associated with renal failure. Because the patient has no localized signs of a structural disturbance (for example, a brain tumor or intracranial hematoma) and pupil responses are normal, a computed tomography scan is not indicated. The BUN level is high because of acute intrinsic renal failure, not dehydration. Because pulmonary artery pressures already are in the high-to-normal range, fluids are contraindicated. Additional haloperidol will not hurt, but it will affect only the patient's symptoms. To reduce agitation, the underlying cause must be treated.
Nursing process step: Implementation
Cognitive level: Analysis

9. This patient will require frequent monitoring for:
   A. Increasing agitation
   B. Fluid overload and pulmonary edema
   C. Obtundation and worsening encephalopathy
   D. Cerebral thrombosis resulting from exacerbation of atherosclerosis

CORRECT ANSWER—C. An agitated patient with uremic encephalopathy eventually becomes obtunded if the BUN level does not decrease and waste products are not removed. If excess fluids are avoided, pulmonary edema is not likely to occur because pulmonary artery pressure is in the high-to-normal range and not yet elevated. Also, the extremely high BUN and subsequent high serum osmolality tend to delay the symptoms typically seen in acute pulmonary edema. Cerebral thrombosis resulting from exacerbation of atherosclerosis is a later complication of chronic, rather than acute, renal failure.
Nursing process step: Implementation
Cognitive level: Application

10. Considering the clinical picture, this patient may be at risk for seizures. To prevent this potential complication, the nurse would do which of the following?
A. Prepare the patient for immediate dialysis and protect him from injury
B. Administer I.V. phenytoin
C. Prepare the patient for intubation and hyperventilation
D. Protect the patient's airway and rapidly reduce the BUN level to normal

CORRECT ANSWER—**B.** Phenytoin is the drug of choice for preventing seizures in this setting, but it will not stop a seizure in progress. Diazepam, lorazepam, or phenobarbital can be used to stop a seizure. Dialysis would reduce the BUN, thus helping the encephalopathy, but it would not prevent seizures. If the BUN is reduced too quickly, rebound cerebral edema may develop. Intubating and hyperventilating a patient would decrease intracranial pressure, but not the potential for seizures.
Nursing process step: Implementation
Cognitive level: Application

11. A female patient was admitted to the medical-surgical unit 4 days ago with fever of unknown origin. Her temperature is 102° F (38.9° C). Her white blood cell count is elevated, yet all X-ray films and cultures are negative. The patient has become unresponsive, and her left pupil is slightly sluggish and 1 mm larger than the right. Nursing management should include which intervention?
A. Elevating the head of the bed, preventing Valsalva's maneuvers, and instituting seizure precautions
B. Preparing for insertion of an intracranial pressure (ICP) monitor
C. Administering anticonvulsants
D. Teaching the patient how to adapt to motor and sensory losses

CORRECT ANSWER—**A.** The patient's signs suggest a potential abscess, which generally produces clinical effects similar to those of a brain tumor. Early symptoms result from increased ICP; the earliest symptom is an altered level of consciousness. The nurse must implement measures to maintain a normal ICP. These include elevating the head of the bed and maintaining the patient's head in alignment to promote venous return. Valsalva's maneuvers increase ICP and should be avoided. Because the patient is at risk for generalized seizures, seizure precautions are necessary. Noting the onset and duration of a seizure can help localize the lesion. An ICP monitor is not indicated at this point. Anticonvulsants would not be started until the diagnosis of a brain abscess is confirmed or a seizure occurs. The patient is not exhibiting any definite motor or sensory losses.
Nursing process step: Implementation
Cognitive level: Application

12. A 24-year-old male playing basketball collapses on the court with a tonic-clonic seizure. In the emergency department, he is responsive and complains of a severe headache involving only the left side of his head. He has photophobia, blurred vision, and nuchal rigidity. A computed tomography scan with contrast media reveals subarachnoid hemorrhage and a large arteriovenous (AV) malformation of the frontal-temporal region measuring 5 to 6 cm. The patient is admitted to the intensive care unit for observation. The nurse would expect to frequently assess this patient for:
A. Neurologic function, blood pressure changes, and need for emotional support
B. Need for sedatives and seizure precautions
C. Neurologic function and need for morphine to relieve the headache
D. Signs of vasospasm

CORRECT ANSWER—A. The patient must be monitored closely for changes in neurologic status and to ensure that his blood pressure remains stable. A patient who learns he has a brain injury will require emotional support. Sedatives and morphine seldom are used in this situation because of the danger of clouding the level of consciousness. However, seizure precautions are necessary because AV malformations are associated with seizures. AV malformations are not associated with vasospasm because the lesion does not involve blood in the basilar cisterns near the major cerebral arteries.
Nursing process step: Assessment
Cognitive level: Application

13. Which spinal cord injury has the best prognosis for return of function?
A. Anterior cord syndrome
B. Brown-Séquard syndrome
C. Central cord syndrome
D. Incomplete cord transection

CORRECT ANSWER—C. Central cord syndrome may resolve because it does not involve transection of the cord. The other spinal cord injuries cause permanent changes.
Nursing process step: Evaluation
Cognitive level: Comprehension

Questions 14 and 15 refer to the following information:
An 87-year-old female patient with mitral valve disease develops a blood clot that becomes an embolus and lodges in the right cerebral artery. She has difficulty swallowing and talking and has significant sensory and motor deficits on the left side.

14. One of the first nursing priorities in the care of this patient is to:

A. Maintain a patent airway and provide nutritional support

B. Prepare for emergency mitral valve replacement

C. Reassure the patient and family that rehabilitation can reduce the patient's motor and sensory deficits

D. Prepare for hypervolemic hemodilution

CORRECT ANSWER—A. Because dysphagia increases the risk of aspiration, maintaining a patent airway is important. Nutritional support is necessary to ensure that the patient receives adequate caloric intake because she may be unable to feed herself. The patient probably is not a candidate for mitral valve replacement because of her age and the major neurologic insult. Hypervolemic hemodilution is of no benefit for an embolus. Reassuring the patient and family that rehabilitation can reduce the patient's deficits is important, but not the first priority.
Nursing process: Implementation
Cognitive level: Application

15. The patient also will need:

A. Mannitol or furosemide to reduce ischemic edema

B. Emotional support to cope with neurologic changes and fear of recurrent emboli

C. Steroid therapy to reduce swelling

D. Digoxin to control atrial fibrillation

CORRECT ANSWER—B. Part of the agony of an embolism is the fear of recurrence. Because the diseased valve cannot be replaced, other thrombi may develop. The patient also must learn to live with the neurologic deficits resulting from the cerebrovascular accident. Because cerebral edema usually is not a serious problem with this type of embolism, mannitol, furosemide, and steroids are not necessary. The patient's embolus occurred because of a diseased mitral valve rather than atrial fibrillation, so digoxin may have no direct benefit.
Nursing process step: Implementation
Cognitive level: Application

16. To enter the cerebral circulation, a cerebral embolus must come from the:

A. Left side of the heart or the systemic arterial circulation

B. Right side of the heart and the systemic venous circulation

C. Cerebral arteries or veins

D. Arteries or veins

CORRECT ANSWER—A. Emboli must enter the brain through the carotid or basilar arteries, which arise from the systemic circulation. They also can originate in the left side of the heart. Emboli from the right side of the heart and the veins would be trapped in the small vessels of the lungs. Although cerebral arteries may produce emboli in the form of plaque, the veins would not.
Nursing process step: Assessment
Cognitive level: Knowledge

Questions 17 and 18 refer to the following information:
A 55-year-old male patient is admitted to the intensive care unit immediately after a coronary artery bypass graft (CABG) and aortic valve replacement for coronary artery disease. Six hours after admission to the unit, the patient is awake and nodding yes and no to questions. However, he does not move his left leg voluntarily or on command.

17. The patient's postoperative condition most likely is due to:
A. Residual effects of anesthesia
B. Embolism of air or debris from the aorta during valve replacement
C. Embolism of clots originating in left ventricle
D. Cerebral infarction resulting from low perfusion during CABG procedure

CORRECT ANSWER—B. After aortic valve replacement or endarterectomy, embolism of air or plaque sometimes occurs. An embolus consisting of air or debris is more likely than one consisting of atherosclerotic plaque. The anesthesia has worn off enough to assess the patient's neurologic status. Because the patient is alert, oriented, and following commands, the weakness is not likely to be caused by residual effects of anesthesia. Cerebral perfusion is carefully maintained during the CABG procedure, so infarction is unlikely. It is less likely that clots were present in the left ventricle before or during surgery.
Nursing process step: Evaluation
Cognitive level: Analysis

18. After the immediate postoperative period, care for this patient must include:
A. Anticoagulant therapy to prevent further emboli
B. Antibiotic therapy to prevent vegetative growth
C. Emotional support and positive attitude toward recovery of function
D. Reassurance that anesthesia will wear off soon

CORRECT ANSWER—C. Emotional support and a positive attitude toward rehabilitation are essential to this patient's care. A patient who has undergone valve replacement will receive anticoagulants to prevent clots from developing on the new valve. Antibiotics are used for a short time, not as continued therapy. The anesthesia has already worn off, as the patient can respond to the questions.
Nursing process step: Planning
Cognitive level: Application

19. Initial measures to rapidly reduce intracranial pressure include:
A. Having the patient lie flat in the bed
B. Elevating the head of the bed and hyperventilating the patient to achieve a partial pressure of carbon dioxide in arterial blood ($PaCO_2$) of 28 to 32 mm Hg
C. Slowly administering 1 g I.V. mannitol
D. Rapidly lowering $PaCO_2$ to 20 mm Hg and administering I.V. dexamethasone

CORRECT ANSWER—B. Intracranial pressure can be lowered quickly by elevating the head of the bed and hyperventilating the patient. Lowering $PaCO_2$ to less than 25 mm Hg can cause ischemia from excess vasoconstriction. Mannitol and dexamethasone reduce intracranial pressure but take longer to work. Hyperventilation may be followed by the administration of mannitol, furosemide, and dexamethasone.
Nursing process step: Implementation
Cognitive level: Application

20. A 37-year-old female victim of domestic violence has a slashing stab wound to the neck that caused hemisection of the spinal cord at the C7 level. She has a Brown-Séquard lesion. After the swelling and edema resolve, the patient will suffer:

A. Loss of sensory function only

B. Loss of motor and sensory function on the same side as the hemisection

C. Upper extremity paralysis more severe than lower extremity paralysis

D. Ipsilateral loss of motor function and contralateral loss of sensory function

CORRECT ANSWER—D. Brown-Séquard syndrome results in loss of motor function on one side and loss of sensory function on the opposite side. Variation in upper and lower motor strength is seen in central cord syndrome.
Nursing process step: Evaluation
Cognitive level: Comprehension

21. Spinal shock, which often lasts for weeks after a spinal cord injury, causes flaccid paralysis and loss of reflex activity. While caring for a patient with this condition, the nurse must watch carefully for:

A. Incontinence and skin breakdown

B. Orthostatic hypotension and bradycardia

C. Depression and tachycardia

D. Decreased metabolic rate and bradycardia

CORRECT ANSWER—B. Loss of vasomotor tone and an inability to constrict vessels in response to sudden changes in blood pressure predispose a patient with spinal shock to hypotension and bradycardia. Although incontinence and skin breakdown are continual concerns, they are directly related to paralysis, not spinal shock. Depression is not limited to the period of spinal shock. Spinal shock does not decrease the metabolic rate.
Nursing process step: Assessment
Cognitive level: Analysis

22. A 56-year-old patient who underwent surgery to repair a cerebral aneurysm will receive dexamethasone 4 mg every 6 hours followed by decreasing doses over the next 3 days to reduce cerebral edema. The nurse caring for this patient should monitor for:

A. Increased susceptibility to infection

B. Ototoxicity

C. Hypotension

D. Glucose intolerance

CORRECT ANSWER—D. Increased glucose levels are common in patients receiving steroid therapy, especially in those who also have diabetes. In some cases, insulin may be necessary to control the glucose level. The short-term administration of this steroid is unlikely to reduce immunity. Ototoxicity is not related to steroid therapy. The sodium retention caused by steroids is more likely to cause hypertension.
Nursing process step: Assessment
Cognitive level: Analysis

23. Which intracranial pressure monitor is the least invasive?

A. Epidural sensor

B. Subdural bolt

C. Subarachnoid screw

D. Intraparenchymal monitor

CORRECT ANSWER—A. An epidural sensor is positioned just underneath the skull and does not penetrate the meninges, whereas a subdural bolt penetrates the dura mater. A subarachnoid screw penetrates one more layer and is in contact with the cerebrospinal fluid. An intraparenchymal monitor slightly enters the brain tissue.
Nursing process step: Implementation
Cognitive level: Comprehension

Questions 24 to 27 refer to the following information:
A 45-year-old male patient with a history of atrial fibrillation is admitted to the intensive care unit from the emergency department, where he was treated for sudden onset of right facial paralysis and numbness and loss of motor function of the right arm. His pupils are equal and reactive to light. His blood pressure is 134/70 mm Hg, and his pulse rate is 75 beats/minute. He has sinus rhythm without ectopy. The patient is a smoker but has no other health problems. The computed tomography scan is inconclusive.

24. What is the most likely cause of the patient's neurologic deficits?
A. Intracerebral hemorrhage with acute cerebral ischemia
B. Cerebral embolus
C. Subarachnoid hemorrhage caused by an aneurysm
D. Cerebral thrombus

CORRECT ANSWER—B. The patient displays no signs of meningeal irritation to indicate a hemorrhage. Therefore, the cause could be either an embolus or a thrombus. Thrombosis is the formation of a blood clot that obstructs a cerebral vessel. It is the most common cause of cerebrovascular accident (CVA) and initially produces transient ischemic attacks secondary to partial occlusion. Thrombotic CVAs are associated with atherosclerosis and arterial narrowing. They manifest over several hours; permanent symptoms appear once the thrombus completely occludes the vessel. Embolism refers to occlusion of a vessel by a fragmented clot, tumor, fat, bacteria, or air. Blockage of an intracerebral artery leads to a localized cerebral infarction. Signs and symptoms develop suddenly, within 1 minute of occlusion. Embolic CVAs are most common in patients with atrial flutter or fibrillation and other forms of heart disease. Because of the patient's health history and sudden onset of symptoms, a cerebral embolus is the most likely cause of his neurologic deficits.
Nursing process step: Evaluation
Cognitive level: Evaluation

25. In addition to magnetic resonance imaging, what other test might help determine the origin of the patient's neurologic deficits?
A. Computed tomography (CT) scan with contrast media
B. Cerebral arteriography
C. Ventilation-perfusion lung scan
D. Echocardiography

CORRECT ANSWER—D. Although CT scan with contrast media and cerebral arteriography might provide valuable information about the site of occlusion, they would not identify the source of the obstruction. Echocardiography is useful for identifying mural thrombi, myxomas, and vegetation on a valve. A ventilation-perfusion lung scan, which is used to detect pulmonary emboli, is not needed based on the clinical assessment.
Nursing process step: Implementation
Cognitive level: Comprehension

26. The patient undergoes mediastinotomy and excision of a left atrial myxoma; he is then sent to the cardiovascular recovery unit. He still has right-sided weakness but is alert and oriented. Postoperatively, the nurse should assess for:
A. Changes in vital signs resulting from herniation of the temporal lobe
B. Changes in neurologic status caused by cerebral edema
C. Changes in neurologic status caused by intraoperative emboli
D. Recurrent intracerebral hemorrhage

CORRECT ANSWER—C. During removal of the myxoma, other pieces could have broken away and entered the arterial circulation, traveling not only to the brain but also to other organs, such as the kidneys, or the mesenteric arteries. Herniation of the temporal lobe is not likely because cerebrovascular accident is an embolic, rather than hemorrhagic, phenomenon. Cerebral edema is less likely to occur than the other options. There is no indication of a hemorrhage.
Nursing process step: Assessment
Cognitive level: Analysis

27. During heparin therapy for mural thrombi secondary to atrial fibrillation, the nurse must monitor:
A. Prothrombin time
B. Partial thromboplastin time
C. Clotting time (Lee-White method)
D. Bleeding time (Ivy method)

CORRECT ANSWER—B. During heparin therapy, the partial thromboplastin time is maintained at 1½ to 2 times the control. The prothrombin time is used to monitor warfarin sodium therapy. The other two tests are not used for monitoring anticoagulant therapy.
Nursing process step: Implementation
Cognitive level: Analysis

28. Possible precipitating causes of autonomic dysreflexia include:
A. Hypertension and tachyarrhythmia
B. Missed doses of antihypertensive medication
C. Spinal cord swelling in the first 24 hours after injury
D. Distended bladder or rectal impaction

CORRECT ANSWER—D. The noxious stimulus for autonomic dysreflexia often is a distended bladder or rectal impaction that leads to massive sympathetic response and severe hypertensive crisis. Autonomic dysreflexia occurs after spinal shock has resolved and is unrelated to antihypertensive therapy. Hypertension and tachycardia are symptoms, not causes, of autonomic dysreflexia.
Nursing process step: Planning
Cognitive level: Comprehension

29. Progressive dementia, a common manifestation of human immunodeficiency virus (HIV) encephalopathy, typically causes:
A. Intractable seizures
B. Hemiparesis and pupillary changes
C. Confusion, disorientation, and psychosis
D. Quadriplegia and peripheral neuropathy

CORRECT ANSWER—C. Although seizures may occur, the most common signs of HIV encephalopathy are confusion, disorientation, and psychosis. Quadriplegia and neuropathy are uncommon. Hemiparesis and pupillary changes occur later in a patient with a space-occupying lesion, which increases intracranial pressure.
Nursing process step: Assessment
Cognitive level: Comprehension

Questions 30 and 31 refer to the following information:
An 84-year-old female patient with non–insulin-dependent diabetes fell and broke her right hip 3 days ago. She underwent a hip replacement 48 hours ago. The patient has been alert and oriented until tonight, when she became confused and progressively less responsive. She appears frail and pale and responds only to deep pain. For the last 24 hours, her fluid intake was 800 ml and fluid output was 350 ml. No drainage or sign of infection is evident. Her laboratory values include serum glucose, 855 mg/dl; potassium, 3.0 mEq/liter; sodium, 155 mEq/liter; and serum osmolality, 365 mOsm/kg.

30. To reverse the metabolic encephalopathy, the nurse would:
A. Administer anticoagulants to prevent further thromboembolisms
B. Institute rehydration therapy and slowly reduce the glucose level to 200 to 300 mg/dl
C. Administer mannitol to reduce cerebral edema caused by hypernatremia
D. Administer calcium channel blockers to relieve cerebral vasospasm

CORRECT ANSWER—**B.** The patient is suffering from hyperosmolar nonketotic syndrome (HNKS). In this condition, enough insulin is being released in the body to prevent ketosis but not enough to prevent hyperglycemia. Older patients with non–insulin-dependent diabetes are especially at risk for HNKS. The high sodium level is a sign of intracellular dehydration. The brain is most sensitive to this dehydration, which is causing the patient's decreased mental status and responsiveness. Lowering the glucose below 200 mg/dl may excessively reduce serum osmolality and cause cerebral edema. Vasospasm is not a part of the patient's problem, and calcium channel blockers are not indicated. Mannitol would worsen the cellular dehydration in this hyperosmolar state. Hydration, rather than anticoagulant therapy, reduces the risk of thromboembolisms.
Nursing process step: Implementation
Cognitive level: Application

31. This patient must be monitored closely for:
A. Cerebral edema as serum osmolality decreases
B. Recurrent cerebral emboli
C. Symptoms of sepsis and infection
D. Cardiac failure caused by cardiac depression

CORRECT ANSWER—**A.** As serum osmolality decreases with the reduction in glucose and dilution of sodium, the patient is at risk for rebound cerebral edema. There is no evidence of cerebral embolus; the encephalopathy results from osmolality changes, not emboli or sepsis. Cardiac depression is unlikely, unless rapid fluid shifts occur.
Nursing process step: Evaluation
Cognitive level: Evaluation

32. A female patient has just undergone arteriography that shows subarachnoid hemorrhage caused by an aneurysm of the middle cerebral artery. Her level of consciousness has been steadily decreasing and her right pupil is sluggishly reactive. The nurse caring for this patient should question which physician order?
A. Prepare the patient for lumbar puncture
B. Perform a bleeding profile
C. Perform a magnetic resonance imaging scan
D. Prepare the patient for elective intubation

CORRECT ANSWER—A. A lumbar puncture is inappropriate. Withdrawing cerebrospinal fluid from the lumbar area can cause herniation in a patient with increased intracranial pressure. A bleeding profile would provide useful information on clotting ability. A magnetic resonance imaging scan could help differentiate between vasospasm or further bleeding from the aneurysm. The physician may choose to place the patient on a mechanical ventilator and hyperventilate the patient to decrease $PaCO_2$, which would decrease intracranial pressure.
Nursing process step: Assessment
Cognitive level: Comprehension

33. Cerebral perfusion pressure should be at least 50 mm Hg. How is it calculated?
A. Mean arterial pressure minus central venous pressure
B. Mean arterial pressure minus intracranial pressure
C. Systemic arterial pressure minus mean arterial pressure
D. Mean arterial pressure minus pulmonary artery wedge pressure

CORRECT ANSWER—B. The correct formula for cerebral perfusion pressure is mean arterial pressure minus intracranial pressure. The normal range for cerebral perfusion pressure is 50 to 130 mm Hg, with a value less than 50 mm Hg indicative of decreased perfusion and a value greater than 130 mm Hg associated with hyperemia. Hyperemia is an increase in cerebral blood flow that exceeds the brain's metabolic needs. It can be detrimental because the increased blood flow results in increased blood volume and, subsequently, increased intracranial pressure. The other calculations are incorrect.
Nursing process step: Assessment
Cognitive level: Knowledge

34. When caring for a patient with a neurologic deficit, the nurse should plan to implement patient-teaching activities:
A. When the patient is ready to learn
B. When family members are available
C. When the patient is admitted
D. After the patient returns from physical therapy

CORRECT ANSWER—A. Patient-teaching activities are vital to the emotional recovery of patients and their families. However, the nurse should implement these activities only after the patient is stable and rested and not distracted by other events. Although family members should be involved, educational efforts should be planned around the patient's needs.
Nursing process step: Implementation
Cognitive level: Synthesis

Questions 35 to 37 refer to the following information:
A 37-year-old male construction worker is admitted to the intensive care unit after falling 15 feet from a scaffold to the floor below. The patient is alert and oriented. His pupils are equal, are reactive to light, and exhibit accommodation. He has no weakness or other deficits. A computed tomography scan shows a frontal bone fracture.

35. Which of the following signs and symptoms are common in a patient with a frontal bone fracture?
A. Headache and progressive muscle weakness
B. Headache and raccoon eyes
C. Headache and photophobia
D. Headache and seizure activity characterized by sensory aura

CORRECT ANSWER—B. Headache commonly is reported by patients with frontal bone fractures because of pneumocephalus. Raccoon eyes (bilateral ecchymoses of the eyes) also are common with frontal bone fractures. Photophobia, muscle weakness, and seizures are less likely to occur, unless intracranial pressure increases or an infection develops.
Nursing process step: Assessment
Cognitive level: Comprehension

36. To decrease intracranial pressure (ICP) and relieve discomfort, what is the position of choice for this patient?
A. Supine position
B. Supine position with head of the bed elevated 30 degrees
C. Left lateral recumbent position
D. Trendelenburg's position

CORRECT ANSWER—B. In the absence of spinal cord injury, the best position for a patient with a head injury is supine with the head of the bed elevated 20 to 30 degrees. This position reduces ICP by promoting cerebrospinal fluid and venous outflow from the head. If a spinal cord injury is present or has not been ruled out, the patient should lie flat on the bed with attention to alignment of the spine. A left lateral recumbent position will not benefit the patient. Trendelenburg's position is contraindicated because it increases ICP and decreases venous return.
Nursing process step: Implementation
Cognitive level: Analysis

37. After 8 hours, the patient complains of a bad headache and appears confused and agitated. About 1 hour later, he becomes sleepy and hard to arouse except with vigorous tactile stimulation. A repeat computed tomography scan is likely to show:

A. Epidural hematoma
B. Subarachnoid hemorrhage
C. Intracerebral hematoma
D. Subdural hematoma

CORRECT ANSWER—D. Although subarachnoid hemorrhage is possible, a subdural hematoma from slower venous bleeding is most consistent with the mechanism of injury. Symptoms of an epidural hematoma would have manifested earlier because this injury usually is caused by arterial damage. An intracerebral hematoma (bleeding within the cerebral tissue or the parenchyma) often results from shearing of small vessels deep within the hemispheres of the brain. Intracerebral hematomas can cause severe generalized headaches, as well as hemiplegia, hemiparesis, abnormal pupil size and response, aphasia, nausea and vomiting, seizures, decorticate or decerebrate posturing, and increased blood pressure.
Nursing process step: Evaluation
Cognitive level: Synthesis

38. The Monroe-Kellie doctrine states that if one of the three volumes (blood, brain tissue, and cerebrospinal fluid) in the skull increases, space for the other two decreases. After compensation ends, what would happen if one volume began to increase again?

A. Intracranial pressure would increase
B. No further increase would occur
C. Pulse and blood pressure would increase to enhance perfusion
D. Blood pressure and pulse would decrease to reduce intracranial pressure

CORRECT ANSWER—A. If the volume continues to increase, intracranial pressure would rise, possibly compromising cerebral perfusion pressure. If vital signs change as a result of brain stem compression, Cushing's phenomenon would result, causing increased blood pressure and a reflex decrease in pulse while the pulse pressure widens.
Nursing process step: Assessment
Cognitive level: Comprehension

39. A patient is admitted for a craniotomy because of an astrocytoma in the left temporal lobe near the tentorial opening. The primary symptom was blurred vision. After surgery, the nurse should carefully evaluate the patient's:

A. Motor function
B. Receptive speech and hearing
C. Visual acuity and pupil reaction
D. Emotional lability and personality changes

CORRECT ANSWER—B. Because the temporal lobe is primarily responsible for receptive speech and hearing, these senses are most likely to be affected. Motor function is associated with the frontal lobe; it is not likely to change unless the patient has a hematoma or swelling large enough to compress the motor tracts. The patient's vision problems should resolve because the tumor is no longer impinging on the optic nerve. Emotional lability often is associated with temporal lobe conditions, but true personality changes would be associated with the frontal lobe.
Nursing process step: Evaluation
Cognitive level: Analysis

40. Blood in the cerebrospinal fluid (CSF) is a positive diagnostic finding in which type of cerebral hemorrhage?
- A. Subarachnoid hemorrhage
- B. Subdural hematoma
- C. Epidural hematoma
- D. Intracerebral hematoma

CORRECT ANSWER—A. Because CSF and the cerebral arteries are located in the subarachnoid space, a subarachnoid hemorrhage would cause bloody CSF. The other conditions would not.
Nursing process step: Evaluation
Cognitive level: Evaluation

41. Which is the solution of choice for mixing phenytoin for a piggyback I.V. infusion?
- A. Dextrose 5% in water
- B. 0.9% sodium chloride solution
- C. Dextrose 5% in 0.9% sodium chloride solution
- D. Dextrose 5% in 0.225% sodium chloride

CORRECT ANSWER—B. Phenytoin precipitates in dextrose. Only 0.9% sodium chloride solution should be used for a piggyback infusion with phenytoin.
Nursing process step: Implementation
Cognitive level: Comprehension

Questions 42 and 43 refer to the following information:
A 65-year-old female patient is admitted to the intensive care unit after transsphenoidal resection of an adenoma of the pituitary gland. She is intubated and placed on mechanical ventilator, and has no neurologic deficits.

---

42. Postoperative care for this patient should include:
- A. Removing nasal packing after 8 hours
- B. Monitoring urine output hourly for polyuria secondary to syndrome of inappropriate antidiuretic hormone secretion (SIADH)
- C. Monitoring blood pressure for hypertension secondary to increased angiotensin level
- D. Monitoring urine output hourly and reporting any output greater than 200 ml in 2 hours

CORRECT ANSWER—D. It is not uncommon for a patient in this situation to require vasopressin postoperatively to prevent hypovolemia resulting from excess urine loss. The packing and stents are left in the nose longer than 8 hours and are removed by the surgeon. SIADH, a condition in which secretion of antidiuretic hormone persists despite low serum osmolality, may be caused by brain tumors and typically results in water intoxication and decreased urine output. Angiotensin is not directly affected by the surgery, only indirectly by stress and hypotension.
Nursing process step: Planning
Cognitive level: Application

43. The patient complains of a frontal headache and has serosanguineous drainage from the right nares. What does this indicate?
A. Bleeding into the sella turcica
B. Recovery from surgery as expected
C. Increasing intracranial pressure (ICP) and impending herniation
D. Increasing ICP and hydrocephalus

CORRECT ANSWER—B. Frontal headache and serosanguineous drainage are normal signs and symptoms following transsphenoidal surgery and require only a drip pad and codeine for the headache. Bleeding into the sella turcica would produce bloody, not serosanguineous, drainage. Both hydrocephalus and increasing ICP would produce a change in level of consciousness and possible pupillary changes, symptoms this patient does not have.
Nursing process step: Evaluation
Cognitive level: Synthesis

44. A 34-year-old male patient diagnosed with acquired immunodeficiency syndrome (AIDS) 2 years ago has been taking zidovudine (also known as azidothymidine or AZT). He is admitted to the intensive care unit after experiencing a tonic-clonic seizure that lasted 1 minute. He is confused, lethargic, and weak on the right side. A computed tomography scan shows multiple abscess lesions in both hemispheres and one very large lesion in the left frontal lobe that is causing increased intracranial pressure. In addition to postoperative care specifically related to the craniotomy, the nurse should include which intervention in the plan of care?
A. Administering barbiturates to control seizures
B. Providing nutritional support to prevent anabolism
C. Providing emotional support because of the terminal nature of the disease
D. Administering acyclovir to prevent secondary viral infections

CORRECT ANSWER—C. Development of neurologic problems in a patient with AIDS often is distressing to both the patient and family members; emotional support for all involved is mandatory. Nutritional support prevents catabolism, not anabolism. Seizures would be controlled with anticonvulsants other than barbiturates (for example, phenytoin, a hydantoin derivative) because barbiturates have more of an effect on the level of consciousness. Acyclovir is not indicated unless a herpes infection develops.
Nursing process step: Planning
Cognitive level: Application

Questions 45 to 49 refer to the following information:
A 34-year-old male patient who had been straining to have a bowel movement becomes unresponsive. In the emergency department, he is lethargic and has left-sided weakness. His right pupil is dilated and sluggishly reactive to light. A computed tomography scan shows an intracerebral hematoma with a shift in midline structures. He is hypertensive with a blood pressure of 178/100 mm Hg.

---

45. What is the immediate goal of care for this patient?

A. Protecting the airway and reducing blood pressure to prevent further hemorrhage

B. Administering mannitol and furosemide to decrease intracranial pressure

C. Preparing for emergency ventriculostomy

D. Reducing blood pressure to increase cerebral perfusion pressure

CORRECT ANSWER—**A.** Blood pressure must be reduced to prevent further hemorrhage. Because of the patient's lethargy, intubation may be needed to protect the airway. Mannitol and furosemide may be used later to decrease cerebral edema, but would not be first-line therapy. A ventriculostomy is not indicated for this patient. Reducing blood pressure will not help increase cerebral perfusion pressure; in fact, cerebral perfusion pressure would not increase unless intracranial pressure also is reduced.
Nursing process step: Planning
Cognitive level: Analysis

46. After his blood pressure is controlled by nitroprusside, the patient is taken to the operating room for emergency craniotomy and hematoma evacuation. Postoperatively, the patient is intubated and hyperventilated to achieve a $PaCO_2$ of 25 to 30 mm Hg. This is necessary to:

A. Reduce swelling of the injured cells

B. Increase functional residual capacity

C. Increase oxygenation

D. Reduce intracranial pressure and prevent hemorrhage

CORRECT ANSWER—**D.** Because carbon dioxide acts as a potent vasodilator within the brain, reducing the CO_2 level to between 25 and 30 mm Hg would cause vasoconstriction and decrease microscopic bleeding. More importantly, total blood volume in the skull would be reduced, thereby decreasing intracranial pressure and increasing cerebral perfusion pressure. Postoperative ventilation would maintain functional residual capacity and oxygenation. Decreased levels of $PaCO_2$ would not directly reduce swelling.
Nursing process step: Implementation
Cognitive level: Comprehension

47. Which finding is crucial to the patient's postoperative assessment?

A. Pupil response

B. Motor function

C. Sensory function

D. Level of consciousness

CORRECT ANSWER—**D.** Level of consciousness is the most important part of the postoperative assessment because it requires the highest level of brain functioning, including input, integration, and response. Assessment of this parameter provides information about postoperative brain functioning. Pupillary changes are due to compression of cranial nerves. Because the pupils were dilated and sluggishly responsive preoperatively, they may still be dilated and sluggishly reactive postoperatively, depending on the amount of damage to the cranial nerves. Motor and sensory function are not the first indicators of increasing intracranial pressure or deterioration.
Nursing process step: Assessment
Cognitive level: Evaluation

48. Because the hematoma involved the frontal lobe, what neurologic deficits might occur in this patient?
A. Sensory changes
B. Ataxia and dyskinesia
C. Personality changes
D. Vision disturbances

CORRECT ANSWER—C. Frontal lobe functions include motor function, motor speech, personality, and judgment. Sensory changes are associated with the parietal lobe. Ataxia and dyskinesia would involve the basal ganglia and cerebellum. Vision disturbances result from cranial nerve or occipital lobe problems.
Nursing process step: Assessment
Cognitive level: Comprehension

49. While removing the hematoma, the neurosurgeon found a metastatic tumor that caused the abnormal vessels which predisposed the patient to hemorrhage. The patient's prognosis is poor, and his family has been told he probably has only a few weeks to live. The nursing plan must include:
A. Emotional support and information
B. Chemotherapy to reduce tumor size
C. Rehabilitation services
D. Telling the patient the prognosis after he recovers from surgery

CORRECT ANSWER—A. This prognosis is devastating for someone with no previous indication of a health problem. Supportive care and emotional support are imperative. Referral to a hospice may be appropriate, but rehabilitation services may have little to offer someone with a short life expectancy. Chemotherapy usually is not as effective for metastatic brain tumors. Families and patients have individual ways of coping with such news, and respecting their needs is important. All questions asked by a patient should be honestly answered, regardless of the timing.
Nursing process step: Planning
Cognitive level: Synthesis

50. Photophobia and headache are common symptoms of meningitis. To relieve discomfort for a patient with meningitis, it is helpful to:
A. Close the blinds to darken the room
B. Provide eye pads to block out light
C. Administer pilocarpine hydrochloride eye drops to constrict the pupils
D. Keep the head of the bed flat

CORRECT ANSWER—A. Darkening the room is better than providing eye pads, which have to be applied and removed. Pilocarpine hydrochloride is used to treat glaucoma. Keeping the head of the bed elevated, not flat, can help relieve the patient's headache.
Nursing process step: Implementation
Cognitive level: Comprehension

Questions 51 to 53 refer to the following information:
A 20-year-old female college student stopped taking her anticonvulsant medication because she was short of money and did not want her friends to know she had epilepsy. She is admitted to the emergency department (ED) after having a tonic-clonic seizure in her dorm room; she has another seizure in the ED. After the seizure is controlled with diazepam and phenytoin, the patient is admitted to the intensive care unit.

51. After waking up, the patient complains of general soreness and weakness on the left side. What does this indicate?

A. Cerebrovascular accident from prolonged seizures

B. Phenytoin toxicity

C. Electrolyte deficit from prolonged seizures

D. Postictal weakness that probably will resolve

CORRECT ANSWER—**D.** It is not uncommon for patients to experience weakness and even transient paralysis after a tonic-clonic seizure. When the adenosine triphosphate (ATP) and other phosphate stores are replenished, the weakness resolves. Phenytoin toxicity usually manifests as nystagmus, excess sedation, and ataxia. Also, the patient's phenytoin level probably is low because her seizures were triggered by drug discontinuation. A cerebrovascular accident is unlikely. Electrolyte levels are not depleted by seizures.
Nursing process step: Assessment
Cognitive level: Analysis

52. When assessing the patient, the nurse notes that the urine is the color of dark tea or cola. This probably indicates:

A. Myoglobin precipitation caused by rhabdomyolysis

B. Discoloration caused by phenytoin

C. Concentration resulting from dehydration

D. Occult hematuria

CORRECT ANSWER—**A.** Prolonged seizures can cause muscle breakdown and increase the risk of acute renal failure caused by obstruction of the tubules by myoglobin. Phenytoin and carbamazepine color cause a reddish brown tint to the urine, not a dark discoloration. Concentrated urine is amber, not the color of tea. Hematuria is a possibility and must be ruled out by urinalysis; however, considering the clinical picture, the discoloration is more likely to be caused by myoglobin precipitation.
Nursing process step: Assessment
Cognitive level: Analysis

53. To reduce the precipitation of myoglobin in the urine, the patient may be given:

A. Albumin or hetastarch to increase urine output

B. Dopamine I.V. at a rate of 2 mcg/kg/minute

C. Mannitol to decrease myoglobin precipitation and furosemide to dilute myoglobin

D. Lactated Ringer's solution to decrease myoglobin precipitation

CORRECT ANSWER—**C.** Mannitol can reduce the precipitation of myoglobin in the urine. It sometimes is used in combination with furosemide to increase dilution and elimination. However, furosemide can cause hypokalemia and hyponatremia, which may lower the seizure threshold. When a patient is given furosemide, electrolytes should be monitored closely. Dopamine increases renal blood flow but would not significantly affect myoglobin excretion. Lactated Ringer's solution would increase urine volume without directly affecting myoglobin. Albumin and hetastarch increase blood volume, which indirectly increases urine output; crystalloids are used more often because they are excreted directly.
Nursing process step: Implementation
Cognitive level: Analysis

54. In a patient in the early stages of encephalitis or meningitis, the nurse must initially assess for:
A. Seizure activity
B. Change in level of consciousness
C. Change in vital signs
D. Change in respiratory pattern

CORRECT ANSWER—**B.** One of the first signs of increasing intracranial pressure is a change in level of consciousness. Coma is an ominous sign in patients with encephalitis and usually results from temporal lobe herniation. Later changes include altered respiratory pattern and vital signs; these changes occur after the level of consciousness has decreased. Seizures may occur in the later stages of encephalitis or meningitis.
Nursing process step: Assessment
Cognitive level: Evaluation

55. Infection of the brain by human immunodeficiency virus causes human immunodeficiency virus (HIV) encephalopathy, which is characterized by:
A. Progressive cognitive, behavioral, and motor deficits
B. Cerebral edema as shown on a computed tomography (CT) scan
C. Hemiparesis and progressive decrease in level of consciousness
D. Confusion, disorientation, and violent outbursts

CORRECT ANSWER—**A.** HIV encephalopathy progresses over several months. In advanced stages, it can cause mutism, incontinence, ataxia, and tremors. A CT scan would reveal cortical atrophy. Focal neurologic deficits are rare. Cognitive changes are more likely to occur than violent outbursts.
Nursing process step: Assessment
Cognitive level: Evaluation

56. What is the drug of choice for treating acquired human immunodeficiency virus (HIV) encephalopathy?
A. Corticosteroids
B. Acyclovir
C. Zidovudine
D. No drug is effective

CORRECT ANSWER—**C.** Zidovudine can slow the development of HIV encephalopathy. Steroids are of little benefit unless the patient has a tumor and cytotoxic edema. Acyclovir is used for other viral infections, such as herpes.
Nursing process step: Implementation
Cognitive level: Comprehension

57. A 53-year-old female carrying a load of laundry falls while descending stairs. She does not lose consciousness but complains of severe headache. No neurologic deficits are apparent. A computed tomography (CT) scan is negative for hematoma or skull fracture. Based on these findings, what is the probable cause of the patient's headache?
  A. Cerebral concussion
  B. Cerebral contusion
  C. Acute cervical strain
  D. Sinusitis

CORRECT ANSWER—A. A concussion is a microscopic injury to brain tissue that results in temporary neurologic dysfunction. Loss of consciousness does not necessarily occur; if it does, it usually resolves within a few minutes. Transient symptoms of concussion include headache, changes in respiratory pattern and vital signs, loss of reflexes, vision disturbances, dizziness, giddiness, confusion, gait changes, drowsiness, irritability, and nausea. If present, these symptoms typically resolve within 48 hours. A cerebral contusion would be seen on the CT scan. Although the patient will have neck pain and general musculoskeletal pain, the headache is due to the concussion. Sinusitis is a possible concurrent problem but would be unrelated to the fall.
Nursing process step: Implementation
Cognitive level: Synthesis

58. A patient with a cerebral aneurysm is at risk for tonic-clonic seizures. Immediate nursing interventions for this possible complication would include:
  A. Restraints to prevent excess movement
  B. Positioning the patient to prevent aspiration
  C. Emergency tracheostomy and hyperventilation
  D. Administration of mannitol and furosemide to decrease swelling

CORRECT ANSWER—B. Aspiration is a serious complication of seizure activity. A patient experiencing seizures should not be restrained. Mannitol and furosemide can help prevent seizures by reducing edema, but administration of these drugs would not be an initial intervention. Intubation may be helpful, but emergency tracheostomy often is not required.
Nursing process step: Planning
Cognitive level: Application

Questions 59 to 61 refer to the following information:
A 17-year-old male patient suffered a C5 to C6 spinal cord injury from a diving accident. He is admitted to the surgical intensive care unit with Gardner-Wells tongs in place. He has no paralysis initially, but has weakness and loss of sensory function in his arms and hands. Ten pounds of traction are added to the traction attached to the tongs.

---

59. The patient complains of pain. The nurse's best response would be to:
A. Reposition the patient and prepare him for intubation
B. Notify the neurosurgeon of the patient's pain
C. Administer analgesics or muscle relaxants as ordered
D. Reduce the traction to 5 lb

CORRECT ANSWER—C. Analgesics or muscle relaxants commonly are administered as traction is increased; respiratory function also should be monitored closely. Pain is not an indication for intubation. Because of the patient's injury, a tracheostomy, if necessary, would be more likely to be performed than intubation. Increased pain is a common response of muscles in severe spasm as the traction pulls against them. Reducing the traction would delay recovery and might not relieve the pain. The neurosurgeon should be notified only if medications are ineffective.
Nursing process step: Implementation
Cognitive level: Application

60. Because of the potential for complications related to immobility, the nurse would perform which of the following interventions?
A. Logroll the patient every 2 hours
B. Keep the patient flat while traction is in place
C. Place the patient in Trendelenburg's position to increase traction
D. Tilt the patient side to side every 2 hours

CORRECT ANSWER—D. Tilting the patient side to side every 2 hours, while maintaining alignment and keeping the sequential compression device on both legs at all times, can help prevent atelectasis and venous stasis. Incentive spirometry also is an important intervention because complete logrolling would not decrease the risk of atelectasis. Trendelenburg's position does not increase traction and may decrease it.
Nursing process step: Implementation
Cognitive level: Application

61. The patient complains of increased numbness in his legs, and he can no longer move his arms. His blood pressure is normal and his heart rate is 110 beats/minute and regular. His vital capacity has decreased to 750 ml. What might this clinical picture indicate?
A. Spinal cord swelling
B. Autonomic dysreflexia
C. Impending spinal shock
D. Inadequate traction on the Gardner-Wells tongs

CORRECT ANSWER—A. Although traction may need to be increased, spinal cord swelling probably is the primary problem, as evidenced by the patient's symptoms. Autonomic dysreflexia causes hypertension, whereas spinal shock would decrease the blood pressure.
Nursing process step: Assessment
Cognitive level: Synthesis

Questions 62 and 63 refer to the following information:
A 76-year-old female patient who underwent left carotid endarterectomy 2 hours ago awakens with ptosis of the right eyelid. Her right hand grip is weaker than the left, with sensory loss as well.

62. The patient's signs and symptoms are consistent with occlusion of the:
   A. Anterior cerebral artery
   B. Internal carotid artery
   C. Basilar artery
   D. Middle cerebral artery

CORRECT ANSWER—**D.** The signs and symptoms are consistent with occlusion of the middle cerebral artery. The left middle cerebral artery is most likely to be affected because this relatively straight vessel provides the path of least resistance for the embolus. Occlusion of the anterior cerebral artery causes similar symptoms, but mental impairment and deficits of the leg and foot would be more severe. Occlusion of the internal carotid artery also results in similar symptoms but with additional aphasia, apraxia, and agnosia. Basilar artery occlusion results in quadriplegia, dysfunction of cranial nerves III to XII, cerebellar dysfunction, and loss of proprioception.
Nursing process step: Assessment
Cognitive level: Evaluation

63. This patient might benefit from treatment with:
   A. Tissue plasminogen activator (alteplase)
   B. Anticoagulants
   C. Nimodipine (to reduce vasospasm)
   D. Dextran

CORRECT ANSWER—**B.** Regardless of whether the embolus consists of air, plaque, or a clot, anticoagulants will prevent the obstruction from expanding. Because the type of embolus is unknown, tissue plasminogen activator would not be used because it could cause bleeding while dissolving the clot. Vasospasm is unlikely because the patient has not suffered a subarachnoid hemorrhage. Dextran is not used if the source of the embolus is unknown.
Nursing process step: Planning
Cognitive level: Comprehension

64. Which of the following symptoms are associated with subarachnoid hemorrhage?
A. Decreased level of consciousness, narrowed pulse pressure, and tachycardia
B. Agitation, headache, and confusion
C. Narrowed pulse pressure, photophobia, and hypotension
D. Positive Kernig's and Brudzinski's signs, photophobia, and seizures

CORRECT ANSWER—D. Subarachnoid hemorrhage often causes signs of meningeal irritation because of blood in the cerebrospinal fluid. A positive Kernig's sign, which is diagnostic of meningitis or meningeal irritation, is characterized by lower back pain and resistance when, after flexing the leg at the hip and the knee, the leg is extended while the thigh is flexed on the abdomen. A positive Brudzinski's sign is an involuntary flexion of the hip and knee when the neck is passively flexed; this also is seen in patients with meningitis or meningeal irritation. Other symptoms associated with subarachnoid hemorrhage include photophobia, seizures, altered level of consciousness, hypertension, and bradycardia. If the pulse pressure changes, it would become wider rather than narrower. Although the patient's level of consciousness may change, the patient with a subarachnoid hemorrhage is more likely to be obtunded than agitated.
Nursing process step: Assessment
Cognitive level: Knowledge

65. The air reference stopcock of a transducer attached to a ventricular catheter should be placed:
A. On the midaxillary line, fifth intercostal space, at the level of the right atrium
B. At the level of the third ventricle, halfway between the tragus of the ear and the corner of the eye
C. In alignment with the base of the skull
D. Just below the angle of the jaw at the bifurcation of the carotid artery

CORRECT ANSWER—B. The air reference stopcock of a transducer is placed at the level of the third ventricle (foramen of Monro) for appropriate calibration and pressure measurement, as well as for directly measuring and draining cerebrospinal fluid. A central venous pressure line or pulmonary artery catheter is placed at the level of the right atrium. The air reference stopcock would not be placed in alignment with the base of the skull or the jaw.
Nursing process step: Implementation
Cognitive level: Application

66. After removal of a large grade III astrocytoma from the cerebellum, a patient should be positioned:
A. With the head of the bed elevated 30 degrees
B. On the opposite side, with the head of the bed elevated 30 degrees
C. With the head of bed flat initially, with gradual elevation over the next few days
D. With the head of the bed elevated 45 degrees

CORRECT ANSWER—C. After removal of a large infratentorial lesion, the patient should remain supine initially to reduce pressure from the brain above the tentorium. As fluid gradually fills the space, the head of the bed is gradually elevated, as tolerated by the patient. A 45-degree angle is not allowed for several days.
Nursing process step: Implementation
Cognitive level: Application

67. Which of the following is one of the earliest, most important indications of deteriorating neurologic function?
  A. Projectile vomiting
  B. Change in level of consciousness
  C. Hypertension and widening pulse pressure
  D. Bradycardia and hyperthermia

CORRECT ANSWER—**B.** A change in the level of consciousness is one of the earliest, most important signs of altered neurologic function. A change in level of consciousness will occur before changes in vital signs or temperature, which are associated with brain stem dysfunction. Projectile vomiting may be seen in meningeal irritation, but it is not always associated with deteriorating neurologic function.
Nursing process step: Assessment
Cognitive level: Knowledge

68. Nursing care for a patient suffering an embolic event must include which intervention?
  A. Maintaining oxygenation and protecting injured and ischemic cells
  B. Reducing blood pressure to prevent breakthrough bleeding
  C. Promoting early rehabilitation and adaptation to permanent disability
  D. Monitoring for complications of steroid therapy

CORRECT ANSWER—**A.** The goal of care for a patient with a brain injury is to protect injured and ischemic cells and to give the patient every chance to recover as much function as possible. Not all patients require a reduction in blood pressure. Early rehabilitation is important, but not all deficits are permanent and many patients regain some lost function as the ischemia resolves and other cells acquire new functions. Steroids are not commonly used for embolic injury.
Nursing process step: Planning
Cognitive level: Application

Questions 69 to 71 refer to the following information:
A 45-year-old male postal worker suffers a severe headache and collapses. In the emergency department, the patient is obtunded and has flaccid paralysis of the right arm and weakness in the right leg. His pupils are unequal, with deviation of the eyes to the left. A computed tomography scan shows a large hematoma of the left frontal lobe that extends into the subdural space. His blood pressure is 220/160 mm Hg on admission. His family reports that the patient has not been taking his blood pressure medication because he felt good and did not think he needed it.

69. What is the first priority in caring for this patient?

   A. Controlling malignant hypertension and maintaining a patent airway

   B. Controlling seizure activity

   C. Preparing him for immediate craniotomy to remove the hematoma

   D. Keeping the patient quiet and sedated

CORRECT ANSWER—A. Severe hypertension will lead to herniation of brain tissue caused by expansion of the hematoma, with devastating effects on vital functions. A patent airway is essential for preserving oxygen to compromised cells and removing carbon dioxide to prevent increased intracranial pressure. If the blood pressure is not controlled preoperatively, intracranial pressure will increase significantly and viable tissue may be lost. A craniotomy would be considered if the hematoma was large enough to cause a mass effect. The patient should remain quiet and may require sedation if agitated. However, because this patient is obtunded, sedation could interfere with assessment of the level of consciousness. Seizures may occur secondary to hypertension and brain tissue herniation; controlling blood pressure and the airway often prevents seizures in a patient experiencing a hypertensive crisis.

Nursing process step: Implementation

Cognitive level: Application

70. After surgery, the patient awakes from anesthesia visibly agitated, fighting his restraints and tossing his head wildly. Two people are needed to further restrain him. He moves all extremities, and his pupils are equal and reactive to light. His systolic blood pressure rose to 260 mm Hg while he was receiving nitroprusside I.V. at a rate of 5 mcg/kg/minute. What should the nurse do first?

   A. Sedate the patient with I.V. diazepam and increase the I.V. nitroprusside drip rate

   B. Explain to the patient what has happened and increase the I.V. nitroprusside drip rate

   C. Hyperventilate the patient to achieve a $PaCO_2$ of 20 mm Hg to reduce intracranial pressure

   D. Administer a barbiturate to induce coma

CORRECT ANSWER—A. The patient should be immediately sedated with diazepam and the nitroprusside I.V. infusion titrated to control the blood pressure. Before another pharmacologic agent is administered, nitroprusside can be titrated up to 10 mcg/kg/minute without toxic effects. This incoherent patient would be unable to understand any explanations given by the nurse. A $PaCO_2$ of 20 mm Hg is too low and could cause excessive vasoconstriction. A barbiturate-induced coma is not indicated.

Nursing process step: Implementation

Cognitive level: Application

71. The patient continues to be combative and hypertensive each time the diazepam level drops. The surgeon orders pancuronium to control the blood pressure and prevent the increased intracranial pressure caused by the patient's fighting the restraints. While the patient is receiving pancuronium, the nurse must remember to:
A. Assess airway and pulmonary status frequently
B. Explain all movements and procedures to the patient and continue the sedation
C. Evaluate renal and hepatic function
D. Monitor central venous pressure

CORRECT ANSWER—B. Because pancuronium is a peripherally acting neuromuscular blocker, it has no effect on the central nervous system and does not influence mental function. Although the patient may be frightened, angry, or panicked, there is no way of knowing because of the paralysis. A patient needs frequent explanations and reassurance when receiving neuromuscular blockers. A patient receiving pancuronium would be intubated and mechanically ventilated, so his airway would already be protected. Increased renal or hepatic activity is not an expected effect of pancuronium. Pulmonary status and central venous pressure should continue to be monitored regardless of whether pancuronium is administered.
Nursing process step: Implementation
Cognitive level: Comprehension

72. A patient with central cord syndrome would experience a loss of:
A. Motor function in the lower extremities
B. Pain sensation in the lower extremities
C. Motor function in the upper extremities
D. Pain sensation in the upper extremities

CORRECT ANSWER—C. Central cord syndrome is an incomplete spinal cord injury involving the central gray matter of the cord. Motor function of the lower extremities is preserved, while motor function of the upper extremities is impaired. Pain sensation is not affected.
Nursing process step: Assessment
Cognitive level: Comprehension

73. A male patient is admitted with a T3 to T4 spinal cord injury. Two hours later, he complains of shortness of breath and chest pain; he has concomitant cyanosis, pallor, and supraventricular tachycardia with 155 beats/minute. What is a possible explanation for the ineffective breathing pattern?
A. Respiratory depression resulting from high spinal cord injury
B. Pneumothorax or fractured ribs
C. Splinting of respirations caused by muscle spasm
D. Anxiety and hyperventilation

CORRECT ANSWER—B. Spinal cord injuries are associated with a high incidence of thoracic injuries. The pain and cyanosis point to a pulmonary problem. Splinting seldom causes cyanosis unless it continues to the point of causing atelectasis. Although respiratory depression is a possibility with such a high spinal cord injury, it would not cause acute chest pain and dyspnea. Anxiety, pain, and hypoxia are the probable causes of the tachycardia.
Nursing process step: Assessment
Cognitive level: Evaluation

74. A 74-year-old male slipped on icy steps and fell 2 weeks ago. He still has a large ecchymotic area on his right flank, where he sustained a retroperitoneal hemorrhage that is slowly resolving without surgery. This morning, he awoke confused and disoriented and had left-sided weakness. What is the probable cause of this deficit?

A. Cerebrovascular accident (CVA)

B. Cerebral embolism from the resolving hematoma

C. Chronic subdural hematoma

D. Epidural hematoma

CORRECT ANSWER—C. This clinical picture is commonly seen with chronic subdural hematoma, especially in an elderly patient. A computed tomography scan is essential for ruling out each of the three causes of CVA: thrombus, embolus, and intracerebral hemorrhage. An epidural hematoma would cause symptoms associated with increased intracranial pressure within hours. Hematoma resolution does not cause cerebral embolism.

Nursing process step: Evaluation

Cognitive level: Analysis

75. A patient with subarachnoid hemorrhage caused by an aneurysm develops obstructive (non-communicating) hydrocephalus from the red blood cells' occlusion of cerebrospinal fluid (CSF) circulation and decreased CSF reabsorption. In this patient, what would be the earliest sign of increased intracranial pressure?

A. Decreased level of consciousness

B. Dilated pupils that react sluggishly to light

C. Distended neck veins

D. Increased seizure activity

CORRECT ANSWER—A. Although seizures and pupil dilation can result from increased intracranial pressure, these signs usually occur after changes in the level of consciousness have occurred. Distended neck veins are unrelated to increased intracranial pressure.

Nursing process step: Planning

Cognitive level: Comprehension

76. A patient with an L4 to L5 spinal cord injury becomes anxious and complains of chest pain and pain in the back between the scapulae. The patient has been receiving dexamethasone. After notifying the physician, what should the nurse do next?

A. Expect an order for a nasogastric tube to evaluate gastric pH and to rule out GI bleeding

B. Prepare the patient for arteriography to rule out dissecting aortic aneurysm

C. Administer pain medication because the pain is caused by the vertebral injury

D. Prepare the patient for arterial blood gas analysis and ventilation-perfusion lung scan to rule out pulmonary embolus

CORRECT ANSWER—D. In some patients, a pulmonary embolus causes vague, nonspecific symptoms. In other patients, it may trigger the sudden onset of dyspnea, tachypnea, restlessness, anxiety, pleuritic pain, and tachycardia. The pain is too high to be related to the original injury. Although an ulcer can result from steroid therapy, the pain is more likely to be epigastric. An aneurysm is a rare possibility; a pulmonary embolus is more likely because of the patient's immobility and poor venous tone, which is secondary to level of injury.

Nursing process step: Implementation

Cognitive level: Analysis

Questions 77 and 78 refer to the following information:
A 20-year-old male patient arrives in the emergency department after the three-wheeled all-terrain vehicle he was riding flipped after hitting a log buried in the mud. The patient was thrown against a tree and has a contusion over the right temporal area. His friends say he was unconscious for 10 to 15 minutes before the ambulance arrived.

77. The nurse would institute measures to prevent which potential problem in this patient?
A. Epidural hematoma
B. Concussion and frontal bone fracture
C. Rhinorrhea and potential encephalitis
D. Bilateral cerebral contusions

CORRECT ANSWER—A. Given the site of injury and the brief period of unconsciousness, the nurse should monitor closely for signs of deterioration caused by epidural hematoma. The patient is less likely to have suffered concussion, rhinorrhea, or bilateral cerebral contusions because the blow to the head did not involve the frontal bone.
Nursing process step: Implementation
Cognitive level: Analysis

78. The patient is alert and moving all extremities on admission. Thirty minutes later, he is obtunded. A computed tomography scan shows a right temporal epidural hematoma. The nurse should prepare the patient for:
A. Intubation and hyperventilation with a mechanical ventilator for the next 4 hours
B. Insertion of a ventricular catheter to decrease intracranial pressure
C. Possible paralysis and loss of receptive speech
D. Emergency craniotomy to evacuate the hematoma

CORRECT ANSWER—D. The patient exhibits the classic signs of epidural hematoma. Because an epidural hematoma is an arterial hemorrhage, immediate surgery is necessary to prevent uncal herniation and death from compression of the vital centers in the brain stem. Intubation and hyperventilation can slow herniation, but the patient cannot wait 4 hours for surgery. A ventricular catheter would not help, although it might be inserted for postoperative monitoring on rare occasions. Paralysis involves the frontal lobe, not the temporal lobe.
Nursing process step: Planning
Cognitive level: Synthesis

79. A 43-year-old female is involved in a motor vehicle accident after suffering a seizure while driving to the hospital to seek treatment for the persistent nausea and vomiting she had been experiencing over the past several days. The patient is admitted to the intensive care unit complaining of pain, stiff neck, and frontal headache. A computed tomography scan and X-ray films show a mass in the vicinity of the fourth ventricle but no spinal cord injury. In addition to monitoring vital signs and performing frequent neurologic assessments (including monitoring level of consciousness), the nurse should assess for:
A. Aspiration resulting from impaired gag and swallowing reflexes
B. Secondary meningitis
C. Metastasis to the spinal cord and hemiparesis
D. Loss of vision from compression of the optic nerve

CORRECT ANSWER—A. Maintaining a patent airway may be difficult given the proximity of the mass to the brain stem. Although metastasis and meningitis are unlikely, they must be ruled out if the mass is an abscess. The optic tracts connected to the brain stem control eye movements and head turning. Brain tumors in this region are more frequently associated with blurred vision than blindness.
Nursing process step: Assessment
Cognitive level: Analysis

80. According to the Monroe-Kellie doctrine, a brain tumor that increases in size will decrease the space available for blood, brain tissue, and cerebrospinal fluid (CSF) and eventually lead to increased intracranial pressure. Which intervention is appropriate for decreasing intracranial pressure before surgery?
A. Keeping the patient in a supine position in bed
B. Administering dexamethasone, mannitol, and furosemide
C. Administering vasopressin to constrict cerebral arteries
D. Intubating and mechanically ventilating the patient to maintain $PaCO_2$ above 35 mm Hg

CORRECT ANSWER—B. Dexamethasone, mannitol, and furosemide would effectively reduce vasogenic edema around the mass and decrease CSF production. Keeping the patient in a supine position would increase intracranial pressure, whereas elevating the head of the bed would decrease it. Vasopressin would be ineffective because the increased intracranial pressure results from a lesion, not bleeding. Decreasing $PaCO_2$ to between 25 and 30 mm Hg can rapidly lower intracranial pressure. A $PaCO_2$ level above 35 mm Hg would not decrease intracranial pressure because hypocapnia is necessary for cerebrovascular constriction.
Nursing process step: Implementation
Cognitive level: Analysis

Questions 81 to 83 refer to the following information:
A 24-year-old male patient contracted hepatitis B after receiving coagulation factors for hemophilia. He has been ill for 3 days and is admitted to the intensive care unit with bleeding esophageal varices. The patient is jaundiced, and his liver is enlarged and hard. Currently, he is hypotensive and lethargic and has tremors in his arms and legs. His pupils are equal and reactive at 4 mm.

---

81. The patient's lethargy most likely is due to:
A. Hepatic encephalopathy resulting from ammonia intoxication
B. Inadequate cerebral blood flow secondary to hypotension
C. Dehydration and malnutrition
D. Possible cerebrovascular accident resulting from coagulopathy

CORRECT ANSWER—A. As blood is digested in the colon, ammonia is released and absorbed into the portal circulation. The patient's damaged liver cannot detoxify the blood, and the ammonia produces encephalopathy. Hypotension can result from hypovolemic shock caused by GI bleeding, but encephalopathy typically is related to ammonia levels. Cerebrovascular accident, dehydration, and malnutrition are less likely causes of the patient's lethargy.
Nursing process step: Assessment
Cognitive level: Evaluation

82. The patient may undergo bowel evacuation and sterilization to:
A. Reduce intestinal toxins and distended varices
B. Reduce abdominal distention
C. Reduce ammonia levels created by the breakdown of blood by bacteria
D. Increase vitamin K production

CORRECT ANSWER—C. Bowel evacuation increases peristalsis, allowing less time for absorption of ammonia created by the bacterial breakdown of blood. By sterilizing the intestines with antibiotics, less ammonia is created. The liver is not producing a normal amount of vitamin K because of cirrhosis, not because of blood in the bowel. Bowel evacuation and sterilization would not decrease abdominal distention caused by presence of ascitic fluid. Evacuation of the colon may reduce intestinal toxins, but has little effect on venous pressure.
Nursing process step: Implementation
Cognitive level: Comprehension

83. The patient is at highest risk for:
A. Inadequate cardiac output resulting from further bleeding
B. Ineffective breathing caused by respiratory acidosis
C. Further deterioration in neurologic function and possible seizures
D. Ineffective airway maintenance and possible aspiration

CORRECT ANSWER—D. Although inadequate cardiac output and hypovolemic shock are concerns, the patient is at greatest risk for aspiration. Consequently, maintaining and protecting the airway is the immediate priority. The encephalopathy and decreased level of consciousness predispose the patient to inadequate airway clearance and ineffective airway maintenance. This lethargic patient may have decreased respirations, leading to hypoventilation and subsequent respiratory acidosis. The ineffective breathing is not caused by the acidosis; rather, the acidosis results from the ineffective breathing. The patient is not at increased risk for seizures.
Nursing process step: Assessment
Cognitive level: Comprehension

84. A 72-year-old female is found unresponsive by family members at her house around 7 p.m. Her right pupil is sluggishly reactive to light. She withdraws to pain more on the right side of her body than the left side. Her admitting blood pressure is 220/140 mm Hg. A computed tomography scan is negative for cerebral hemorrhage. Which immediate measures should the nurse plan for this patient?

A. Protecting the airway and decreasing systolic blood pressure to 150 mm Hg

B. Elevating the head of the bed, implementing seizure precautions, and monitoring blood pressure for further increases

C. Helping the patient's family realize that her condition probably is terminal

D. Protecting the airway and monitoring blood pressure for further increases

CORRECT ANSWER—A. Protecting the airway is essential in a patient with a decreased level of consciousness. Reducing the blood pressure also is crucial to prevent hypertensive encephalopathy and seizures. Because the patient's blood pressure is not expected to increase, the nurse shouldn't monitor for increased blood pressure. The patient's condition is not necessarily terminal.
Nursing process step: Planning
Cognitive level: Analysis

85. What is the primary nursing diagnosis for a patient with seizures?

A. Ineffective breathing pattern

B. Ineffective airway clearance

C. Decreased cardiac output secondary to cardiac ischemia

D. Risk for injury

CORRECT ANSWER—D. Seizures can cause injury, especially if the patient falls or bites the tongue. Prolonged seizures can cause cerebral ischemia and may prevent the patient from maintaining a patent airway, thereby increasing the risk of aspiration. Not all patients experience respiratory problems or cardiac ischemia.
Nursing process step: Planning
Cognitive level: Application

Questions 86 to 89 refer to the following information:
A 24-year-old female patient with a history of seizures since infancy sometimes has tonic-clonic seizures just before her menstrual period. She is admitted to the neurologic intensive care unit after an episode of three seizures 30 minutes apart. She has not awakened between seizures, and aspiration pneumonia is a possibility. A continuous electroencephalogram shows continuous subclinical seizure activity. Despite phenytoin and benzodiazepine therapy, the seizures continue. The decision is made to place the patient in a barbiturate-induced coma.

---

86. While in a barbiturate-induced coma, the patient will require:
  A. Total systems support (complete life support)
  B. Continuous positive airway pressure
  C. Total parenteral nutrition
  D. Minimal oxygen concentration to prevent toxicity

CORRECT ANSWER—A. While in a coma, the patient is susceptible to injury in many ways. Because all systems may be compromised, the patient will require respiratory support, nutritional support, and, possibly, circulatory support. The oxygen concentration must be sufficient to maintain a PaO_2 level of 80 to 100 mm Hg, with the goal of providing the minimal oxygen concentration necessary to achieve this PaO_2 level. Continuous positive airway pressure requires spontaneous breathing, and a patient in a barbiturate-induced coma typically has a reduced or suppressed respiratory drive.
Nursing process step: Implementation
Cognitive level: Application

87. Barbiturates can cause:
  A. Acute renal failure
  B. Acute pancreatitis
  C. Liver failure
  D. Cardiac depression

CORRECT ANSWER—D. Cardiac depression (decreased cardiac contractility) and hypotension are common adverse effects of barbiturates. Acute renal failure typically is related to myoglobin released from stressed muscles. Pancreatitis is not associated with barbiturate use. Liver enzyme levels may be increased by anticonvulsants, but not usually to the point of liver failure.
Nursing process step: Evaluation
Cognitive level: Comprehension

88. What is the most common acid-base disturbance in a patient with a seizure disorder?
  A. Respiratory alkalosis
  B. Metabolic alkalosis
  C. Respiratory acidosis
  D. Metabolic acidosis

CORRECT ANSWER—D. The continuous muscle spasm of seizure activity causes anaerobic metabolism, which results in metabolic acidosis. Respiratory alkalosis and metabolic alkalosis are uncommon. Respiratory acidosis usually is not seen unless the patient aspirates.
Nursing process step: Assessment
Cognitive level: Evaluation

89. Continuous seizure activity, as with status epilepticus, can cause:
  A. Hyperthermia
  B. Hypothermia
  C. Hyperglycemia
  D. Hypocapnia

CORRECT ANSWER—A. The increased metabolic rate caused by the continuous muscle contraction that occurs in status epilepticus can lead to hyperthermia. Hypothermia does not occur. Not only can seizures be triggered by hypoglycemia, but they also can cause hypoglycemia through increased glucose consumption. Hypocapnia can cause seizures, but seizures do not cause hypocapnia.
Nursing process step: Evaluation
Cognitive level: Comprehension

90. After an aneurysm repair, a patient experiences apraxia, which means he:
A. Cannot use a common object correctly
B. Cannot express thoughts in writing
C. Cannot recognize a body part
D. Has increased cutaneous sensitivity to touch and temperature

CORRECT ANSWER—A. Apraxia is an impaired ability to perform purposeful acts or manipulate objects. Sensory (ideational) apraxia is an impaired ability to perceive how an object is used. Motor apraxia is an impaired ability to use an object or perform a task, although the patient recognizes how the object should be used. Amnestic apraxia is an impaired ability to perform a task because the patient cannot remember how to do it. Agraphia is an inability to express thoughts in writing. Atopognosia is an inability to recognize a body part. Hyperesthesia is an increased cutaneous sensitivity to touch, temperature, and pain.
Nursing process step: Assessment
Cognitive level: Knowledge

91. What is the most common location for spinal cord tumors?
A. Cervical area
B. Thoracic area
C. Lumbar area
D. Cauda equina

CORRECT ANSWER—B. Spinal cord tumors most commonly are located in the thoracic spine. Approximately 50% of all spinal cord tumors occur in this area.
Nursing process step: Assessment
Cognitive level: Knowledge

92. A patient undergoes laser surgery for an acoustic neuroma involving cranial nerve VII. The postoperative interventions for this patient must include assessment of:
A. Ocular movement
B. Oculocephalic (doll's eyes) reflex
C. Facial nerve weakness
D. Swallowing and hoarseness

CORRECT ANSWER—C. Facial nerve weakness is the most likely deficit resulting from edema or damage to cranial nerve VII. The other options would be appropriate when assessing cranial nerves I, II, III, and IX.
Nursing process step: Assessment
Cognitive level: Analysis

Questions 93 and 94 refer to the following information:
A 74-year-old female patient has been taking furosemide for hypertension and heart failure. She also takes digoxin 0.125 mg P.O. daily. On Friday evening, she calls 911 and asks for help. While talking on the phone, she has a tonic-clonic seizure and becomes unconscious. When the paramedics arrive, she is responsive to pain and mumbling incoherently. En route to the emergency department, she has another tonic-clonic seizure and aspirates. She is intubated, placed on a mechanical ventilator, and admitted to the intensive care unit, where she responds to deep pain by withdrawing.

Her neurologic assessment reveals dilated pupils sluggishly reactive to light and an inability to follow commands. The patient continues to respond to pain by withdrawing all extremities with +3 strength. A computed tomography scan shows no specific lesions or deviations; an arteriogram shows

100% occlusion of the left internal carotid artery and 90% occlusion of the right internal carotid artery. There is questionable spasm of the vertebrobasilar artery because of hypoxia.

The patient's electrolyte report includes sodium, 124 mEq/liter; potassium, 2.5 mEq/liter; and chloride, 100 mEq/liter. Her arterial blood gas values on 100% oxygen are pH, 7.48; $PaCO_2$, 34 mm Hg; HCO_3^-, 28 mEq/liter; and PaO_2, 48 mm Hg. Her blood CO_2 level is 20 mEq/liter.

---

93. The seizure activity and coma most likely are due to:
A. Hyponatremia and excess intracellular fluid
B. Hypokalemia and alkalosis
C. Hypoxia and acidosis
D. Hypokalemia and hypoxia

CORRECT ANSWER—A. The severe hyponatremia contributes to cerebral edema and increased intracranial pressure. Encephalopathy developed secondary to hypoxia caused by both aspiration pneumonitis and ischemia resulting from vascular narrowing or constriction. The alkalosis may contribute to hypoxia by constricting blood vessels and worsening the ischemia, which can lead to seizures. This patient has metabolic alkalosis, not acidosis. Hypokalemia does not directly contribute to encephalopathy, although it reduces cardiac output and may decrease oxygen flow to the brain.
Nursing process step: Assessment
Cognitive level: Comprehension

94. What is the first nursing priority in managing this patient's care?
A. Controlling intracranial pressure and improving oxygenation of brain tissue
B. Implementing measures to dilate the carotid arteries and performing frequent neurologic assessments
C. Replacing sodium and potassium and performing frequent neurologic assessments
D. Further reducing $PaCO_2$ to 30 mm Hg to decrease intracranial pressure (ICP)

CORRECT ANSWER—A. Oxygenation is essential to protect injured or ischemic brain cells in a patient with severe hypoxia and constriction of the carotid arteries. Providing optimum ventilation and pulmonary toilet can help improve brain tissue oxygenation. However, the nurse must avoid further increasing ICP with treatment that is too vigorous. The increased ICP must be treated and controlled to prevent herniation. Elevating the head of the bed 30 degrees and ensuring proper neck position can decrease ICP. Although replacing electrolytes and monitoring neurologic function are essential, the first priority is to increase oxygenation and maintain respiratory support. The cerebral vessels are already constricted because of vascular narrowing and alkalosis; further vasoconstriction by decreasing $PaCO_2$ would not be beneficial. Surgery and anticoagulant therapy to dilate the stenosed cerebral arteries may be necessary, but these interventions are not immediate priorities.
Nursing process step: Implementation
Cognitive level: Application

95. After suffering a subarachnoid hemorrhage resulting from an arteriovenous malformation, a patient should be monitored closely for vasospasm. Early symptoms of vasospasm include:
A. Meningeal irritation
B. Hemiplegia or hemiparesis
C. Asystole
D. Respiratory arrest

CORRECT ANSWER—B. Vasospasm compromises blood flow to one area of the brain, resulting in hemiplegia, pupillary changes, or change in level of consciousness. Meningeal irritation commonly is caused by blood in the cerebrospinal fluid, not vasospasm. Asystole and respiratory arrest are not directly related to vasospasm, but may occur with recurrent major hemorrhage.
Nursing process step: Assessment
Cognitive level: Evaluation

96. A male patient is admitted with a diagnosis of syndrome of inappropriate antidiuretic hormone (SIADH). He is confused, disoriented, and combative. His pupils are equal and reactive to light at 4 mm. He moves all extremities with +5 strength. His family reports that he has become progressively more confused over the last 4 days and has not eaten. He gained 5 lb, however, over the last 4 days. An indwelling urinary (Foley) catheter is inserted and drains only 100 ml of concentrated, dark amber urine with a normal urine sodium level. The laboratory report shows serum sodium, 120 mEq/liter; serum potassium, 5.5 mEq/liter; blood urea nitrogen (BUN), 25 mg/dl; and serum creatinine, 1.8 mg/dl. What is the goal of care for this patient?
A. Monitoring for lateralizing signs or mass effect
B. Increasing fluid intake to reduce uremic encephalopathy by decreasing BUN and creatinine levels
C. Restricting fluid intake to reduce the encephalopathy caused by intracellular fluid excess by allowing sodium level to increase
D. Initiating seizure precautions and administering nimodipine to reduce the vasospasm causing the encephalopathy

CORRECT ANSWER—C. The low sodium level is caused by dilutional hyponatremia and water retention. Hyponatremia reflects dilution from water retention, not sodium loss. The water retention results from the inappropriate release of antidiuretic hormone. Confusion and disorientation result from subsequent hypo-osmolality caused by intracellular fluid excess. Restricting fluids and treating the cause of SIADH are the goals of treatment. Correct management of this patient would include fluid restriction with 3.0% sodium chloride solution for severe hyponatremia; lithium also might be helpful in blocking the renal response to antidiuretic hormone. A focal lesion is unlikely because the patient's pupils are normal, and his clinical picture fits the abnormal electrolyte findings common to SIADH. Seizure precautions are warranted because of the electrolyte imbalance, but there is no reason to suspect vasospasm as the cause of the problem.
Nursing process step: Planning
Cognitive level: Application

97. Altered thermoregulation in a patient with a spinal cord injury results from:
  A. Vasodilation and inability to shiver secondary to spinal shock
  B. Direct brain stem injury associated with cervical spine injuries
  C. Abnormal autonomic reflexes
  D. Reflex vasoconstriction

CORRECT ANSWER—**A.** Sympathetic nervous system responses are blocked when the spinal cord is injured; therefore, the patient's blood vessels cannot constrict to reduce heat loss or dilate to reduce temperature. The patient also cannot shiver below the level of the injury; this produces excess heat loss and hypothermia. Although head injuries often accompany cervical spine injuries, they do not routinely damage the thermoregulatory centers in the medulla. Abnormal autonomic reflexes may be present secondary to spinal shock, not altered thermoregulation.
Nursing process step: Planning
Cognitive level: Analysis

98. Toxic levels of anticonvulsants can cause:
  A. Nystagmus or excess sedation
  B. Nausea and vomiting
  C. Status epilepticus
  D. Acute renal failure

CORRECT ANSWER—**A.** Anticonvulsants, especially phenytoin and phenobarbital, can cause excess sedation, which is particularly severe when toxic levels are reached. Nystagmus is common when anticonvulsant blood levels rise. Nausea and vomiting are possible adverse reactions but not signs of toxicity. Status epilepticus also is not a sign of toxicity. Anticonvulsants are more hepatotoxic than nephrotoxic.
Nursing process step: Evaluation
Cognitive level: Comprehension

99. During status epilepticus, a patient may be intubated and:
  A. Hyperventilated to achieve a $PaCO_2$ of 25 to 30 mm Hg
  B. Sedated with pentobarbital, phenobarbital, or thiopental
  C. Paralyzed with atracurium or pancuronium
  D. Sedated with morphine or meperidine

CORRECT ANSWER—**B.** Sedating a patient with barbiturates reduces seizure activity. Hyperventilation can lower the seizure threshold in susceptible patients. However, even though hyperventilation reduces intracranial pressure, it could potentiate the seizures. Paralysis with peripherally acting muscle relaxants stops muscle movement but not neuronal firing. Morphine and meperidine are less effective than benzodiazepines and barbiturates in reducing seizure activity.
Nursing process step: Implementation
Cognitive level: Application

Questions 100 to 103 refer to the following information:

A 63-year-old female patient has been in the intensive care unit for 5 days after suffering a subarachnoid hemorrhage resulting from an aneurysm of the posterior communicating artery. She has no focal neurologic deficits but still complains of headache, nuchal rigidity, photophobia, and intermittent nausea. She has been alert and oriented to person, place, and time during previous assessments.

100. The patient's symptoms may be categorized as a:
A. Grade I hemorrhage
B. Grade II hemorrhage
C. Grade III hemorrhage
D. Grade IV hemorrhage

CORRECT ANSWER—B. Given the continued symptoms of meningeal irritation, a classification of grade II hemorrhage is appropriate. A grade II hemorrhage is characterized by minimal neurologic deficits, mild to severe headache, and nuchal rigidity; the patient typically is alert and has no vasospasm. A grade I hemorrhage is characterized by minimal headache and slight nuchal rigidity. A grade III hemorrhage causes confusion and drowsiness; the patient may have mild focal deficits and nuchal rigidity. With a grade IV hemorrhage, the patient is unresponsive and has hemiplegia, with or without vasospasm. A grade V hemorrhage is ominous; the patient is comatose and moribund and has decerebrate posturing.
Nursing process step: Assessment
Cognitive level: Knowledge

101. The patient has been stable for the last 6 days with minimal deficits. At midnight, the night-shift nurse has trouble waking her and notes that she is confused and disoriented. The patient has weakness on the right side and cannot speak clearly. Her pupils are equal and reactive. These symptoms are consistent with:
A. Oversedation caused by sleeping medication
B. Onset of cerebral edema
C. Excess vasodilation and hypotension caused by antihypertensive medication
D. Onset of vasospasm

CORRECT ANSWER—D. About 4 to 14 days after a subarachnoid hemorrhage, cerebral vasospasm may occur, possibly because of spasmogenic by-products as the clots in the basal cisterns or cerebral fissures break down. The other possibility is rebleeding from the aneurysm. A computed tomography scan is needed to differentiate between the two. The patient probably would not have received a sleeping medication because of the risk of altering the neurologic assessment. Cerebral edema is more likely to occur soon after the initial insult occurred. Excess vasodilation is unlikely to cause the focal neurologic symptoms exhibited by the patient.
Nursing process step: Assessment
Cognitive level: Analysis

102. A repeat computed tomography scan shows no other reason for the patient's neurologic deterioration, and vasospasm is diagnosed. When hypervolemic, hypertensive hemodilution is begun, the nurse must monitor the patient carefully for:
A. Increase in hematocrit to 38% and decrease in pulmonary artery wedge pressure (PAWP) to 10 mm Hg
B. Decrease in hematocrit to 25% and decrease in PAWP to 12 mm Hg
C. Decrease in hematocrit to 30%, decrease in systolic blood pressure to 160 mm Hg, and increase in PAWP to 18 mm Hg
D. Increase in systolic blood pressure to 150 mm Hg and decrease in PAWP to 8 mm Hg

CORRECT ANSWER—C. Hypertensive, hypervolemic hemodilution is designed to increase cerebral perfusion pressure while making the blood more dilute and thus easier to move past the narrowed blood vessels. The goals are to reduce the hematocrit to between 30% and 33% using crystalloid or colloid solutions, such as albumin and mannitol; to increase systolic blood pressure to between 150 and 170 mm Hg; and to raise cardiac output to between 7 and 8 liters/minute with a PAWP of 14 to 18 mm Hg.
Nursing process step: Implementation
Cognitive level: Evaluation

103. In response to the photophobia caused by meningeal irritation, the nurse caring for this patient should:
A. Patch the affected eye
B. Instill 0.9% sodium chloride eye drops every 4 hours
C. Elevate the head of the bed 30 degrees
D. Darken the room

CORRECT ANSWER—D. Darkening the room decreases stimulation of the optic nerve and reduces the discomfort of photophobia. Eye drops and patching the eye will not help. Elevating the head of the bed would relieve the headache and decrease intracranial pressure but would not alleviate the photophobia.
Nursing process step: Implementation
Cognitive level: Application

104. A 26-year-old female has a T1 to T2 spinal cord injury. While in the hospital for a respiratory tract infection, she complains of severe headache and blurred vision. Her blood pressure is 220/120 mm Hg, and her pulse rate is 47 beats/minute. She is perspiring profusely on her arms and face; her face is flushed and her pupils are dilated. The nurse's immediate intervention should be to:
A. Obtain blood samples for cultures, monitor blood pressure closely, and evaluate for septic shock secondary to respiratory tract infection
B. Monitor blood pressure closely and prepare the patient for pacemaker insertion
C. Assess for aspiration, elevate the head of the bed, and prepare the patient for intubation
D. Monitor blood pressure closely, elevate the head of the bed, and check the bladder catheter for kinks or clamps

CORRECT ANSWER—D. The patient exhibits the classic signs and symptoms of autonomic dysreflexia, which often is triggered by bladder distention or rectal impaction. The massive autonomic nervous system stimulation causes hypertension and vagal stimulation, which leads to bradycardia and pupil dilation. Sepsis is a danger but is not indicated by these autonomic symptoms. The key in this situation is to find the cause. Intubation would have no effect on blood pressure or autonomic dysreflexia and might worsen the situation because the head of the bed would have to be lowered. Autonomic dysreflexia is not a cardiac problem and therefore does not require a pacemaker.
Nursing process step: Implementation
Cognitive level: Application

105. Cardiac irregularities, hypoxemia, and hypoglycemia must be avoided during a seizure because:
A. Seizure threshold would be lowered
B. Postictal period would be prolonged
C. Myocardial damage might occur after the seizure
D. Oxygen demand in the brain increases 250% during a seizure

CORRECT ANSWER—D. During a seizure, a phenomenal increase occurs in the energy and oxygen requirements of the neurons, primarily those in the brain. This can quickly lead to ischemia. If the patient is hypoxic or hypoglycemic or has an arrhythmia that decreases cardiac output, the cells tolerate the deficit poorly. If cells are ischemic, hypoxia can continue into the postictal period; however, the postictal period would not necessarily be prolonged. The seizure threshold will remain low until medications are given. Although myocardial ischemia is possible, the primary concern is the prevention of cerebral ischemia.
Nursing process step: Implementation
Cognitive level: Analysis

Questions 106 and 107 refer to the following information:
A 35-year-old female patient is admitted with a temperature of 103° F (39.4° C), severe headache, and nuchal rigidity. She had a sinus infection 2 weeks ago and reports that she took only half of the prescribed antibiotic. She has a fine rash across her chest and petechiae in the mucous membranes. A lumbar puncture is performed, and the results show an elevated white blood cell count and protein in the cloudy cerebrospinal fluid (CSF). CSF cultures are pending.

---

106. What type of precautions are necessary for this patient?
A. Strict isolation
B. Universal precautions and respiratory isolation
C. Universal precautions only
D. None

CORRECT ANSWER—B. Bacterial meningitis is possible given the patient's symptoms and the presence of white blood cells in the cerebrospinal fluid. The history of a recent sinus infection supports this diagnosis. If the culture is negative, respiratory isolation can be discontinued. However, universal precautions should be used for all patients. Because bacterial meningitis commonly is transmitted via droplets from the nasopharynx, the nurse should wear a mask until the culture results are available. Strict isolation, which includes wearing gowns and goggles, is not necessary in bacterial meningitis.
Nursing process step: Planning
Cognitive level: Comprehension

107. As the patient becomes more confused and disoriented, which nursing intervention must be implemented?
   A. Protecting the patient from injury
   B. Administering anticonvulsants to prevent seizures
   C. Increasing the frequency of neurologic assessments
   D. Reorienting the patient and avoiding restraints

CORRECT ANSWER—**A.** Injury is more likely to occur as confusion increases. Restraints may be necessary, but their use must be weighed against the resulting increase in intracranial pressure if the patient fights them. Seizures are possible but not directly related to the altered level of consciousness. Frequent neurologic assessments would already have been implemented as a means of monitoring for potential bacterial meningitis.
Nursing process step: Planning
Cognitive level: Application

108. To prevent an increase in intracranial pressure, the nurse should ask staff and family members at the bedside of a comatose patient to:
   A. Freely discuss all aspects of the patient's condition
   B. Touch the patient when talking about his condition
   C. Keep quiet and not talk at the bedside
   D. Talk to the patient, not about the patient

CORRECT ANSWER—**D.** Although talking to and touching the patient are important, talking about the patient's condition when he can hear has been shown to elevate intracranial pressure. The patient needs to know he is not in a vacuum. If others are present in the room, the patient may hear them even if he is comatose.
Nursing process step: Implementation
Cognitive level: Application

Questions 109 and 110 refer to the following information:
A 21-year-old male patient is admitted to the critical care unit with bacterial endocarditis. He has a history of I.V. drug abuse. The patient has developed a heart murmur since admission and remains febrile despite 4 days of antibiotic therapy. His white blood cell count is 25,000/mm^3. Repeat blood cultures are pending. At 2 a.m., when awakened by the nurse for vital signs assessment, he is unable to move his right side. His face droops on the right side.

109. What do the patient's symptoms indicate?
   A. Embolism of vegetative growth to the left frontal lobe
   B. Decreased cardiac output and inadequate cerebral perfusion
   C. Embolism of a mural thrombus from the right atrium
   D. Thrombosis of a cerebral vessel caused by dehydration secondary to fever

CORRECT ANSWER—**A.** The most likely cause of the patient's symptoms, and one of the most serious complications of endocarditis, is the embolism of vegetation from the damaged valves. Decreased cardiac output would cause obtundation but no focal symptoms. A thrombus from the right atrium would migrate to the lungs, not the brain. Thrombosis from dehydration is not likely 4 days after admission.
Nursing process step: Assessment
Cognitive level: Comprehension

110. Treatment for the patient's cerebral emboli would include:

A. Continued antibiotic therapy and, eventually, valve replacement

B. Inotropic agent therapy to increase cardiac output

C. Anticoagulant therapy to reduce clots in the atrium

D. Fluid resuscitation to rehydrate the patient and increase perfusion

CORRECT ANSWER—A. Control of bacterial growth is critical in preventing the formation of emboli. Replacing the damaged valves before bacterial growth is controlled is risky. Inotropic agent therapy would be needed if the embolus entered the coronary artery instead of the brain. Use of anticoagulants would not resolve the vegetation. Fluid balance is essential for maintaining perfusion but will not prevent vegetative emboli.
Nursing process step: Implementation
Cognitive level: Application

111. Simple partial motor seizures are characterized by:

A. Twitching of fingers or toes on one side of the body

B. Causative lesion in the prerolandic gyrus

C. Brain stem involvement only

D. Maintenance of consciousness

CORRECT ANSWER—B. Simple partial motor seizures, also known as focal or Jacksonian seizures, occur when the focal point is in the prerolandic gyrus (motor strip area). A typical simple partial seizure begins with twitching on one side of the body that spreads until the entire side is completely involved. Consciousness is maintained unless the seizure becomes generalized and spreads to the rest of the body. Consciousness is lost if the brain stem, hypothalamus, or thalmus is involved. Simple partial sensory seizures are caused by lesions in the postrolandic gyrus (the sensory strip between the frontal and parietal lobes).
Nursing process step: Assessment
Cognitive level: Comprehension

Questions 112 to 114 refer to the following information:
A 42-year-old female patient is admitted to the intensive care unit with a tentative diagnosis of Guillain-Barré syndrome. Weakness and tingling sensations are present in both legs. Although not a true nervous system infection, Guillain-Barré syndrome often follows a recent viral infection. In this case, the patient had an upper respiratory tract infection 2 weeks ago that has since resolved. The polyneuritis caused by Guillain-Barré syndrome will lead to progressive motor, sensory, and cranial nerve dysfunction.

112. The primary assessment of this patient must include:

A. Neurologic assessment for increased intracranial pressure

B. Respiratory monitoring of vital capacity and tidal volume

C. Nutritional assessment to prevent catabolism and vitamin deficiency

D. Management of pain and discomfort

CORRECT ANSWER—B. When the thoracic nerves are involved, the most serious complication of Guillain-Barré syndrome is respiratory failure. Frequent assessments of vital capacity, tidal volume, and negative inspiratory force are essential to prevent respiratory failure caused by the ascending paralysis associated with this disease. In some cases, the patient requires prolonged ventilatory support. Because polyneuritis is a peripheral nerve disorder, intracranial pressure does not increase. Although nutritional support is essential, Guillain-Barré syndrome is unlikely to cause a vitamin deficiency. Maintaining respiratory function is more important initially than managing pain and discomfort.
Nursing process step: Assessment
Cognitive level: Analysis

113. The disease extensively involves the nervous system. The patient suffers respiratory failure and is placed on a mechanical ventilator. The nurse caring for this patient should monitor for what other potential problems?

A. Further deterioration in vital capacity

B. Deep vein thrombosis or ileus

C. Electrolyte imbalance

D. Delayed return of function as evidenced by electromyograms

CORRECT ANSWER—B. Because the patient will be on bed rest for an extended time, deep vein thrombosis and pulmonary embolism are concerns. Sequential compression devices for the lower extremities typically are not used because of the painful, sensitive, demyelinated peripheral nerves. Vital capacity would already be monitored because of the patient's respiratory failure. Electrolyte imbalance can be prevented by adequate, early nutritional support. Electromyography is not a part of the early acute care of a patient with Guillain-Barré syndrome.
Nursing process step: Evaluation
Cognitive level: Application

114. A patient with polyneuritis may experience pain, fear, and anxiety. Which of the following statements about polyneuritis must the nurse consider when developing a plan of care?
A. Polyneuritis causes no cognitive loss, only reversible peripheral nerve failure
B. Polyneuritis causes no sensory loss, only motor loss
C. Polyneuritis causes permanent motor and sensory losses
D. Polyneuritis is associated with inevitable complications of paralysis

CORRECT ANSWER—**A.** A patient with polyneuritis experiences no cognitive loss but is almost completely dependent on nursing care for survival. The patient may be unable to move even the eyes, yet remains completely alert and oriented. The patient also may be terrified and unable to express fear. The complications of paralysis can be prevented by excellent nursing care. Although the loss is primarily motor in nature, sensory neurons may cause pain and hyperesthesia. Consideration of the patient's feelings, anticipation of pain, and gentle treatment to prevent complications are the mainstays of care for a patient with Guillain-Barré-induced polyneuritis. In most patients, return of motor function occurs proximally and extends distally.
Nursing process level: Implementation
Cognitive level: Application

115. A patient has just undergone craniotomy for a glioblastoma (grade IV astrocytoma). He has weakness on the right side of his body and slurred speech, but he is alert and oriented. The nurse finds the patient crying quietly. What action is indicated?
A. Reassure the patient that symptoms will subside and the tumor is benign
B. Call the surgeon for a sedation order
C. Reassure the patient that depression is a normal response to craniotomy and encourage him to express his concerns
D. Encourage the patient to express his concerns about dying and possibly request additional help from social services

CORRECT ANSWER—**C.** Depression is common after craniotomy, and emotions often are labile. A glioblastoma is a malignant tumor, and the patient probably faces chemotherapy or radiation treatment. Light sedation may help, but allowing the patient to talk about his problems rather than masking the symptoms is preferable. Social services would be of benefit later in the course of treatment.
Nursing process step: Implementation
Cognitive level: Synthesis

116. A 49-year-old male patient had a large glioblastoma multiforme of the frontal lobe with hemorrhagic areas. Most of the tumor was removed, but cerebral edema is extensive and intracranial pressure (ICP) has been hard to control. Debulking of the tumor with a craniectomy is then performed to reduce ICP. Postoperatively, the nurse would plan to do which of the following?

A. Prevent trauma to the unprotected brain tissue

B. Measure ICP repeatedly and turn and suction the patient every 2 hours

C. Avoid turning the patient to the operative side

D. Prepare for insertion of a ventriculoperitoneal shunt if ICP remains elevated

CORRECT ANSWER—A. The nurse must protect the brain tissue and prevent trauma because part of the cranium has been removed. Although turning the patient and measuring ICP are important, suctioning every 2 hours is not required. The patient can be turned to the operative side if the unprotected tissue is supported by soft foam or other supports. A ventriculoperitoneal shunt probably would not be useful because the increased intracranial pressure is related to tumor growth and size, not obstructive hydrocephalus. **Nursing process step:** Planning **Cognitive level:** Application

117. A patient with idiopathic epilepsy may have a genetic predisposition to seizures. The nurse should plan to teach this patient to:

A. Not have children to avoid passing on the genetic predisposition·

B. Take phenytoin if a seizure develops

C. Understand that epilepsy is an abnormality of the electrical rhythm of the brain, not a contagious disease

D. Live quietly and not socialize extensively

CORRECT ANSWER—C. Epilepsy is an abnormality of the electrical rhythm of the brain, just as atrial fibrillation is an abnormality of the electrical activity of the heart. Most persons with seizure disorders live normal, productive lives. They need not restrict their activities, although they should avoid alcohol and becoming overly tired. Some patients must avoid flashing lights or excessive loss of sleep. A predisposition to a seizure disorder is not a contraindication to having children. Patients should be taught about the prophylactic use anticonvulsants, such as phenytoin or phenobarbital; these drugs can effectively control seizures in 75% of patients. **Nursing process step:** Planning **Cognitive level:** Synthesis

---

Questions 118 to 121 refer to the following information:
A 32-year-old male patient is admitted to the neurologic intensive care unit with severe headache, nuchal rigidity, projectile vomiting, photophobia, and expressive aphasia. Apparently well until about 12 hours ago, he has not been out of the country and has no evidence of insect bites. However, he has a purulent sore in his left ear and a draining fever blister on his lower lip.

---

118. What do these symptoms suggest?
- **A.** Viral meningitis
- **B.** Bacterial meningitis
- **C.** Herpes simplex encephalitis
- **D.** Human immunodeficiency virus (HIV) encephalopathy

CORRECT ANSWER—**C.** All viral forms of encephalitis have a similar clinical picture, including sudden onset of fever, headache, and vomiting, and signs and symptoms of meningeal irritation (such as stiff neck) and neuronal damage (such as drowsiness, decreasing level of consciousness, focal deficits, and paralysis). Herpes simplex encephalitis attacks the frontal and temporal lobes, causing cerebral edema and, sometimes, hemorrhagic necrosis. The patient's symptoms are consistent with temporal lobe dysfunction and increased intracranial pressure. Encephalitis is difficult to differentiate from meningitis, but the herpetic lesions support the diagnosis of herpes simplex encephalitis. The information provided does not suggest HIV encephalopathy.
Nursing process step: Assessment
Cognitive level: Evaluation

119. What is the drug of choice for treating herpes simplex encephalitis?
- **A.** Acyclovir
- **B.** Zidovudine
- **C.** Vancomycin hydrochloride
- **D.** Cefotaxime sodium

CORRECT ANSWER—**A.** Acyclovir often is used to control herpes simplex virus. It can be started prophylactically while waiting for the culture results from the lumbar puncture. Vidarabine also is used to treat herpes encephalitis. Zidovudine is used for human immunodeficiency virus infections. Vancomycin hydrochloride and cefotaxime sodium would only be used for bacterial infections superimposed on the viral infection.
Nursing process step: Implementation
Cognitive level: Comprehension

120. This patient will require:
  A. Enteric isolation
  B. Respiratory isolation
  C. Strict isolation
  D. Universal precautions

CORRECT ANSWER—**D.** All hospitalized patients require universal precautions, which include good hand washing and use of gloves for any contact or potential contact with body secretions and blood. In essence, there is nothing to isolate if the virus is contained within the skull. The virus probably travels through the blood or along the path of the nerve. If the external herpetic lesion is still draining, it is infectious and should not be touched without gloves. Respiratory isolation (which includes having health care personnel wear masks and providing the patient with a private room), enteric isolation (which requires health care personnel to handle waste or contaminated articles in a special manner), and strict isolation (which requires a private room; use of mask, gown, and gloves; and special procedures for disposing of waste and contaminated articles) are not indicated for this patient.
Nursing process step: Implementation
Cognitive level: Comprehension

121. Corticosteroids may be administered to reduce cerebral edema in the temporal or frontal lobe. If corticosteroids are used, the nurse should monitor for:
  A. Hyperglycemia and GI bleeding
  B. Hypoglycemia
  C. Syndrome of inappropriate antidiuretic hormone (SIADH)
  D. Abscess formation

CORRECT ANSWER—**A.** Hyperglycemia and GI bleeding are known complications of corticosteroid therapy. Steroids often lead to fluid retention, which results from the release of aldosterone, not antidiuretic hormone. An abscess may develop, but not as a result of steroid therapy.
Nursing process step: Evaluation
Cognitive level: Evaluation

122. A 56-year-old male is admitted with a metastatic spinal cord tumor at the T12 level. He is in severe pain and has motor weakness resulting from compression of the spinal cord and meninges and from traction on the nerve roots. Management of this patient will include:
  A. Performing immediate laminectomy
  B. Providing cervical traction and intrathecal analgesics
  C. Using transcutaneous electrical nerve stimulation (TENS) combined with repositioning the patient from side to side
  D. Elevating the head of the patient's bed to relieve traction on the nerves and administering epidural or systemic analgesics

CORRECT ANSWER—**D.** Elevating the head of the bed will reduce pressure on the nerve roots, and systemic analgesics will help control the pain. TENS is of little value because of the severity of the pain. Cervical traction is not beneficial for a thoracic condition, and a laminectomy is not indicated.
Nursing process step: Implementation
Cognitive level: Application

Questions 123 and 124 refer to the following information:
A 76-year-old female patient with a history of poorly controlled hypertension is found lying in bed, incontinent, and with facial drooping on the left side. She did not respond to her name when her son called her. In the emergency department, the patient exhibits decerebrate posturing only in response to painful stimuli. Her right pupil is completely dilated and unresponsive to light; her left pupil is sluggishly reactive. She has a positive Babinski's reflex on the left side. Vital signs include blood pressure, 180/112 mm Hg; pulse, 64 beats/minute; and respirations, 14 breaths/minute and irregular. A computed tomography scan shows an intracerebral hemorrhage in the temporoparietal region with a shift in the midline structures.

123. Which intervention should the intensive care unit nurse plan to implement for this patient?
A. Elevating the head of the bed 30 degrees, maintaining oxygenation, controlling blood pressure, and providing emotional support for the family
B. Administering mannitol and furosemide to decrease intracranial pressure
C. Hyperventilating the patient to decrease intracranial pressure
D. Providing nutritional support and administering nitroprusside to reduce systolic blood pressure to between 90 and 100 mm Hg

CORRECT ANSWER—**A.** This devastating intracerebral hemorrhage is traumatic for the family as well as the patient. The nurse should encourage family members to talk to the patient even though she will be unable to respond. Elevating the head of the bed can decrease intracranial pressure and improve oxygenation, although it may be of little benefit for this patient. The use of mannitol and furosemide to decrease intracranial pressure is less critical than controlling the blood pressure. However, lowering systolic blood pressure to between 90 and 100 mm Hg could cause relative hypotension and trigger a sympathetic nervous system response, leading to vasoconstriction and tachycardia. A systolic blood pressure of 120 to 130 mm Hg would be better tolerated. Nutritional support is important for all patients but would not be an initial intervention. Hyperventilation will not be enough to help this patient.
Nursing process step: Planning
Cognitive level: Analysis

124. After 4 hours, the patient has a tonic-clonic seizure lasting 1 minute. Afterward, both pupils are fixed and dilated, and the patient does not respond to painful stimuli. There is no Babinski's reflex on either side. Her blood pressure is 220/64 mm Hg, pulse is 45 beats/minute, and respirations are 38 breaths/minute. What does this situation represent?

A. Postictal changes that may resolve

B. Herniation of the temporal lobe into the tentorial opening

C. Rebleeding and herniation of the brain stem

D. Acute cerebral edema with herniation of the temporal lobe

CORRECT ANSWER—C. The most likely cause of this event is recurrent hemorrhage and herniation of the brain stem, resulting in Cushing's phenomenon of hypertension, widening pulse pressure, and bradycardia. These symptoms are more severe and more graphic than those caused by temporal lobe herniation, cerebral edema, or postictal state.
Nursing process step: Evaluation
Cognitive level: Analysis

125. Vasogenic cerebral edema caused by a brain tumor often dramatically responds to:

A. Calcium channel blockers, such as nimodipine

B. Osmotic diuresis and intracranial pressure monitoring

C. Corticosteroids, such as dexamethasone

D. Hypervolemic hemodilution

CORRECT ANSWER—C. Vasogenic edema is highly responsive to steroid therapy. Osmotic diuresis sometimes helps by dehydrating normal cells and allowing edematous tissue more room to expand. Hypervolemic hemodilution and calcium channel blockers are used for vasospasm.
Nursing process step: Implementation
Cognitive level: Comprehension

126. The earliest, most important indication of a change in neurologic status and intracranial pressure is:

A. Decreased level of consciousness

B. Change in pupillary reaction

C. New onset of decorticate posturing

D. New onset of decerebrate posturing

CORRECT ANSWER—A. The first indication of increased intracranial pressure and worsening neurologic function often is a decrease in the level of consciousness. Change in pupillary reaction and decorticate or decerebrate posturing are later signs of deteriorating neurologic function.
Nursing process step: Evaluation
Cognitive level: Knowledge

127. A 39-year-old female has fever of unknown origin. All cultures and X-ray films are negative, but her white blood cell count is 19,600/μliter. On the patient's fourth day in the hospital, the nurse finds her unresponsive and her left pupil is slightly sluggish and 1 mm larger than the right. Nursing management should include which intervention?
A. Elevating the head of the bed, preventing Valsalva's maneuvers, and instituting seizure precautions
B. Preparing for insertion of an intracranial pressure (ICP) monitor
C. Administering anticonvulsants
D. Teaching the patient how to adapt to motor and sensory losses

CORRECT ANSWER—A. The patient has a fever, infection, and increased white blood cell count, as well as neurologic deficits, unequal pupils, and decreased level of consciousness. She must be evaluated for a potential brain abscess, which typically produces a clinical picture similar to that of a brain tumor. Early symptoms of brain abscess result from increased ICP; the earliest sign is altered level of consciousness. All efforts must be made to maintain a normal ICP. This includes elevating the head of the bed and maintaining the head in alignment to promote venous return. Valsalva's maneuvers increase ICP and must be avoided. The patient is at risk for generalized seizures; therefore, seizure precautions are necessary to protect her from injury. Noting the onset and duration of a seizure can help localize the lesion. At this point, an ICP monitor is not indicated. Anticonvulsants would not be started until the diagnosis of a brain abscess is confirmed or a seizure occurs. The patient currently displays no definite motor or sensory losses.
Nursing process step: Implementation
Cognitive level: Application

128. After trauma or surgery, blood flow in the spinal cord can slow because of cellular dysfunction in injured areas. To offset free-radical damage and to increase spinal cord nerve impulse generation and transmission, which of the following medications might be given within 8 hours of injury?
A. Methylprednisolone in high doses
B. Epinephrine
C. Levarterenol
D. Furosemide and mannitol

CORRECT ANSWER—A. The drug of choice in this early phase is a high-dose steroid, such as methylprednisolone. Epinephrine might indirectly increase perfusion by raising mean arterial pressure, but it would not directly prevent damage. Levarterenol would decrease spinal cord perfusion through alpha-receptor stimulation. Furosemide and mannitol might be used, but they are not the drugs of choice.
Nursing process step: Implementation
Cognitive level: Application

129. Tentorial herniation will most likely cause:
 A. Changes in vital signs
 B. Ataxic breathing
 C. Altered level of consciousness only
 D. Decreased level of consciousness and ipsilateral pupil dilation

CORRECT ANSWER—D. Herniation through the tentorial opening compresses the reticular activating system, causing a decreased level of consciousness and a nonreactive or sluggishly reactive pupil on the same side as the lesion. Vital sign changes are more likely to occur with herniation through the foramen magnum at the base of the skull. Ataxic breathing is seen when the brain stem is compressed near the foramen magnum.
Nursing process step: Assessment
Cognitive level: Evaluation

130. After sustaining a depressed skull fracture resulting from a motor vehicle accident, a 17-year-old high school student is admitted for debridement and left frontal craniectomy. Four days after surgery, the patient is intubated and mechanically ventilated; neurologic and vital signs are stable. The current nursing plan should include:
 A. Administering mannitol and furosemide to reduce intracranial pressure (ICP)
 B. Monitoring for signs of diabetes insipidus
 C. Hyperventilating the patient to achieve a $PaCO_2$ of 20 mm Hg
 D. Instituting range-of-motion exercises and using splints to prevent complications related to immobility

CORRECT ANSWER—D. Now that the patient is stable, the nurse must seek to prevent complications related to immobility. The nursing plan of care also must include adequate nutrition to promote recovery of injured cells and prevent catabolism. Diabetes insipidus is seen in cases of head trauma or neurosurgery in which neurohypophysial damage occurs; this is unlikely with a craniectomy. If symptoms of diabetes insipidus did occur, they would have appeared within the first 1 to 2 days after surgery. Because there are no signs of increased ICP, diuretics are not needed. Hyperventilation effectively reduces ICP, but $PaCO_2$ should not be lower than 25 mm Hg to prevent ischemia. Also, the patient underwent surgery 4 days ago, and hyperventilation works best in the first 24 to 48 hours after surgery.
Nursing process step: Planning
Cognitive level: Application

131. A patient with a spinal cord injury may require a suprapubic catheter for:
 A. Bladder training
 B. Intermittent catheterization
 C. High-level quadriplegia with poor motor coordination
 D. Early stages of injury during spinal shock

CORRECT ANSWER—C. Suprapubic catheters are used for quadriplegic patients with poor hand coordination and arm weakness who cannot undergo normal catheterization. To prevent infection and maintain bladder tone, bladder training and intermittent catheterization are preferable to leaving the catheter in place. The only exception to intermittent catheterization is during the initial period of spinal shock before spinal reflexes return. A suprapubic catheter is not necessary during this early period.
Nursing process step: Implementation
Cognitive level: Application

132. A 38-year-old patient is prescribed sublingual nimodipine and I.V. phenytoin. Nimodipine is used to:
A. Reduce intracranial pressure
B. Control seizures
C. Reduce cerebral edema resulting from hypo-osmolality
D. Reduce vasospasm and increase cerebral blood flow

CORRECT ANSWER—D. Phenytoin increases the seizure threshold. Nimodipine, a calcium channel blocker, is widely used to reduce vasospasm. Nimodipine indirectly contributes to the control of seizures by reducing ischemia; it does not control cerebral edema or intracranial pressure.
Nursing process step: Implementation
Cognitive level: Comprehension

133. Carbamazepine is particularly effective for:
A. Status epilepticus
B. Simple partial and complex partial seizures
C. Absence (petit mal) seizures
D. Pregnant patients who have epilepsy

CORRECT ANSWER—B. Carbamazepine is the drug of choice for treating simple partial and complex partial seizures. Carbamazepine also is used to treat generalized tonic-clonic seizures and to relieve the pain of trigeminal neuralgia. The drug may control seizures by inhibiting the spread of seizure activity or neuromuscular transmission in general and by increasing the discharge of noradrenergic neurons. Carbamazepine also has sedative, anticholinergic, antidepressant, muscle relaxant, antiarrhythmic, and antidiuretic properties. Diazepam is used to treat status epilepticus. Absence seizures are controlled with valproic acid and ethosuximide. Phenobarbital is used for pregnant patients with seizure disorders.
Nursing process step: Implementation
Cognitive level: Comprehension

RENAL SYSTEM

CHAPTER 4

Renal System

Questions 1 to 5 refer to the following information:
A 55-year-old female patient with diabetes is being treated with antibiotics for cellulitis of the right foot. Oliguria develops on the fourth day of treatment. The patient's laboratory values are as follows:
- serum potassium, 6 mEq/liter
- blood urea nitrogen, 75 mg/dl
- serum creatinine, 4 mg/dl
- serum sodium, 131 mEq/liter
- serum chloride, 98 mEq/liter.

Vital signs include temperature, 99° F (37.2° C); pulse rate, 110 beats/minute and irregular; respirations, 28 breaths/minute; and blood pressure, 200/100 mm Hg. Renal function was normal before oliguria occurred.

1. Which type of acute renal disorder is the most likely cause of the patient's renal failure?
- **A.** Prerenal failure
- **B.** Intrarenal failure
- **C.** Postrenal failure
- **D.** Diabetic nephropathy

CORRECT ANSWER—B. Intrarenal failure results from damage to the capillaries and tubules of the kidney and is associated with increases in blood urea nitrogen (BUN) and serum creatinine. Intrarenal failure frequently is caused by antibiotic therapy. Prerenal failure, a result of hypoperfusion of the kidneys, leads to an increase in BUN that is greater than the increase in serum creatinine (ratio greater than 10:1). Postrenal failure, caused by urinary outflow obstruction, is associated with no urine flow. Diabetic nephropathy is a chronic process that develops over months to years and can lead to chronic renal failure by causing progressive kidney damage.
Nursing process step: Assessment
Cognitive level: Analysis

2. The patient's hypertension probably results from:
A. Dehydration and anxiety
B. Dehydration and action of the renin-angiotensin system
C. Fluid retention and sepsis
D. Fluid retention and renin-angiotensin mechanism

CORRECT ANSWER—**D.** Fluid retention caused by decreased secretion of urine is one cause of the patient's hypertension. The renin-angiotensin system's attempt to increase the glomerular filtration rate also causes hypertension in intrarenal failure. Hypotension more commonly is seen in dehydration. Anxiety, which may or may not be present in this patient, could lead to hypertension if severe. Sepsis typically leads to hypotension.
Nursing process step: Assessment
Cognitive level: Analysis

3. The patient's blood urea nitrogen and serum creatinine levels continue to rise, and she remains oliguric. What additional physical assessment finding would *not* be attributable to her renal status?
A. Bilateral crackles in the middle and lower lung fields
B. Peripheral edema
C. Vision changes
D. Lethargy

CORRECT ANSWER—**C.** Vision changes are not a sign of uremia or of the electrolyte imbalances of acute renal failure. Crackles and peripheral edema indicate fluid retention. Lethargy is related to uremia and anemia.
Nursing process step: Assessment
Cognitive level: Analysis

4. Which ECG changes are related to the patient's electrolyte profile?
A. Peaked T waves
B. Prolonged PR interval
C. U wave
D. ST-segment depression

CORRECT ANSWER—**A.** Peaked T waves, indicating ventricular repolarization, are an early sign of hyperkalemia. The PR interval shortens as the potassium level rises. A U wave occurs in hypokalemia. ST-segment depression is a sign of pharmacologic or ischemic effects on the heart.
Nursing process step: Assessment
Cognitive level: Analysis

5. Which of the following urinalysis findings most commonly are associated with intrarenal failure?
A. Urine sodium level of 10 mEq/liter, no red blood cells or protein present
B. Urine sodium level of 60 mEq/liter, no red blood cells or protein present
C. Urine sodium level of 60 mEq/liter, red blood cells and protein present
D. Urine sodium level of 10 mEq/liter, red blood cells and protein present

CORRECT ANSWER—**C.** In intrarenal failure, the tubules lose their ability to retain sodium. Consequently, the urine sodium level typically ranges from 40 to 80 mEq/liter. Because the injured glomerulus loses its ability to retain red blood cells and protein, these substances are found in the urine of patients with intrarenal failure.
Nursing process step: Assessment
Cognitive level: Analysis

6. The most reliable indicator of fluid balance is:
A. Intake and output
B. Daily weight
C. Blood urea nitrogen (BUN) level
D. Hemoglobin level

CORRECT ANSWER—B. Daily weight, measured on the same scale at the same time of day, is the most reliable method of assessing fluid balance. Intake and output is open to error and cannot account for insensible loss, which varies from patient to patient. BUN and hemoglobin levels can be affected by fluid balance, but they also are affected by other processes common to critically ill patients, such as renal failure or bleeding. Therefore, BUN and hemoglobin are not reliable indicators of fluid balance.
Nursing process step: Assessment
Cognitive level: Comprehension

7. If corrected, which arterial blood gas values can reverse hypokalemia?
A. pH, 7.50; partial pressure of carbon dioxide in arterial blood ($PaCO_2$), 30 mm Hg; HCO_3^-, 24 mEq/liter
B. pH, 7.30; $PaCO_2$, 55 mm Hg; HCO_3^-, 24 mEq/liter
C. pH, 7.42; $PaCO_2$, 45 mm Hg; HCO_3^-, 24 mEq/liter
D. pH, 7.24; $PaCO_2$, 45 mm Hg; HCO_3^-, 13 mEq/liter

CORRECT ANSWER—A. A pH above 7.45 and a $PaCO_2$ below 35 mm Hg indicate respiratory alkalosis, which leads to loss of potassium in the distal tubules of the kidneys. Option B indicates respiratory acidosis, in which the pH is low and the carbon dioxide level is high. Option C consists of normal arterial blood gas values. Option D indicates metabolic acidosis, with a low pH and low HCO_3^- level.
Nursing process step: Evaluation
Cognitive level: Analysis

8. Which calcium value would be expected if a patient's phosphate level is 6.0 mg/dl?
A. 7.0 mg/dl
B. 8.5 mg/dl
C. 9.5 mg/dl
D. 10.5 mg/dl

CORRECT ANSWER—A. As phosphate level increases, the body responds by lowering the calcium level via decreased absorption in the intestine and decreased stimulation of the bone to release calcium. A phosphate level of 6.0 mg/dl is high, so a low calcium level is expected. A normal calcium level ranges from 8.5 to 10.5 mg/dl; thus, a calcium level of about 7.0 mg/dl would be expected with a high phosphate level.
Nursing process step: Assessment
Cognitive level: Analysis

9. Which finding does *not* indicate the need for surgery in a patient with renal trauma?
A. Hematocrit of 40% on admission, 35% 2 hours later, and 30% 4 hours later
B. Lower abdominal pain with increasing abdominal girth
C. Hematoma over the flank area that increases in size 12 hours after injury
D. Increase in blood urea nitrogen (BUN) from 10 mg/dl to 50 mg/dl 10 hours after injury

CORRECT ANSWER—D. An increase in BUN above the normal range of 10 to 20 mg/dl should be examined in relation to the serum creatinine value. If the serum creatinine value is 1.0 mg/dl or less, the increasing BUN reflects prerenal failure. If the serum creatinine value is greater than 1.0 mg/dl, intrarenal failure exists; however, this does not indicate a need for surgery. A continually decreasing hematocrit, urinary extravasation, or an increase in the size of a hematoma indicate the need for surgical repair.
Nursing process step: Evaluation
Cognitive level: Analysis

10. Which patient is at *least* risk for hypercalcemia?
A. 21-year-old patient with hypophosphatemia resulting from malnutrition
B. 72-year-old patient with metastatic cancer to the bone
C. 55-year-old patient with multiple myeloma
D. 80-year-old patient with arthritis of the hip

CORRECT ANSWER—D. An 80-year-old patient with arthritis of the hip has the lowest risk of hypercalcemia. Hypophosphatemia leads to a reciprocal increase in calcium level. Tumors of the bone, both metastatic and primary, release calcium into the bloodstream as they grow.
Nursing process step: Assessment
Cognitive level: Analysis

11. Which life-threatening event is related to hypercalcemia?
A. Heart block and cardiac arrest
B. Prolonged QT interval
C. Seizures
D. Laryngospasm

CORRECT ANSWER—A. Heart block and cardiac arrest can result when the calcium level reaches 18 mg/dl or higher. A prolonged QT interval, seizures, and laryngospasm may lead to the life-threatening consequences associated with hypocalcemia.
Nursing process step: Assessment
Cognitive level: Comprehension

12. Which of the following interventions are useful in correcting hypercalcemia?
A. Implementation of bed rest, administration of phosphorus supplements, and administration of a hypotonic solution
B. Diuresis, administration of phosphorus supplements, and administration of 0.9% sodium chloride solution
C. Implementation of bed rest, diuresis, and I.V. administration of dextrose 5% in water (D5W)
D. Diuresis, administration of vitamin D supplements, and fluid restriction

CORRECT ANSWER—B. Diuretics and 0.9% sodium chloride solution are used in hypercalcemia to promote calcium loss via the renal system. Phosphorus supplements increase phosphate level and thus lead to lower calcium level because of the reciprocal relationship between phosphate and calcium. The immobility of bed rest may increase the calcium level as bone demineralizes. Administration of a hypotonic solution, such as D5W, would not cause a significant loss of calcium. Vitamin D would increase calcium absorption and thus raise the calcium level.
Nursing process step: Implementation
Cognitive level: Application

13. In a patient with a phosphate level of 6.0 mg/dl, the nurse would monitor for signs and symptoms of:

A. Hypercalcemia
B. Hyperkalemia
C. Hypokalemia
D. Hypocalcemia

CORRECT ANSWER—**D.** Imbalances of calcium and phosphate typically cause abnormalities in the central nervous system, muscles, and heart. Hyperphosphatemia leads to an inversely proportional decrease in calcium. Because hyperphosphatemia typically is asymptomatic, the nurse would monitor for signs and symptoms of hypocalcemia, which include rapid and irregular pulse, tachycardia, hypotension, tremors, hyperreflexia, hallucinations, mood swings, and syncope.
Nursing process step: Planning
Cognitive level: Comprehension

14. During which phase of intrarenal failure should fluid intake be most severely restricted?

A. Onset phase
B. Oliguric phase
C. Nonoliguric phase
D. Recovery phase

CORRECT ANSWER—**B.** The oliguric phase reflects severe tubular damage as manifested by a urine output of 400 ml/day. Fluid intake should be limited to the previous 24-hour total output plus 500 ml for insensible loss. The onset phase precedes the actual injury and is not necessarily treated with fluid restriction. Nonoliguric renal failure may require fluid replacement because urine output can exceed 1 liter/hour. During the recovery phase, renal function returns and fluid restriction is not required unless significant renal damage has occurred.
Nursing process step: Planning
Cognitive level: Analysis

15. The plan of care for a patient with postrenal failure might include which of the following?

A. Preparing for surgery after acute management
B. Using drug therapy to enhance cardiac output
C. Using aggressive diuretic therapy to manage fluid overload
D. Using aggressive fluid resuscitation to avoid intrarenal failure

CORRECT ANSWER—**A.** Patients with postrenal failure have no urine flow. Postrenal failure is caused by obstructive processes, such as ruptured bladder, interruption of ureteral or urethral integrity, or pressure from hematomas or displaced organs. One of the more common obstructive processes is prostatic hypertrophy of a tumor, which may require surgical correction. Drug therapy and fluid resuscitation are used with prerenal processes. Diuretic therapy is a component of treatment for oliguric intrarenal failure.
Nursing process step: Planning
Cognitive level: Application

Questions 16 to 25 refer to the following information:
A 21-year-old lumberyard worker was trapped beneath a fallen board. His abdomen, pelvis, and lower extremities took the weight of the fall. In the emergency department, abdominal paracentesis reveals bloody fluid. An indwelling urinary (Foley) catheter is inserted, and bloody urine is drained. Pelvic X-ray films reveal multiple pelvic fractures. The patient undergoes exploratory laparotomy, during which a fractured spleen and left kidney laceration are repaired. When the patient returns to the intensive care unit, his vital signs are blood pressure, 100/50 mm Hg; heart rate, 110 beats/minute with sinus rhythm; and respirations, 24 breaths/minute on a 50% Venturi mask. Breath sounds are decreased at the bases of the lungs and no crackles or rhonchi are heard. A nasogastric tube is connected to intermittent suction, and bile-colored fluid is draining. The Foley catheter is draining pink-tinged urine at a rate of 30 to 50 ml/hour. Dextrose 5% and 0.45% sodium chloride are being infused at a rate of 100 ml/hour.

16. Which of the following parts of the kidney are involved in the patient's injury?
A. Kidney capsule
B. Parenchyma and collecting system
C. Urethra
D. All of the above

CORRECT ANSWER—B. Laceration of the kidney involves the parenchyma or kidney tissue and the collecting system. This type of injury occurs in about 10% of all such kidney injuries. The more common injury, a contusion, occurs in 85% of such cases and involves the kidney capsule, not the collecting system. Urethral damage is a separate injury and not part of the laceration profile.
Nursing process step: Assessment
Cognitive level: Comprehension

17. During the postoperative assessment, the nurse would plan to evaluate all of the following *except:*
A. Urine output
B. Hemoglobin level
C. Blood urea nitrogen and serum creatinine levels
D. I.V. pyelogram results

CORRECT ANSWER—D. An I.V. pyelogram is performed before surgery to delineate lacerations and renal function. Postoperative kidney function and potential bleeding would be determined by evaluating urine output and blood urea nitrogen, serum creatinine, and hemoglobin levels.
Nursing process step: Planning
Cognitive level: Analysis

18. The patient initially had extremely red, gross hematuria. Which statement correctly identifies the relationship between degree of hematuria and injury?

A. No association exists between amount of hematuria and extent of injury

B. Increased hematuria is associated with significant renal laceration

C. Increased hematuria is associated with extensive renal contusion

D. Increased hematuria is associated with renal vascular injury

CORRECT ANSWER—A. The degree of hematuria is not directly related to the extent of renal injury. Renal laceration, renal contusion, and renal vascular injury produce varying amounts of hematuria independent of the degree of injury.

Nursing process step: Assessment

Cognitive level: Analysis

19. The patient's potassium level is 6.5 mEq/liter. Which electrolyte disorder does this level represent?

A. Hypokalemia caused by diuresis

B. Hyperkalemia caused by crush injury

C. Hypokalemia caused by stress

D. Hyperkalemia caused by stress

CORRECT ANSWER—B. A normal potassium level is 3.5 to 5.5 mEq/liter. The patient's increased level represents hyperkalemia caused by the release of potassium from multiple crushed cells.

Nursing process step: Evaluation

Cognitive level: Analysis

20. The patient's blood urea nitrogen (BUN) level has increased from 20 mg/dl to 50 mg/dl. What is the most likely explanation for the patient's electrolyte disturbance?

A. Hemorrhage within the kidney

B. Hypovolemia and catabolism

C. Decreased perfusion caused by heart failure

D. Clot within the kidney

CORRECT ANSWER—B. Elevated BUN occurs in renal disease, reduced renal blood flow (such as in dehydration), urinary tract obstruction, and increased protein metabolism. Hypovolemia and the catabolic state of this trauma victim are the most likely reasons for the prerenal failure exhibited by this patient. Hemorrhage would cause renewed hematuria but would not increase the BUN level. Heart failure is unlikely in a 21-year-old patient, and the available data do not support this explanation. A clot within the kidney could cause postrenal failure and an increase in BUN; however, pain usually accompanies this process.

Nursing process step: Planning

Cognitive level: Analysis

21. Which ECG change would indicate hyperkalemia?

A. Peaked T waves
B. Tachycardia
C. Premature ventricular contractions
D. Shortened QT interval

CORRECT ANSWER—A. Peaked T waves indicate hyperkalemia. Additional findings might include a widened QRS complex, short or absent P waves, and bradycardia. Tachycardia can result from various physiologic conditions, including fever and anxiety. Premature ventricular contractions are more likely to occur in patients with hypokalemia. A shortened QT interval may indicate hypercalcemia.
Nursing process step: Assessment
Cognitive level: Comprehension

22. Which treatment would be appropriate for the patient's hyperkalemia?

A. Increasing I.V. fluids
B. Administering 20 mg furosemide I.V.
C. Starting dialysis
D. Administering sodium polystyrene sulfonate (Kayexalate)

CORRECT ANSWER—D. Sodium polystyrene sulfonate, a sodium exchange resin that acts in the GI tract, helps promote potassium loss. Increasing I.V. fluids would not be as effective in clearing the excess potassium. A diuretic, such as furosemide, would lead to hypovolemia, which should be avoided in a patient with renal trauma. Dialysis is unnecessary unless more conservative treatments, such Kayexalate, do not work or cannot be used. Another conservative approach is dextrose 50% in water with insulin, which would move the potassium intercellularly and temporarily reduce the elevated and potentially lethal potassium level.
Nursing process step: Implementation
Cognitive level: Application

23. On the second postoperative day, the patient's blood urea nitrogen (BUN) level is 35 mg/dl and serum creatinine level is 1.0 mg/dl. His urine output drops to 20 ml/hour and remains slightly pink. His heart rate is 110 beats/minute with sinus tachycardia and his blood pressure is 100/80 mm Hg. His lungs are clear. He has no additional pain aside from incisional pain. His hemoglobin level is 10 g/dl. What condition does this represent?

A. Prerenal failure
B. Intrarenal failure
C. Postrenal failure
D. Renal contusion

CORRECT ANSWER—A. Normal BUN level is 10 to 20 mg/dl, and normal serum creatinine level in men ranges from 0.8 to 1.2 mg/dl. An increase in BUN with a normal creatinine resulting in a BUN:creatinine ratio greater than 20:1 indicates prerenal failure. Intrarenal failure elevates both BUN and serum creatinine levels because of a decreased glomerular filtration rate. Postrenal failure resulting from obstruction is associated with no urine output. Renal contusion alone would not raise the BUN or serum creatinine level.
Nursing process step: Assessment
Cognitive level: Evaluation

24. Which of the following is the treatment of choice for correcting the patient's hypovolemia?
   A. Dialysis
   B. Colloid solutions
   C. Blood products
   D. Crystalloid solutions

CORRECT ANSWER—D. Crystalloid solutions, especially 0.9% sodium chloride or lactated Ringer's solution, are the treatment of choice for hypovolemia. Dialysis would be used in intrarenal failure when the blood urea nitrogen approaches 100 mg/dl with a concurrent rise in creatinine. Colloid solutions usually are not used for hypovolemia because of their expense and the effectiveness of crystalloid solutions. Blood products are reserved for treating significant decreases in hemoglobin.
Nursing process step: Implementation
Cognitive level: Comprehension

25. The patient receives 2 liters of 0.9% sodium chloride solution over 8 hours. Which finding would be *least* helpful in evaluating the effectiveness of therapy?
   A. Urine output of 35 ml/hour
   B. Serum creatinine less than 1.0 mg/dl
   C. Blood urea nitrogen (BUN) of 18 mg/dl
   D. Decrease in amount of hematuria

CORRECT ANSWER—D. The degree of hematuria is least helpful in evaluating improvement in a patient with prerenal failure. Urine output should increase to more than 30 ml/hour, the serum creatinine level should remain below 1.0 mg/dl, and the BUN level should decrease to less than 20 mg/dl as perfusion of the kidney increases as a result of increased intravascular volume.
Nursing process step: Evaluation
Cognitive level: Evaluation

26. Which of the following would *not* cause hypernatremia?
   A. Hypotonic solution
   B. Potassium level of 2.5 mEq/liter
   C. Diabetes insipidus
   D. Loop diuretics

CORRECT ANSWER—D. Loop diuretics inhibit sodium and chloride retention in the renal tubules and inhibit sodium and chloride reabsorption in the proximal tubules, thus leading to hyponatremia. Hypotonic solutions, hypokalemia, and diabetes insipidus are potential precipitating factors for hypernatremia.
Nursing process step: Assessment
Cognitive level: Comprehension

27. Which nursing measure would be appropriate for treating hypernatremia?
   A. Administering a hypotonic solution or diuretics
   B. Administering diuretics or restricting water intake
   C. Replacing free water or initiating dialysis
   D. Restricting free water or initiating dialysis

CORRECT ANSWER—A. A hypotonic solution can be used to treat hypernatremia resulting from excessive water loss; diuretics are used to prevent sodium retention. Restricting free water would increase hypernatremia. Dialysis usually is not necessary because the other measures are effective.
Nursing process step: Implementation
Cognitive level: Application

28. Which patient is at *least* risk for hypocalcemia?
A. 45-year-old patient who underwent thyroidectomy
B. 55-year-old patient with acute pancreatitis
C. 65-year-old patient with coronary artery disease
D. 30-year-old patient with acute renal failure

CORRECT ANSWER—C. Coronary artery disease does not predispose a patient to calcium imbalances. A 45-year-old post-thyroidectomy patient should be observed for hypocalcemia; the parathyroid glands, which are responsible for regulating calcium and phosphate, may have been removed during surgery. A patient with acute pancreatitis may experience hypocalcemia secondary to precipitation of calcium in the inflamed pancreas. Because of decreased excretion of phosphate, patients in acute renal failure experience hyperphosphatemia, which leads to reciprocal hypocalcemia.
Nursing process step: Assessment
Cognitive level: Analysis

29. Which intervention is *not* appropriate for a patient with a serum magnesium level of 3.0 mEq/liter?
A. Avoiding magnesium-containing laxatives and antacids
B. Inducing diuresis to promote magnesium loss if no evidence of renal failure exists
C. Monitoring the ECG for peaked T waves
D. Using sorbitol to promote loss of magnesium via bowel evacuation

CORRECT ANSWER—D. A serum magnesium level of 3.0 mEq/liter indicates hypermagnesemia; normal serum magnesium level is 1.5 to 2.5 mEq/liter. Because magnesium is excreted via the kidneys, administration of a laxative would not cause magnesium loss. Avoiding magnesium-containing medications, inducing diuresis, and monitoring for peaked T waves are appropriate interventions for hypermagnesemia.
Nursing process step: Implementation
Cognitive level: Application

30. A 55-year-old alcoholic patient has arrived at the emergency department; he is confused and is having seizures. His laboratory values reveal a serum magnesium level of 0.8 mEq/liter and a serum potassium level of 3.8 mEq/liter. Which nursing intervention is *not* appropriate given these data?
A. Monitoring for prolonged QT interval
B. Correcting the magnesium level before correcting the potassium level
C. Restricting intake of magnesium-containing antacids and laxatives
D. Administering magnesium supplements intravenously

CORRECT ANSWER—C. A magnesium level of 0.8 mEq/liter indicates hypomagnesemia related to decreased intake and absorption in the alcoholic patient. Magnesium-containing medications should not be restricted because they may help increase the magnesium level. Prolonged QT intervals are associated with hypomagnesemia and should be monitored during therapy. If hypokalemia exists along with hypomagnesemia, the magnesium level should be corrected first. The low level of magnesium should be corrected rapidly through intravenous means to prevent the cardiovascular and neurologic problems associated with hypomagnesemia.
Nursing process step: Implementation
Cognitive level: Application

Questions 31 to 34 refer to the following information:
A 72-year-old male patient arrives at the emergency department with his wife, who states that her husband has been increasingly confused over the last several days and has not eaten or voided in the last 24 hours. His vital signs are temperature, 102° F (38.9° C); heart rate, 130 beats/minute and irregular; respirations, 10 breaths/minute and deep; and blood pressure, 90/60 mm Hg while supine and 60/60 mm Hg while sitting. Laboratory values include serum sodium, 110 mg/dl; serum chloride, 79 mg/dl; serum potassium, 3.0 mEq/liter; and serum glucose, 520 mg/dl. The patient's peripheral pulses are not palpable. His oral cavity is dry and his tongue is furrowed. His pupils are equal and reactive to light. All muscle responses are present but dulled. His arterial blood gas values are pH, 7.08; partial pressure of oxygen in arterial blood (PaO_2), 60 mm Hg; $PaCO_2$, 32 mm Hg; and HCO_3^-, 13 mEq/liter.

31. The patient's ECG shows sinus tachycardia with frequent premature ventricular contractions (PVCs). The most likely explanation for this is:
A. Dehydration, fever, and hypokalemia
B. Heart failure and hyponatremia
C. Dehydration, hypernatremia, and hyperglycemia
D. Sepsis and hyponatremia

CORRECT ANSWER—A. The sinus tachycardia is directly related to hypovolemia as the heart attempts to maintain an adequate cardiac output. The PVCs are related to hypokalemia. The patient's blood pressure changes, decreased pulses, dry tongue, glucose level, and metabolic acidosis (evidenced by pH and HCO_3^- level) are indicative of diabetic ketoacidosis. There is no evidence of heart failure in this patient, whose lungs are clear. Hyponatremia, hypernatremia, and hyperglycemia have no direct effect on the heart's conduction system.
Nursing process step: Assessment
Cognitive level: Analysis

32. All of the following nursing actions would be appropriate during treatment of the patient's electrolyte imbalances *except:*
A. Monitoring the ECG during potassium correction
B. Taking measures to correct hyponatremia over several days
C. Monitoring potassium level frequently as the acidosis is corrected
D. Administering calcium to antagonize the effect of potassium on the heart

CORRECT ANSWER—D. Calcium is used to stimulate the heart in a patient with hyperkalemia. This patient has hypokalemia, for which ECG monitoring is appropriate to detect rhythms related to potassium repletion. As acidosis is corrected, additional potassium will be lost as potassium enters the cell in exchange for hydrogen ions. Therefore, frequent checks of the potassium level are important. Hyponatremia should be corrected over several days to prevent cerebral edema.
Nursing process step: Implementation
Cognitive level: Application

33. Which finding would alert the nurse to the need for caution during continued potassium replacement?
  A. Blood pressure of 100/60 mm Hg
  B. Blood urea nitrogen (BUN) of 40 mg/dl
  C. Urine output of 10 ml/hour
  D. Arterial pH of 7.32

CORRECT ANSWER—C. A urine output that remains low after vigorous fluid and potassium replacement have been initiated may reflect intrinsic renal damage. If urine output is only 10 ml/hour, potassium should be replaced cautiously to prevent hyperkalemia until the output increases. Blood pressure has no direct effect on potassium repletion. A BUN level of 40 mg/dl must be evaluated in relation to the serum creatinine level to diagnose acute renal failure; if the serum creatinine value is low with a BUN of 40 mg/dl, the patient may be experiencing prerenal failure secondary to hypovolemia. An arterial pH of 7.32 indicates partial correction of the acidosis and a decreasing need for potassium replacement.
Nursing process step: Implementation
Cognitive level: Evaluation

34. Which body system exhibits the most signs and symptoms of hyponatremia?
  A. Renal system
  B. Cardiac system
  C. Central nervous system
  D. Peripheral vascular system

CORRECT ANSWER—C. The central nervous system manifests most signs and symptoms of hyponatremia, which can include altered level of consciousness (ranging from confusion to coma), headache, muscle weakness, and seizures. These signs and symptoms are life-threatening components of hyponatremia. In the renal system, hyponatremia can cause alterations in the urine sodium level, which probably will be less than 20 mEq/liter. In the cardiac system, hyponatremia can cause changes in central venous pressure and jugular venous pressure, depending on whether the imbalance is accompanied by fluid volume excess or fluid volume deficit. The peripheral vascular system is not affected by hyponatremia.
Nursing process step: Assessment
Cognitive level: Analysis

35. A patient arrives in the emergency department in acute renal failure with oliguria. Which value is *most* helpful in differentiating prerenal failure from intrarenal failure?
   A. Blood urea nitrogen (BUN) of 33 mEq/dl
   B. Urine sodium of 8 mEq/dl
   C. Blood pressure of 120/80 mm Hg
   D. Urine specific gravity of 1.010

CORRECT ANSWER—B. The urine sodium level is most helpful in determining whether the new onset of oliguria is caused by prerenal failure or intrarenal failure. In prerenal failure, the urine sodium level is less than 10 mEq/liter as the kidneys attempt to retain sodium and fluid to correct hypoperfusion. In intrarenal failure, the urine sodium level ranges from 40 to 80 mEq/liter as the nephrons lose the ability to hold sodium because of tubular damage. The BUN and serum creatinine levels increase with either type of renal failure, although the BUN level can increase secondary to other causes, such as blood in the GI tract. Therefore, the BUN value should be viewed in relation to serum creatinine level. Blood pressure changes are not necessarily related to prerenal or intrarenal failure. Urine specific gravity may be helpful because concentrated urine is more likely to be seen in prerenal failure, whereas a urine specific gravity of 1.010 to 1.020 is found consistently in intrarenal failure.
Nursing process step: Evaluation
Cognitive level: Evaluation

36. A patient in acute renal failure with a phosphate level of 5.5 mg/dl and a calcium level of 7 mg/dl should be treated with:
   A. I.V. calcium
   B. Oral aluminum hydroxide gels
   C. I.V. phosphate
   D. Oral phosphate

CORRECT ANSWER—B. A phosphate level of 5.5 mg/dl indicates hyperphosphatemia; normal phosphate level is 3.0 to 4.5 mg/dl. Oral aluminum hydroxide gels bind phosphate in the intestines, thereby decreasing absorption and lowering the phosphate level. As a reciprocal relationship between the calcium and phosphate levels exists, lowering the phosphate level will allow calcium to rise to normal value (8.9 to 10 mg/dl). Administration of I.V. calcium should not be necessary in this case. Because I.V. calcium can trigger arrhythmias, this treatment is used to correct a high phosphate level only when a life-threatening calcium level is present. I.V. and oral phosphates are used to treat hypophosphatemia.
Nursing process step: Implementation
Cognitive level: Application

37. A patient with hypocalcemia will have ECG changes. Which of the following ECG changes would indicate the effectiveness of treatment for hypocalcemia?
  A. Shortened ST segment and QT interval
  B. Shortened PR and QT intervals
  C. Prolonged QT interval and premature ventricular contractions (PVCs)
  D. Shortened QT interval and PVCs

CORRECT ANSWER—A. A prolonged ST segment and QT interval are associated with calcium level below 8.5 mg/dl. Hypocalcemia does not cause premature ventricular contractions or shortened QT or PR intervals.
Nursing process step: Planning
Cognitive level: Comprehension

38. The nurse is planning to administer a sodium polystyrene sulfonate (Kayexalate) enema to a patient with a potassium level of 5.9 mEq/liter. Correct administration and the effects of this enema would include:
  A. Having the patient retain the enema for 30 minutes to allow for sodium exchange; afterward, the patient should have diarrhea
  B. Having the patient retain the enema for 30 minutes to allow for glucose exchange; afterward, the patient should have diarrhea
  C. Having the patient retain the enema for 60 minutes to allow for sodium exchange; diarrhea is not necessary to reduce the potassium level
  D. Having the patient retain the enema for 60 minutes to allow for glucose exchange; diarrhea is not necessary to reduce the potassium level

CORRECT ANSWER—A. Kayexalate is a sodium exchange resin. Thus the patient will gain sodium as potassium is lost in the bowel. For the exchange to occur, Kayexalate must be in contact with the bowel for at least 30 minutes. Sorbitol in the Kayexalate enema causes diarrhea, which increases potassium loss and decreases the potential for Kayexalate retention.
Nursing process step: Planning
Cognitive level: Comprehension

39. Which electrolyte imbalance will not enhance the effects of digitalis glycosides and cause arrhythmias indicative of digitalis toxicity?
  A. Hypomagnesemia
  B. Hypercalcemia
  C. Hypocalcemia
  D. Hypokalemia

CORRECT ANSWER—C. Hypocalcemia is not associated with digitalis toxicity. Low serum magnesium level, high serum calcium level, and low serum potassium level are associated with arrhythmias related to digitalis toxicity.
Nursing process step: Assessment
Cognitive level: Comprehension

Questions 40 to 47 refer to the following information:
A 68-year-old male patient is admitted to the hospital with a 2-week history of nocturia, urinary hesitancy and dribbling, and straining during urination. For the past 2 days, he has complained of malaise, anorexia, and nausea. Bilateral flank pain recently developed. His admitting laboratory values include:
  • blood urea nitrogen (BUN), 180 mg/dl
  • serum creatinine, 11 mg/dl
  • serum sodium, 130 mEq/liter
  • serum potassium, 6 mEq/liter
  • serum calcium, 7 mg/dl
  • white blood cell count, 12/mm^3.

Vital signs are temperature, 98.6° F (37° C); heart rate, 90 beats/minute and irregular with an S_3 gallop; respirations, 26 breaths/minute and deep; and blood pressure, 160/90 mm Hg. Arterial blood gas values include pH, 7.25; $PaCO_2$, 30 mm Hg; PaO_2, 65 mm Hg; and HCO_3^-, 16 mEq/liter.

---

40. The patient's arterial blood gas values are indicative of which process?
A. Respiratory alkalosis resulting from hypoxia
B. Metabolic acidosis resulting from excess organic acids
C. Respiratory acidosis resulting from hypoventilation
D. Metabolic alkalosis resulting from excess bicarbonate

CORRECT ANSWER—B. Metabolic acidosis resulting from excess organic acids that are not being excreted by the damaged kidney is the typical acid-base disturbance seen in acute renal failure. A pH less than 7.35 and a bicarbonate value less than 22 mEq/liter are signs of metabolic acidosis. The patient's carbon dioxide is low because his respiratory system is attempting to compensate for the excess acid by eliminating carbon dioxide. Metabolic alkalosis is characterized by a pH greater than 7.35 and a bicarbonate value greater than 26 mEq/liter. Respiratory alkalosis is indicated by a pH greater than 7.35 and a PaCO2 less than 35 mm Hg. Respiratory acidosis manifests as a pH less than 7.35 and a PaCO2 greater than 45 mm Hg.
Nursing process step: Implementation
Cognitive level: Application

41. The patient requires hemodialysis. Which of the following drugs should be withheld before this procedure?
A. Phosphate binders
B. Insulin
C. Antibiotics
D. Digoxin

CORRECT ANSWER—D. Digoxin should be withheld before hemodialysis. Hypokalemia is one of the electrolyte shifts that occur during dialysis, and a hypokalemic patient is at risk for arrhythmias secondary to digitalis toxicity. Phosphate binders and insulin can be administered because they are not removed from the blood by dialysis. Some antibiotics are removed by dialysis and should be administered after the procedure to ensure their therapeutic effects. The nurse should check a formulary to determine if a particular antibiotic should be administered before or after dialysis.
Nursing process step: Implementation
Cognitive level: Comprehension

42. The dosage of which drug does not need to be adjusted in a patient with acute renal failure?
A. Digoxin
B. Vancomycin hydrochloride
C. Acetaminophen
D. Cimetidine

CORRECT ANSWER—**C.** Because acetaminophen is metabolized in the liver, adjustments in dosage are not necessary in a patient with acute renal failure. Digoxin and cimetidine are excreted by the kidneys, and dosage should be adjusted. Dosage for vancomycin should be adjusted according to serum peak and trough levels of the drug because high and potentially toxic serum concentrations of vancomycin can occur in patients with renal insufficiency.
Nursing process step: Implementation
Cognitive level: Comprehension

43. Because of difficulties with hemodialysis, peritoneal dialysis is initiated to treat the patient's uremia. Which finding signals a significant problem during this procedure?
A. Blood glucose level of 200 mg/dl
B. White blood cell count of 20,000/mm^3
C. Potassium level of 3.5 mEq/liter
D. Hematocrit of 35%

CORRECT ANSWER—**B.** An increased white blood cell count indicates infection, probably resulting from peritonitis, which may have been caused by insertion of the peritoneal catheter into the peritoneal cavity. Peritonitis can cause the peritoneal membrane to lose its ability to filter solutes; therefore, peritoneal dialysis would no longer be a treatment option for this patient. Hyperglycemia occurs during peritoneal dialysis because of the high glucose content of the dialysate; it is readily treatable with sliding-scale insulin. A potassium level of 3.5 mEq/liter can be treated by adding potassium to the dialysate solution. A hematocrit of 35% is lower than normal. However, in this patient, the value is not abnormally low because of the daily blood samplings. A lower hematocrit is common in patients with chronic renal failure because of the lack of erythropoietin.
Nursing process step: Assessment
Cognitive level: Evaluation

44. Which symptom is associated with peritonitis?
A. Blood-tinged dialysate outflow with abdominal pain
B. Brown dialysate outflow with an urge to move the bowels
C. Amber dialysate outflow with urinary incontinence
D. Cloudy dialysate outflow with abdominal pain

CORRECT ANSWER—**D.** Cloudy dialysate outflow with abdominal pain indicates peritonitis. Blood-tinged outflow may indicate abdominal bleeding or uremic coagulopathy. Brown outflow is associated with bowel perforation and usually occurs in the first exchange of dialysate fluid. Amber outflow is a sign of bladder perforation and occurs during the first exchange of dialysate fluid.
Nursing process step: Implementation
Cognitive level: Comprehension

45. The patient develops sepsis and is hypotensive. His blood urea nitrogen (BUN) continues to increase during peritoneal dialysis. Continuous arteriovenous hemodialysis (CAVHD) is initiated via large-bore catheters in the femoral artery and in the femoral vein. Which statement would best explain this form of dialysis to the patient and his family?

A. "CAVHD combines the properties of diffusion with convection to remove creatinine, urea, and body water."

B. "CAVHD removes extra water and body wastes faster than peritoneal dialysis without causing the blood pressure changes associated with hemodialysis."

C. "CAVHD removes extra water and body wastes better than peritoneal dialysis and hemodialysis."

D. "CAVHD uses an external filter, which works like the kidney to replace substances lost by the body during peritoneal dialysis and hemodialysis."

CORRECT ANSWER—B. Option B correctly identifies the properties of CAVHD in language appropriate for the layperson. Option A uses terminology inappropriate for a patient and family members, although it correctly describes the CAVHD process. Option C is incorrect because hemodialysis is the most effective form of dialysis. Option D is incorrect because the purpose of CAVHD is to remove substances, not replace them.
Nursing process step: Implementation
Cognitive level: Synthesis

46. The nurse would plan to use which fluid as the dialysate in CAVHD?

A. Peritoneal dialysate fluid
B. Lactated Ringer's solution with bicarbonate
C. 0.9% sodium chloride solution with bicarbonate
D. Lactated Ringer's solution

CORRECT ANSWER—A. Peritoneal dialysate fluid is used to promote diffusion across the hemofilter. Lactated Ringer's and 0.9% sodium chloride solutions do not contain glucose, the osmotic agent that leads to diffusion.
Nursing process step: Planning
Cognitive level: Application

47. The patient's hypotension resolves after treatment with appropriate antibiotics. Continuous arteriovenous hemodialysis (CAVHD) continues for 1 week, after which the patient begins the diuretic phase of intrarenal failure. What should the nurse tell the patient's wife regarding CAVHD?

A. "CAVHD will end when the wastes in the blood decrease to safe levels; even though your husband is producing urine, his kidneys are readjusting to their normal way of filtering wastes."

B. "CAVHD will end when the osmotic diuretic effect of urea ends; recovery could take several months."

C. "CAVHD will end now because your husband can produce urine; the wastes in his blood will decrease from now on. "

D. "CAVHD will be continued indefinitely because your husband's kidneys are damaged for life."

CORRECT ANSWER—A. The diuretic phase of acute intrarenal failure signals the beginning of the return of renal function. Although massive quantities of water are excreted, blood urea nitrogen (BUN) and serum creatinine levels may continue to increase for several days as the kidneys regain their ability to effectively filter these waste products. CAVHD may need to continue until the BUN and creatinine levels decrease and remain below acceptable levels on consecutive days. Option B is incorrect because the terminology is inappropriate for a layperson; also, the diuretic effect continues for several days to weeks, not months. Option C is incorrect because even though the patient is producing urine, the BUN and creatinine levels may continue to rise; these waste products must cleared by dialysis until the values stay below acceptable levels on consecutive days. Option D is incorrect because the kidneys may regain full or partial function, and CAVHD may not necessarily be required.
Nursing process step: Implementation
Cognitive level: Synthesis

48. Which action is *not* appropriate during correction of hypocalcemia?
A. Monitoring for decreased cardiac output
B. Implementing seizure precautions
C. Administering I.V. calcium gluconate or calcium chloride rapidly at a rate of 10 ml/minute
D. Monitoring for Chvostek's and Trousseau's signs

CORRECT ANSWER—C. Calcium gluconate or calcium chloride should be administered slowly over 1 ml/minute, not 10 ml/minute. Decreased cardiac output and seizures are potential complications of hypocalcemia. Chvostek's and Trousseau's signs are positive in a patient with hypocalcemia and should be used to evaluate the effectiveness of therapy.
Nursing process step: Implementation
Cognitive level: Evaluation

49. Which problem can develop as a result of too-rapid correction of hypernatremia?
A. Pulmonary edema
B. Cerebral edema
C. Arrhythmias
D. Renal failure

CORRECT ANSWER—B. Cerebral edema can occur when hypernatremia is corrected, as water moves into cerebral cells because of increased amounts of sodium in the brain cells. Slow correction of hypernatremia allows sodium to equilibrate between the vascular space and the brain cells. Pulmonary edema, arrhythmias, and renal failure are not associated with correction of hypernatremia.
Nursing process step: Implementation
Cognitive level: Comprehension

50. Which laboratory data would be expected for a patient with intrarenal failure whose oliguria was corrected?
A. Urine output greater than 60 ml/hour, blood urea nitrogen less than 100 mg/dl
B. Urine output greater than 50 ml/hour, serum creatinine less than 10 mg/dl
C. Urine output greater than 40 ml/hour, diastolic blood pressure less than 90 mm Hg
D. Urine output greater than 30 ml/hour, weight stable

CORRECT ANSWER—D. The nonoliguric phase of renal failure is characterized by a urine output greater than 30 ml/hour with minimal weight gain. To achieve this goal of therapy, diuretics and low-dosage dopamine are administered; these agents cause renal vessel dilation and increase blood flow to the kidneys. The nonoliguric phase of intrarenal failure is associated with improved patient outcome. Blood urea nitrogen and creatinine levels may continue to increase in nonoliguric intrarenal failure. Lowering blood pressure is not associated with conversion of oliguric to nonoliguric intrarenal failure.
Nursing process step: Evaluation
Cognitive level: Evaluation

51. Which of the following are appropriate evaluation criteria for a patient with an initial phosphate level of 2.5 mg/dl?
A. Phosphate level of 1.0 mg/dl, absence of muscle weakness
B. Phosphate level of 3.0 mg/dl, absence of cardiac arrhythmias
C. Phosphate level of 3.0 mg/dl, absence of muscle weakness
D. Phosphate level of 1.0 mg/dl, absence of cardiac arrhythmias

CORRECT ANSWER—C. A phosphate level of 2.5 mg/dl indicates hypophosphatemia; normal phosphate level is 3.0 to 4.5 mg/dl. Evaluation criteria would include achieving a phosphate level of 3.0 mg/dl and the absence of symptoms associated with hypophosphatemia, which include muscle weakness but not arrhythmias.
Nursing process step: Evaluation
Cognitive level: Analysis

52. Which of the following values for urine creatinine is normal for a 24-hour collection?
A. 1 g
B. 0.5 g
C. 0.25 g
D. 0.125 g

CORRECT ANSWER—A. For an average-sized person, 1 g of creatinine in the urine is the normal amount in a 24-hour collection. A value of less than 1 g/day indicates an inability of the renal system to filter wastes.
Nursing process step: Assessment
Cognitive level: Knowledge

53. Which findings would indicate a successful outcome of therapy for hypercalcemia?

A. Calcium 10.5 mg/dl, ECG with heart block, and patient is awake and alert

B. Calcium 11 mg/dl, ECG with premature atrial contractions, and patient is lethargic but oriented

C. Calcium 10.5 mg/dl, ECG with premature atrial contractions, and patient is awake and alert

D. Calcium 12 mg/dl, ECG with heart block, and patient is lethargic and confused

CORRECT ANSWER—**C.** A calcium level of 10.5 mg/dl is the upper limit of normal; normal serum calcium level ranges from 8.5 to 10.5 mg/dl, or 4.0 to 5.5 mEq/liter. Calcium causes excitation and contraction of cardiac muscle. In a patient with hypercalcemia, the nurse would initially observe a shortened QT interval and tachycardia, and, eventually, bradycardia and cardiac arrest. As hypercalcemia is corrected, the nurse may observe cardiac irritability as represented by premature atrial contractions; these usually are not treated unless there is a subsequent decrease in cardiovascular stability. Neuromuscular involvement in a patient with hypercalcemia includes changes in level of consciousness, lethargy, and muscle weakness.
Nursing process step: Evaluation
Cognitive level: Evaluation

54. Which statement best describes the therapeutic action of loop diuretics?

A. They block reabsorption of potassium in the collecting tubule

B. They promote sodium secretion into the distal tubule

C. They block sodium reabsorption in the ascending loop and dilate renal vessels

D. They promote potassium secretion into the distal tubule and constrict renal vessels

CORRECT ANSWER—**C.** Loop diuretics block sodium reabsorption in the ascending loop of Henle, which promotes water diuresis. They also dilate renal vessels. Loop diuretics block potassium reabsorption, but this is not a therapeutic effect. Thiazide diuretics promote sodium secretion into the distal tubule.
Nursing process step: Implementation
Cognitive level: Comprehension

55. Which of the following antihypertensive drugs is a sympathetic blocker?

A. Nitroprusside sodium

B. Minoxidil

C. Hydralazine hydrochloride

D. Clonidine hydrochloride

CORRECT ANSWER—**D.** Clonidine acts in the central nervous system to block the sympathetic response of hypertension. Nitroprusside, minoxidil, and hydralazine are direct vasodilators.
Nursing process step: Implementation
Cognitive level: Comprehension

56. Which arrhythmia would be the final rhythm to occur if hyperkalemia is not treated?
A. Ventricular fibrillation
B. Junctional rhythm
C. Asystole
D. Bradycardia

CORRECT ANSWER—**C.** Asystole is the final rhythm in progressive hyperkalemia. This arrhythmia usually occurs at a potassium level of 7 mEq/liter or higher and depends on how rapidly hyperkalemia develops. Junctional rhythm and bradycardia can occur when the potassium level progressively increases; however, asystole would be the final rhythm seen. Ventricular fibrillation is an uncommon rhythm in hyperkalemia because potassium exerts a depressant effect on the conduction system.
Nursing process step: Assessment
Cognitive level: Comprehension

57. Which body system most commonly is affected in patients with electrolyte imbalances?
A. Cardiovascular system
B. Neuromuscular system
C. Renal system
D. Endocrine system

CORRECT ANSWER—**B.** The neuromuscular system is extremely sensitive to changes in electrolyte balance and therefore is most commonly affected. Whether it involves changes in level of consciousness (as with sodium) or changes in muscle functioning (as with potassium and calcium), the neuromuscular system serves as a warning system to the nurse to assess electrolyte levels.
Nursing process step: Assessment
Cognitive level: Comprehension

58. Which is the most appropriate method of monitoring access sites in a patient undergoing continuous arteriovenous hemodialysis (CAVHD)?
A. Check proximal pulses and monitor for bleeding and swelling at the arterial and venous sites every hour
B. Check proximal pulses and monitor for bleeding and swelling at the catheter site every hour
C. Check distal pulses and monitor for bleeding and swelling at the arterial and venous sites every hour
D. Check distal pulses and monitor for bleeding and swelling at the catheter site every hour

CORRECT ANSWER—**C.** Distal pulses should be checked every hour to ensure that circulation to the legs is not impeded. Proximal pulses provide no information about circulation affected by the catheters. Two catheters are used in CAVHD—an arterial and a venous access catheter. Blood fills the filter from the arterial catheter and returns via the venous catheter. Consequently, both catheter sites should be checked for bleeding and swelling throughout the CAVHD process.
Nursing process step: Implementation
Cognitive level: Application

59. A 47-year-old patient with chronic renal failure is admitted to the intensive care unit with a blood pressure of 190/110 mm Hg. The admitting nurse is aware that, besides hypertension, a patient with renal failure is susceptible to all of the following complications *except:*

A. Metabolic acidosis
B. Anemia
C. Respiratory alkalosis
D. Esophagitis

CORRECT ANSWER—C. A patient with chronic renal failure experiences many physiologic body system changes. Metabolic acidosis occurs because of the elevated concentration of hydrogen ions and decreased pH. The serum bicarbonate level decreases as the body tries unsuccessfully to compensate for metabolic acidosis. Although the patient may hyperventilate to compensate for the low pH, the primary acid-base disturbance is metabolic acidosis, not respiratory alkalosis. Anemia results from bone marrow suppression and decreased level of erythropoietin. Gastritis and esophagitis are caused by the accumulation of waste products resulting from chronic renal failure.
Nursing process step: Assessment
Cognitive level: Comprehension

60. The nurse is caring for a male patient undergoing peritoneal dialysis. He is 20 kg heavier than he was preoperatively; this weight gain is secondary to massive fluid resuscitation related to excessive blood loss during surgery. The physician orders exchanges of 4.25% dialysate solution alternated with 1 liter of 2.5% dialysate solution every 2 hours. The nurse will need to monitor for which of the following potential complications that may be caused by this dialysate regimen?

A. Hypervolemia and hypoglycemia
B. Hypovolemia and hypoglycemia
C. Hypervolemia and hyperglycemia
D. Hypovolemia and hyperglycemia

CORRECT ANSWER—D. Because of the high concentration of glucose in the dialysate, this patient may become hyperglycemic. This complication can be treated by adding regular insulin to the dialysate before administration or by administering sliding-scale regular insulin to control the glucose level; for either treatment, the patient's glucose level must be monitored closely. The high concentration of dialysate fluid will remove more fluid from the patient, placing him at risk for intravascular dehydration and hypovolemia. The patient's intake and output must be assessed every 2 hours to check for this potential complication.
Nursing process step: Evaluation
Cognitive level: Analysis

61. Peritoneal fluid specimens from a patient receiving peritoneal dialysis are obtained every 8 hours and sent to the laboratory for analysis. The nurse would consider all of the following findings normal *except:*

A. Odorless fluid
B. Glucose level between 70 and 100 mg/dl
C. Clear, pale yellow fluid
D. White blood cell count less than 600/µliter

CORRECT ANSWER—D. A white blood cell count greater than 300/µliter in peritoneal fluid as well as a cloudy, turbid, or foul-smelling peritoneal fluid specimen may indicate peritonitis. A glucose level of 70 to 100 mg/dl is considered a normal finding.
Nursing process step: Evaluation
Cognitive level: Analysis

62. Which of the following statements is correct regarding the hematopoietic effects of acute renal failure?
A. Decreased red blood cell count
B. Increased white blood cell count
C. Decreased platelet count
D. Increased erythropoietin production

CORRECT ANSWER—**A.** Acute renal failure causes decreased production of erythropoietin, which is produced by the kidneys. A decrease in erythropoietin leads to a decrease in red blood cell production. The decreased red blood cell count contributes to the patient's anemic state; hemodialysis, which causes a decreased red blood cell life span as well as the loss of red blood cells, also contributes to the patient's anemic state. In a patient in acute renal failure, platelets become dysfunctional secondary to the uremic toxins present in the blood; however, they are not necessarily decreased in number. Dysfunctional platelets contribute to bleeding tendencies in this patient. A patient in acute renal failure is in an immunocompromised state and is prone to infection. An increased white blood cell count may occur secondary to the patient's immunocompromised state, not secondary to acute renal failure.
Nursing process step: Comprehension
Cognitive level: Analysis

GASTROINTESTINAL SYSTEM

CHAPTER 5

Gastrointestinal System

Questions 1 to 5 refer to the following information:
A 72-year-old male patient develops acute upper GI bleeding. He is admitted to the intensive care unit after having vomited 550 ml of bloody fluid. He has a history of osteoarthritis and has been taking 10 aspirins a day for pain relief.

1. Which diagnostic test would be used first to evaluate a patient with upper GI bleeding?
   A. Endoscopy
   B. Upper GI series
   C. Hemoglobin and hematocrit values
   D. Arteriography

CORRECT ANSWER—A. Endoscopy permits direct evaluation of the upper GI tract and can detect 90% of bleeding lesions. An upper GI series, or barium study, usually is not the diagnostic method of choice, especially in a patient with acute active bleeding who is vomiting and unstable. An upper GI series also is less accurate than endoscopy. Although an upper GI series might confirm the presence of a lesion, it would not necessarily reveal whether the lesion is bleeding. Hemoglobin and hematocrit values, which indicate loss of blood volume, are not always reliable indicators of GI bleeding because a decrease in these values may not be seen for several hours. Arteriography is an invasive study associated with life-threatening complications and would not be used for an initial evaluation.
Nursing process step: Assessment
Cognitive level: Comprehension

2. What would be the earliest sign exhibited by this patient in response to the acute loss of blood?
   A. Hypotension
   B. Pallor
   C. Cool, clammy skin
   D. Tachycardia

CORRECT ANSWER—D. Hypotension, pallor, cool and clammy skin, and tachycardia are all signs of hypovolemia resulting from acute GI bleeding. However, tachycardia is the earliest manifestation of hypovolemia; the other signs would occur later.
Nursing process step: Assessment
Cognitive level: Comprehension

3. In planning the patient's care, the nurse's primary concern would be to:
A. Control bleeding
B. Replace fluids
C. Increase gastric pH
D. Assist with diagnostic studies

CORRECT ANSWER—B. Fluid replacement to maintain homeostasis and to prevent shock is the primary nursing objective. Identifying the source of bleeding through diagnostic studies would be the next step. This would be followed by interventions to control the bleeding lesion and prevent further bleeding, such as increasing the gastric pH level.
Nursing process step: Planning
Cognitive level: Analysis

4. The nurse administers famotidine intravenously. This drug achieves its effect by:
A. Neutralizing gastric acid
B. Forming a complex that adheres to the ulcer
C. Blocking histamine receptors
D. Increasing production of gastric mucus

CORRECT ANSWER—C. Famotidine, a histamine$_2$ (H$_2$)-receptor antagonist, inhibits histamine at H$_2$-receptor sites, thereby decreasing gastric secretions. Gastric acids are neutralized by antacids. Protectants, such as sucralfate, cover ulcers with an adherent complex. Prostaglandin E$_1$ analogues, such as misoprostol, inhibit gastric acid secretion and may increase mucus production to protect the gastric mucosa.
Nursing process step: Implementation
Cognitive level: Comprehension

5. The patient has a nasogastric (NG) tube in place, and the physician orders gastric lavage. This is performed for all of the following reasons *except:*
A. Cleansing the stomach for endoscopy
B. Providing an indication of the rate of bleeding
C. Allowing the walls of the stomach to collapse and contribute to hemostasis
D. Providing gastric aspirate for pH testing

CORRECT ANSWER—D. Gastric aspirate would provide no useful information at this time. Because blood is alkaline, its presence in aspirate would cause the gastric pH to be alkaline, thereby negating pH testing, especially if the patient's condition is related to gastric acidity. Cleansing the stomach for endoscopy is accepted practice to allow removal of clots and observation of the lesion. Performing gastric lavage via the NG tube until it is clear provides an indication of the rate of bleeding. Emptying the stomach by removing as many clots and intragastric material as possible allows the walls of the stomach to collapse, thereby contributing to hemostasis.
Nursing process step: Implementation
Cognitive level: Comprehension

6. When evaluating a patient for complications of acute pancreatitis, the nurse would observe for:
A. Increased intracranial pressure
B. Decreased urine output
C. Bradycardia
D. Hypertension

CORRECT ANSWER—**B.** Acute pancreatitis can cause decreased urine output, which results from the renal failure that sometimes accompanies this condition. Intracranial pressure neither increases nor decreases in a patient with pancreatitis. Tachycardia, not bradycardia, usually is associated with pulmonary or hypovolemic complications of pancreatitis. Hypotension can be caused by a hypovolemic complication, but hypertension usually is not related to acute pancreatitis.
Nursing process step: Evaluation
Cognitive level: Evaluation

7. Which risk factors are most commonly associated with acute pancreatitis?
A. Hyperlipidemia and family history of pancreatitis
B. Excessive alcohol intake and biliary tract disease
C. Abdominal trauma and biliary tract disease
D. Excessive alcohol intake and bacterial infection

CORRECT ANSWER—**B.** Alcohol intake and biliary tract disease are associated with 65% to 90% of all cases of pancreatitis. Alcohol directly irritates the pancreas, and biliary tract disease may allow bile reflux, which also irritates the pancreas and causes autodigestion. Hyperlipidemia, family history of pancreatitis, abdominal trauma, bacterial infection, drug use, connective tissue disease, and hypercalcemia are less commonly associated with acute pancreatitis.
Nursing process step: Assessment
Cognitive level: Knowledge

8. Treatment for a patient with ascites secondary to hepatic failure should include all of the following *except:*
A. Withholding diuretics
B. Restricting dietary sodium
C. Providing a high-calorie, 50-g protein diet
D. Performing paracentesis

CORRECT ANSWER—**A.** Ascites results from serious pathophysiologic processes. Restricting dietary sodium and fluid intake, performing paracentesis to remove excess fluid, and providing a high-calorie, 50-g protein diet are used to treat a patient with ascites secondary to hepatic failure. Because a diseased liver cannot metabolize protein, moderate restriction of protein can prevent hepatic coma. Diuretics can be administered, particularly when ascites is not controlled by medical management.
Nursing process step: Planning
Cognitive level: Analysis

Questions 9 and 10 refer to the following information:
An 80-year-old female patient with an extensive history of cardiac problems is transferred from a nursing home to the intensive care unit because she is experiencing abdominal distention, cramping abdominal pain, and nausea and vomiting after meals.

---

9. While auscultating the patient's abdomen, the nurse would suspect a partial intestinal obstruction upon hearing which sound?
  A. Slow, rhythmic gurgles every 5 to 15 seconds
  B. Rapid, high-pitched tinkling sounds
  C. Slow, rhythmic gurgles every minute
  D. Longer-duration, low-pitched tinkling sounds

CORRECT ANSWER—B. Rapid, high-pitched tinkling sounds indicate that intestinal fluid and air may be under increased pressure in the dilated proximal bowel. Normal bowel sounds are auscultated as slow, rhythmic gurgles every 5 to 15 seconds. Hypoactive bowel sounds are heard as slow, rhythmic gurgles every minute. Longer-duration, low-pitched tinkling sounds are indicative of a distal obstruction.
Nursing process step: Assessment
Cognitive level: Knowledge

10. The patient undergoes a double-barrel colostomy because of the intestinal obstruction. The proximal end of the colostomy will drain:
  A. Fecal material
  B. Minimal amounts of blood and mucus
  C. Minimal amounts of fecal material
  D. Blood and mucus

CORRECT ANSWER—A. A double-barrel colostomy is a temporary procedure commonly performed in hopes of eventually restoring bowel continuity. In this procedure, the colon is divided and two skin openings—the proximal end and the distal end or mucous fistula—are formed. The proximal end drains fecal material; the distal end drains a minimal amount of blood and mucus.
Nursing process step: Implementation
Cognitive level: Evaluation

11. When assessing a patient with pancreatic trauma, the nurse notes ecchymosis in the umbilical area. This is known as:
  A. Rovsing's sign
  B. Turner's sign
  C. Coopernail's sign
  D. Cullen's sign

CORRECT ANSWER—D. Cullen's sign is associated with pancreatic trauma; it manifests as ecchymosis in the umbilical area caused by intra-abdominal bleeding. Rovsing's sign occurs when pain is felt at McBurney's point as pressure is exerted on the left side of the abdomen; it is associated with appendicitis. Turner's sign manifests as ecchymosis in the flank area; it suggests retroperitoneal bleeding. Coopernail's sign manifests as ecchymosis of the scrotum or labia and indicates pelvic bleeding.
Nursing process step: Assessment
Cognitive level: Comprehension

12. Postoperative care of a patient with a stab wound of the colon includes administration of antibiotics. These drugs are administered to:
A. Prevent nosocomial infections
B. Combat postoperative pneumonia
C. Prevent wound dehiscence
D. Treat the contaminated peritoneum

CORRECT ANSWER—D. In a patient with a stab wound of the colon, antibiotics are given not only postoperatively but also preoperatively and intraoperatively. This decreases the amount of colon bacteria that may have infiltrated the peritoneum after the injury. Because of the emergency nature of the surgery, there is no time for bowel evacuation or sterilization; consequently, antibiotics help control contamination of the peritoneum when the bowel is surgically manipulated. Antibiotics are not administered to prevent nosocomial infections, postoperative pneumonia, or wound dehiscence.
Nursing process step: Implementation
Cognitive level: Comprehension

13. An increase in serum creatinine and blood urea nitrogen levels most likely is due to an adverse effect of which drug?
A. Neomycin
B. Vasopressin
C. Lactulose
D. Famotidine

CORRECT ANSWER—A. Increased serum creatinine and blood urea nitrogen levels result from nephrotoxicity, which is an adverse effect of neomycin. Neomycin eliminates the colonic bacteria that form ammonia and is administered to patients with hepatic failure to lower blood ammonia concentrations. Nephrotoxicity is not associated with vasopressin, lactulose, or famotidine.
Nursing process step: Evaluation
Cognitive level: Comprehension

Questions 14 to 17 refer to the following information:
A 45-year-old female patient is admitted to the hospital with a diagnosis of hepatic failure secondary to hepatitis B. The patient is confused and disoriented. She has recently had bleeding problems.

---

14. Which laboratory study is most helpful in evaluating bleeding tendencies in a patient with liver disease?
A. White blood cell (WBC) count
B. Prothrombin time (PT)
C. Fibrin split products
D. Platelet count

CORRECT ANSWER—B. Bleeding tendencies occur in patients with liver failure because the liver cannot produce prothrombin and clotting factors VII, IX, and X. The PT reflects activity of the extrinsic and common coagulation pathways (prothrombin, fibrinogen, and factors V, VII, IX, and X). Thus, this test directly measures the liver's contribution to clotting. An increased WBC count is a sign of infection, not bleeding. A decreased WBC count may indicate splenomegaly. Fibrin split products and platelet counts do not measure the liver's involvement in bleeding tendencies.
Nursing process step: Assessment
Cognitive level: Comprehension

15. When planning the patient's care, the nurse should plan to implement which type of isolation measure?
   A. Enteric precautions
   B. Universal precautions
   C. Respiratory isolation
   D. Strict isolation

CORRECT ANSWER—**B.** Because hepatitis B is transmitted through blood and other body fluids, universal precautions are indicated. Enteric precautions would be appropriate if the infection was spread via the fecal or oral route. Respiratory isolation is used when the infectious organism is spread by airborne droplets alone. Strict isolation requires the use of a mask, gown, and gloves when the infectious organism may be spread by both air droplets and via direct contact; it is unnecessary for this patient.
Nursing process step: Implementation
Cognitive level: Application

16. The patient has a prolonged prothrombin time and several large ecchymotic areas on the extremities. Which medication would the nurse plan to administer to treat the patient's bleeding disorder?
   A. Cryoprecipitate
   B. Albumin
   C. Vitamin K
   D. Protamine sulfate

CORRECT ANSWER—**C.** Vitamin K is necessary for the hepatic synthesis of prothrombin and clotting factors VII, IX, and X. Storage of this vitamin in the liver is impaired by liver disease; this leads to bleeding tendencies. Cryoprecipitate contains factor VIII, which is not lacking in this case. Albumin does not contain coagulation factors, nor does protamine sulfate, which is used to neutralize the effects of heparin.
Nursing process step: Planning
Cognitive level: Application

17. In assessing for signs and symptoms of hepatitis B, the nurse knows that the finding most consistent with the patient's diagnosis is:
   A. Excitability
   B. Ascites
   C. Mahogany-colored urine
   D. Dark-colored stools

CORRECT ANSWER—**C.** Mahogany-colored urine indicates the secretion of excess bilirubin into the kidneys that cannot be broken down chemically by the diseased liver. Clay-colored or light stools occur for the same reason. At this stage, the patient usually suffers from malaise, not excitability. Ascites typically is not seen in hepatitis B; it may occur occur secondary to a complication of hepatitis B.
Nursing process step: Assessment
Cognitive level: Comprehension

18. Which statement about ranitidine is correct?
   A. Administer ranitidine 1 hour before meals
   B. Administer ranitidine for no more than 4 weeks at a time
   C. Administer ranitidine and antacids 1 hour apart
   D. Administer oral ranitidine with at least 8 ounces of water

CORRECT ANSWER—**C.** Antacids should be administered 1 hour before or 1 hour after ranitidine because they decrease its absorption. Ranitidine should be administered with meals for prolonged effect. Ranitidine can be given for any length of time, and there is no benefit in drinking 8 ounces of water when taking this medication.
Nursing process step: Implementation
Cognitive level: Application

Questions 19 and 20 refer to the following information:
A 53-year-old male patient is admitted to the hospital with cramping, wavelike abdominal pain and vomiting of fecal contents. Bowel sounds are high-pitched and tinkling. The patient's abdomen is distended and exhibits hyperresonance on percussion.

19. These findings are characteristic of:
   A. Small-bowel obstruction
   B. Perforated duodenal ulcer
   C. Paralytic ileus
   D. Bowel infarction

CORRECT ANSWER—**A.** Characteristic signs of bowel obstruction include high-pitched bowel sounds above the area of the obstruction and cramping, wavelike pain that occurs as peristalsis attempts to move the bowel contents past the obstructed area. Vomitus containing fecal matter and abdominal distention with hyperresonance also may occur. In contrast, paralytic ileus produces a more constant, generalized discomfort. Perforated duodenal ulcer causes severe upper abdominal pain that quickly spreads throughout the abdomen; bowel sounds usually are absent, and vomiting rarely occurs. Bowel infarction is indicated by absent or hypoactive bowel sounds, colicky abdominal pain in the periumbilical area, and bloody diarrhea.
Nursing process step: Assessment
Cognitive level: Evaluation

20. Abdominal X-ray films of this patient would reveal:
   A. "Stepladder" pattern with alternating fluid and gas
   B. Air-filled colon
   C. Distended, air-filled colon
   D. Edematous and gaseous distention in the small and large bowels

CORRECT ANSWER—**A.** In a patient with small-bowel obstruction, abdominal X-ray films reveal a characteristic "stepladder" pattern with alternating fluid and gas levels apparent in 3 to 4 hours after obstruction has occurred. Barium enema studies of a patient with large-bowel obstruction would reveal a distended, air-filled colon, rather than just an air-filled colon. Abdominal X-ray films showing edematous and gaseous distention of the small and large bowels suggest peritonitis.
Nursing process step: Assessment
Cognitive level: Evaluation

Questions 21 and 22 refer to the following information:
A 32-year-old male patient was admitted to the intensive care unit 1 week ago after a diving accident. He sustained a spinal cord injury and is now quadriplegic, intubated, and mechanically ventilated.

21. This patient is at risk for which of the following ulcers?
   A. Curling's ulcer
   B. Serpiginous ulcer
   C. Barrett's ulcer
   D. Cushing's ulcer

CORRECT ANSWER—D. Cushing's ulcer is a type of stress ulcer caused by increased gastric acid secretion after trauma, spinal cord injury, or intracranial surgery. Barrett's ulcer occurs in the distal esophagus and is common in the elderly. Curling's ulcer is another type of stress ulcer that occurs in the stomach and duodenum after burn injury. Serpiginous ulcer is an ulceration of the skin that heals in one area and extends to another.
Nursing process step: Assessment
Cognitive level: Comprehension

22. The patient is being treated pharmacologically for stress ulcers. Which of the following medications stimulates gastric cytoprotective mechanisms and coats inflamed mucosal areas?
   A. Ranitidine
   B. Omeprazole
   C. Sucralfate
   D. Aluminum carbonate

CORRECT ANSWER—C. Sucralfate stimulates gastric cytoprotective mechanisms. It also coats and protects the inflamed mucosal area from pepsin, acid, and bile and allows the area to heal. Ranitidine is an antiulcer agent that competitively inhibits the action of histamine at receptor sites in the parietal cells, thereby decreasing gastric acid secretion. The antiulcer agent omeprazole inhibits the activity of the acid pump, thereby suppressing gastric acid production. Aluminum carbonate is an antacid that reduces total acid in the GI tract and raises gastric pH to reduce pepsin activity.
Nursing process step: Planning
Cognitive level: Comprehension

23. Which drug is administered to inhibit the release of pancreatic secretions in a patient with acute pancreatitis?
   A. Somatostatin
   B. Pancreatin
   C. Acetylcholine
   D. Nitroglycerin

CORRECT ANSWER—A. Somatostatin inhibits the release of pancreatic secretions and is used to treat acute pancreatitis. Pancreatin is used to replace deficient pancreatic enzymes and is used to treat chronic pancreatitis. Acetylcholine, a cholinergic agent, would increase the release of pancreatic secretions. Nitroglycerin relaxes smooth muscle and decreases pain, but does not affect pancreatic secretions.
Nursing process step: Implementation
Cognitive level: Comprehension

24. Propantheline bromide is used to decrease the volume and concentration of bicarbonate and enzymes released from the pancreas during acute pancreatitis. When this medication is used, the nurse should observe for:
A. Bradycardia
B. Chest pain
C. Ileus
D. Hypotension

CORRECT ANSWER—C. One adverse effect of propantheline bromide is bowel hypomotility, which can lead to ileus. Acute pancreatitis itself also can cause ileus resulting from the effect of enzymes and other chemicals on the bowel. Thus, a patient taking propantheline is at double risk for this complication. Other adverse effects of propantheline bromide include tachycardia and hypertension; bradycardia, chest pain, and hypotension are not associated with this drug.
Nursing process step: Evaluation
Cognitive level: Comprehension

Questions 25 to 27 refer to the following information:
A 45-year-old male patient with a history of alcoholism is admitted to the intensive care unit. Arterial and pulmonary artery lines are inserted. The patient's abdomen is firm and distended; when it is palpated, a positive fluid wave occurs, indicating ascites.

25. When assessing this patient, the nurse keeps in mind that all of the following are signs of hepatic failure *except*:
A. Fetor hepaticas
B. Asterixis
C. Spider angioma
D. Decreased cardiac output

CORRECT ANSWER—D. Fetor hepaticas, asterixis, and spider angioma are signs of hepatic failure. Fetor hepaticas is a sweet, musty odor of the breath caused by abnormal metabolism of sulfur compounds. Asterixis is a tremor of the hand elicited by extending the wrist upward. Spider angioma are small, red telangiectases found on the upper portion of the trunk, face, neck, and arms of patients with cirrhosis. In hepatic failure, cardiac output typically increases as a result of decreased peripheral vascular resistance and expanded blood volume.
Nursing process step: Assessment
Cognitive level: Evaluation

26. Pharmacotherapy for this patient would include:
A. Diazepam and lactulose
B. Ranitidine and methylprednisolone
C. Diazepam and methylprednisolone
D. Ranitidine and lactulose

CORRECT ANSWER—D. This patient would be treated with ranitidine and lactulose. Ranitidine, a histamine$_2$-receptor antagonist, blocks acid secretion and prevents gastric erosion. Lactulose acts as a laxative; it also reduces ammonia absorption by decreasing colon pH. Sedatives, such as diazepam, should be avoided because they contribute to hepatic encephalopathy. Corticosteroids, such as methylprednisolone, are not recommended for patients with cirrhosis.
Nursing process step: Implementation
Cognitive level: Analysis

27. Oliguria, azotemia, and mild hypertension develop in this patient. In addition to collecting a urine specimen for electrolyte level determination, the nurse would perform all of the following *except:*

A. Measuring daily weight and hourly intake and output

B. Preparing for paracentesis

C. Monitoring serum blood urea nitrogen, serum creatinine, and serum potassium values

D. Withholding albumin products

CORRECT ANSWER—D. Hepatorenal syndrome is characterized by oliguria, azotemia, mild systemic hypertension, ascites, and low urine sodium level. This syndrome results from reduced renal perfusion caused by decreased effective plasma volume, ascites, hypoalbuminemia, and portal hypertension. Ascites increases intra-abdominal pressure, which could lead to further hypoperfusion of the kidneys. Mild systemic hypertension results from fluid accumulation. Portal hypertension, or hypertension of the venous system and liver, can further damage the liver and kidneys. When caring for a patient with hepatorenal syndrome, the nurse should measure daily weight and hourly intake and output, prepare for paracentesis, and monitor blood urea nitrogen, serum creatinine, and serum potassium values. Plasma volume expanders, such as albumin, should be administered.

Nursing process step: Implementation

Cognitive level: Analysis

Questions 28 to 30 refer to the following information:

A 44-year-old male patient is admitted to the hospital with acute upper GI bleeding secondary to Zollinger-Ellison syndrome. The patient is receiving a blood transfusion consisting of packed red blood cells.

---

28. During the transfusion, the patient complains of chills. The nurse's initial response would be to:

A. Call the physician

B. Continue to observe the patient

C. Notify the blood bank

D. Stop the transfusion

CORRECT ANSWER—D. Chills may be a sign of a transfusion reaction. Because any additional blood could worsen the reaction, the nurse should stop the transfusion first and then call the physician. The nurse would then continue to observe the patient for further signs of a reaction, including fever, urticaria, tachycardia, dyspnea, nausea, vomiting, hypotension, and bronchospasm. The blood bank must be notified, and the unused portion of red blood cells probably will be returned. Samples of the patient's urine and blood should be sent to the laboratory for analysis.

Nursing process step: Implementation

Cognitive level: Application

29. The patient undergoes total gastrectomy. Several hours after surgery, the nurse notes that the patient's nasogastric tube has stopped draining. How should the nurse respond?
   A. Notify the physician
   B. Reposition the tube
   C. Irrigate the tube
   D. Increase the suction level

CORRECT ANSWER—A. A tube that fails to drain during the postoperative period should be reported to the physician immediately. The tube may be clogged, which could increase pressure on the suture site because fluid is not draining adequately. Repositioning or irrigating a tube in a patient who has undergone gastric surgery can disrupt the anastomosis. Increasing the level of suction may cause trauma to GI mucosa or the suture line.
Nursing process step: Implementation
Cognitive level: Application

30. The patient will require which supplement for the rest of his life?
   A. Pyridoxine
   B. Vitamin C
   C. Thiamine
   D. Vitamin B_{12}

CORRECT ANSWER—D. Removing the proximal portion or all of the stomach results in loss of intrinsic factor, a protein secreted by the stomach's parietal cells that is necessary for absorption of vitamin B_{12}. Consequently, the patient will require vitamin B_{12} supplements. Deficiencies of the other supplements do not occur as a direct result of partial or total gastrectomy; pyridoxine (vitamin B_6), vitamin C, and thiamine (vitamin B_1) do not depend on the stomach for their production.
Nursing process step: Planning
Cognitive level: Analysis

31. A 17-year-old male is admitted to the hospital with upper abdominal pain, colicky symptoms, hematemesis, and jaundice. Two days ago, he was involved in a biking accident in which the bike's handlebars struck him sharply in the abdomen. The patient's vital signs include heart rate, 130 beats/minute with sinus tachycardia; blood pressure, 96/45 mm Hg; and respirations, 30 breaths/minute. The patient is afebrile. Based on these findings, the patient probably has an injury to the:
   A. Liver
   B. Stomach
   C. Pancreas
   D. Small bowel

CORRECT ANSWER—A. The size and location of the liver make it particularly susceptible to injury. The liver is the most commonly injured organ in abdominal trauma caused by both blunt and penetrating injuries. Although bleeding into the biliary tract may be delayed, this patient has the classic signs and symptoms of liver injury—upper or lower GI bleeding, obstructive jaundice, and colicky pain. Bleeding occurs because of the highly vascular composition of the liver. Blunt injury to the stomach usually does not occur because the stomach is mobile and protected by other structures; if the stomach had been injured, the patient would complain of left epigastric pain. Pancreatic injuries cause epigastric pain and increase the amylase level. Symptoms of small bowel injury range from no acute symptoms to nausea and vomiting and signs of peritonitis.
Nursing process step: Assessment
Cognitive level: Evaluation

32. If a patient's peritoneal lavage returns indicate frank bleeding, the nurse should plan for which intervention?
A. Sending the lavage fluid to the laboratory
B. Monitoring vital signs while the physician checks the position of the lavage catheter
C. Transferring the patient to the operating room
D. Preparing for computed tomography scan of the abdomen

CORRECT ANSWER—C. Frank, bloody returns indicate intra-abdominal bleeding, and the patient should be transported to the operating room immediately. Laboratory analysis of the lavage fluid is unnecessary because the results are so grossly positive. Likewise, there is no need to recheck the position of the lavage catheter. Performing a computed tomography scan would delay surgery for up to 1 hour; during this time, the patient could die of shock.
Nursing process step: Planning
Cognitive level: Application

33. All of the following are intestinal tubes *except:*
A. Miller-Abbott tube
B. Levin tube
C. Cantor tube
D. Harris tube

CORRECT ANSWER—B. The Levin tube is a single-lumen nasogastric suction tube. The Miller-Abbott, Cantor, and Harris tubes are intestinal tubes. These nasoenteric tubes, which are introduced into the small intestine using gravity and peristalsis, are used for decompression and to facilitate prevention of aspiration.
Nursing process step: Implementation
Cognitive level: Comprehension

34. A patient with colonic obstruction should be observed for which potential complication?
A. Hepatitis
B. Cirrhosis
C. Bowel necrosis
D. Pancreatitis

CORRECT ANSWER—C. The potential complications of colonic obstruction are bowel necrosis and perforation. Bowel necrosis results from impaired circulation caused by volvulus and closed-loop obstruction. Hepatitis is caused by a virus or hepatotoxic drugs. Cirrhosis can be idiopathic but commonly is caused by alcoholism; it also can occur secondary to biliary duct disease, hemochromatosis, and right-sided heart failure. Pancreatitis typically is caused by alcoholism or biliary tract obstruction.
Nursing process step: Evaluation
Cognitive level: Analysis

Questions 35 to 39 refer to the following information:
A 62-year-old male patient is being treated for hepatic encephalopathy. The patient has liver disease secondary to alcoholism and had been hospitalized previously for bleeding esophageal varices associated with the liver disease.

35. What is one of the earliest signs of hepatic encephalopathy?

A. Forgetfulness and slight personality changes
B. Drowsiness
C. Mental confusion and disorientation
D. Asterixis

CORRECT ANSWER—A. The clinical manifestations of hepatic encephalopathy in stage I (prodromal stage) are so subtle they often are overlooked. Slight personality changes and forgetfulness, as well as reversal of the sleep-wake pattern, are associated with this initial stage. Stage II (impending stage) manifests as drowsiness, mental confusion, disorientation, and asterixis. During stage III (stuporous stage), the patient may be stuporous but on arousal becomes noisy and abusive. Signs of stage IV (comatose stage) include hyperactive reflexes, fetor hepaticus, and coma.

Nursing process step: Assessment
Cognitive level: Comprehension

36. Which type of diet is appropriate for a patient with hepatic encephalopathy?

A. Low-protein, high-carbohydrate diet
B. High-protein, low-carbohydrate diet
C. Low-protein, low-carbohydrate diet
D. High-protein, high-carbohydrate diet

CORRECT ANSWER—A. Because a failing liver cannot manufacture carbohydrates, a high-carbohydrate diet is appropriate for a patient with hepatic encephalopathy. The diet also should be low in protein. Protein is converted to ammonia, which the damaged liver cannot break down. Thus, a high-protein diet would worsen hepatic encephalopathy.

Nursing process step: Implementation
Cognitive level: Application

37. The patient is receiving oral neomycin 3 g daily. This drug is used to:

A. Prevent infection because phagocytosis is decreased in liver failure
B. Inhibit production of ammonia by reducing intestinal bacteria
C. Promote production of prothrombin by activating vitamin K
D. Create an acidic environment in the colon that favors conversion of ammonia to ammonium

CORRECT ANSWER—B. Fermentation in the bowel by bacteria converts urea and amino acids into ammonia. Neomycin, an antibiotic, inhibits production of ammonia by reducing the number of intestinal bacteria. Neomycin does not activate vitamin K and is not used to prevent infection in patients with liver disease. Lactulose creates an acidic environment in the colon that favors the conversion of ammonia to ammonium.

Nursing process step: Implementation
Cognitive level: Comprehension

38. The effectiveness of treatment for hepatic encephalopathy is best evaluated by monitoring which laboratory value?
   A. Serum aspartate aminotransferase (AST)
   B. Bilirubin
   C. Ammonia
   D. Serum alanine aminotransferase (ALT)

CORRECT ANSWER—C. Neomycin and lactulose, along with a low-protein diet, are used to decrease the ammonia level in a patient with hepatic encephalopathy. Therefore, the ammonia level is an appropriate indicator of the effectiveness of treatment. Although liver enzymes (AST and ALT) and bilirubin levels are increased by liver disease, changes in these levels would not be helpful in evaluating treatment effectiveness.
Nursing process step: Evaluation
Cognitive level: Evaluation

39. After undergoing a liver biopsy, the patient would be placed in which position?
   A. Semi-Fowler's position
   B. Right lateral decubitus position
   C. Supine position
   D. Prone position

CORRECT ANSWER—B. After a liver biopsy, the patient is placed on the right side to exert pressure on the liver and prevent bleeding. The other positions would not achieve this goal.
Nursing process step: Implementation
Cognitive level: Application

40. Massive, painless GI bleeding can result from:
   A. Duodenal ulcer
   B. Borborygmus
   C. Mallory-Weiss syndrome
   D. Asterixis

CORRECT ANSWER—C. Massive, painless GI bleeding can result from Mallory-Weiss syndrome. This laceration in the mucous membrane at the junction of the esophagus and stomach is caused by retching, vomiting, or coughing. Duodenal ulcers are the most common type of peptic ulcer. Borborygmus is a rumbling sound heard when auscultating the abdomen; it is caused by hyperperistalsis. Asterixis, also known as flapping tremor, is a motor disturbance commonly associated with metabolic abnormalities.
Nursing process step: Assessment
Cognitive level: Analysis

41. The nurse caring for a patient with small-bowel obstruction would plan to implement which nursing intervention first?
   A. Administering pain medication
   B. Obtaining a blood sample for laboratory studies
   C. Preparing to insert a nasogastric (NG) tube
   D. Administering I.V. fluids

CORRECT ANSWER—D. I.V. infusions containing 0.9% sodium chloride solution and potassium should be given first to maintain fluid and electrolyte balance. For the patient's comfort and to assist in bowel decompression, the nurse should prepare to insert an NG tube next. A blood sample is then obtained for laboratory studies to aid in the diagnosis of bowel obstruction and guide treatment. Blood studies usually include a complete blood count, serum electrolyte levels, and blood urea nitrogen level. Pain medication often is withheld until obstruction is diagnosed because analgesics can decrease intestinal motility.
Nursing process step: Planning
Cognitive level: Application

Questions 42 to 45 refer to the following information:
A 32-year-old female patient is admitted to the critical care unit after being injured in a motor vehicle accident. An unrestrained backseat passenger, she was thrown across the front seat during impact. Her clinical examination reveals:
- blood pressure, 70 mm Hg/palpation
- hemoglobin, 8.2 g/dl
- hematocrit, 24%
- heart rate, 132 beats/minute
- respirations, 38 beats/minute.

42. The patient complains of left upper quadrant abdominal pain referred to the left shoulder. This type of pain suggests injury to the:
A. Pancreas
B. Stomach
C. Spleen
D. Small bowel

CORRECT ANSWER—C. Left upper quadrant abdominal pain referred to the left shoulder, commonly called Kehr's sign, results from irritation of the diaphragm by freely circulating blood and typically is caused by an injured spleen. Injury to the pancreas causes epigastric pain. The stomach usually is not damaged by blunt injury; if the stomach had been injured, the patient would report left upper gastric pain. A small-bowel injury causes pain in the right upper abdominal quadrant.
Nursing process step: Assessment
Cognitive level: Evaluation

43. The patient requests pain medication. The nurse would:
A. Administer 5 mg morphine sulfate subcutaneously
B. Administer 50 mg meperidine intramuscularly
C. Administer 1 mg lorazepam intravenously
D. Not administer any pain medication

CORRECT ANSWER—D. Pain medication would not be given at this time because it could mask specific injuries and interfere with accurate neurologic assessments. Also, because the patient is hemodynamically unstable, pain medication could further decrease her blood pressure.
Nursing process step: Implementation
Cognitive level: Application

44. The nurse would expect to do all of the following during the immediate care of this patient *except:*
A. Administer lactated Ringer's solution
B. Administer blood
C. Apply medical antishock trousers (MAST)
D. Begin a dopamine I.V. infusion

CORRECT ANSWER—D. The vasopressor dopamine would not be used at this time because the patient requires fluids, not vasoconstriction. A balanced salt solution with electrolytes, such as lactated Ringer's solution, should be administered. Blood would be administered to replace blood losses, as indicated by the patient's hemoglobin and hematocrit values. A MAST suit raises blood pressure by increasing systemic vascular resistance.
Nursing process step: Implementation
Cognitive level: Application

45. Which assessment findings would most accurately reflect the patient's fluid status?
A. Mentation, urine output, and abdominal girth
B. Urine output, urine specific gravity, and blood pressure
C. Mentation, urine output, and central venous pressure (CVP)
D. Mentation, abdominal girth, and CVP

CORRECT ANSWER—C. CVP is the most accurate measurement of a patient's fluid status. Urine output and mentation indicate the degree to which the kidneys and brain are being perfused. Adequate perfusion can be accomplished only if the patient has sufficient circulating volume. Although not as accurate as CVP, urine output and mentation are reliable indicators of fluid volume. Blood pressure, urine specific gravity, and measurements of abdominal girth to assess sequestration of blood in the abdomen are inaccurate measures of fluid status.
Nursing process step: Evaluation
Cognitive level: Evaluation

46. A 32-year-old male patient with appendicitis is experiencing excruciating abdominal pain. An abdominal X-ray film reveals intraperitoneal air. The nurse should prepare the patient for:
A. Surgery
B. Colonoscopy
C. Nasointestinal tube insertion
D. Barium enema

CORRECT ANSWER—A. The patient should be prepared for surgery because his signs and symptoms indicate bowel perforation. Appendicitis is the most common cause of bowel perforation in the United States. Because perforation can lead to peritonitis and sepsis, surgery would not be delayed to perform any of the other interventions. Also, none of the other procedures are necessary at this point.
Nursing process step: Implementation
Cognitive level: Application

47. Medical management of a patient with peritonitis includes antibiotics, I.V. fluids, and:
A. Nasogastric suctioning
B. Enemas
C. Clear liquid diet
D. Early ambulation

CORRECT ANSWER—A. Medical treatment for peritonitis consists of antibiotics to fight infection, I.V. fluids to maintain fluid and electrolyte balance, and nasogastric suctioning to decompress the bowel. Enemas are not administered to patients with peritonitis because they could worsen the infection. The patient should be given nothing by mouth to allow the bowel to rest. Bed rest is required until the acute phase has passed.
Nursing process step: Implementation
Cognitive level: Application

Questions 48 to 51 refer to the following information:
A 47-year-old male patient is admitted to the hospital with a diagnosis of acute pancreatitis following a weekend drinking binge. He complains of abdominal pain, nausea, and thirst. His assessment findings are as follows:

- serum aspartate aminotransferase (AST), 79 U/liter
- serum alanine aminotransferase (ALT), 67 U/liter
- hemoglobin, 14 g/dl
- hematocrit, 48%
- serum bilirubin, 8.0 mg/100 ml
- serum amylase, 175 U/ml
- serum lipase, 56 U/ml
- serum glucose, 254 mg/100 ml
- blood pressure, 92/58 mm Hg
- pulmonary capillary wedge pressure, 5 mm Hg.

---

48. In light of the patient's nausea, which nursing intervention would be most appropriate?
A. Providing ice chips
B. Inserting a nasogastric (NG) tube
C. Giving nothing by mouth (NPO status)
D. Administering dextrose 10% in water ($D_{10}W$) intravenously

CORRECT ANSWER—C. The patient would be placed on strict NPO status because anything taken by mouth, even ice chips, could stimulate the pancreas to release more digestive enzymes. Because pancreatitis is an autodigestive disease in which enzymes are released, oral intake would worsen the patient's condition. NG tubes are no longer routinely used; they do not alter the course of the disease and can contribute to fluid and electrolyte imbalance. NG tubes are reserved for patients with ileus, persistent vomiting, or gastric distention. Intravenous therapy would be initiated, but $D_{10}W$ is not the fluid of choice because of the patient's increased blood glucose level.
Nursing process step: Planning
Cognitive level: Application

49. The patient complains of palpitations and numbness and tingling of the lips. The nurse would plan to:
A. Add potassium chloride to the I.V. fluid infusion
B. Administer calcium chloride intravenously
C. Have the patient breathe into a paper bag
D. Administer 2 mg oral lorazepam

CORRECT ANSWER—B. The patient has symptoms of hypocalcemia, a common electrolyte disorder in acute pancreatitis; therefore, I.V. calcium chloride is indicated. Potassium chloride would be administered if the patient had signs and symptoms of hypokalemia, which include muscle weakness, apathy, and irritability. Breathing into a paper bag can alleviate respiratory alkalosis resulting from hyperventilation, but would have no effect on hypocalcemia. Lorazepam is used to decrease agitation.
Nursing process step: Planning
Cognitive level: Application

50. What is the treatment of choice for regulating the patient's blood pressure and pulmonary capillary wedge pressure (PCWP)?
  A. 0.9% sodium chloride solution administered intravenously
  B. Albumin
  C. Dopamine
  D. Blood transfusion

CORRECT ANSWER—B. The patient is hypovolemic, with a PCWP of 5 mm Hg; albumin is the best treatment for restoring the oncotic pressure lost because of pancreatic exudate. The patient also would receive lactated Ringer's solution intravenously to replenish electrolytes. Dopamine is not warranted unless the circulating blood volume is restored and the patient remains hypotensive. A blood transfusion would be required if the patient had hemorrhagic pancreatitis; hemoglobin and hematocrit values indicate that this is not the case.
Nursing process step: Implementation
Cognitive level: Application

51. Which intervention is most appropriate in the initial stages of acute pancreatitis?
  A. Administering prophylactic antibiotics
  B. Administering insulin
  C. Performing peritoneal lavage
  D. Restricting sodium intake

CORRECT ANSWER—B. In acute pancreatitis, an increased amount of glucagon is released from the injured islets of Langerhans; insulin is given to control the resulting increased serum glucose level. Prophylactic antibiotics do not prevent the formation or extension of pseudocysts or abscesses, which are complications of acute pancreatitis. These drugs are used only after infection is documented. Peritoneal lavage is used to remove toxic substances from peritoneal fluid. These substances may cause many of the adverse systemic effects characteristic of pancreatitis, including decreased blood pressure, increased vascular permeability, and respiratory failure. However, peritoneal lavage typically is reserved for patients who do not respond to initial therapy. Sodium is not restricted because hyponatremia often results from extravasation of fluid from the pancreas, vomiting, and diarrhea.
Nursing process step: Implementation
Cognitive level: Analysis

Questions 52 and 53 refer to the following information:
A 26-year-old male patient who ruptured his spleen in a motorcycle accident is admitted to the hospital and requires a splenectomy.

52. A splenectomy is necessary because rupture of the spleen:
  A. Causes severe hemorrhage
  B. Impairs liver and bone marrow function
  C. Damages the largest mass of lymphatic tissue in the body
  D. Causes severe pain

CORRECT ANSWER—**A.** The spleen is a highly vascular organ responsible for various tasks, including immunologic functions, hematopoiesis, blood storage, and destruction of red blood cells and platelets. Rupture of the spleen causes severe intraperitoneal hemorrhage and shock, but it does not impair liver and bone marrow function. In fact, the functions of the ruptured spleen are assumed by other structures, particularly the liver and bone marrow. The spleen is the largest mass of lymphatic tissue in the body and its rupture causes severe pain; however, these are not reasons for its removal.
Nursing process step: Implementation
Cognitive level: Comprehension

53. The nurse should plan to administer which vaccine postoperatively?
  A. Recombivax HB
  B. Attenuvax
  C. Pneumovax 23
  D. Tetanus toxoid

CORRECT ANSWER—**C.** Pneumovax 23, a polyvalent pneumococcal vaccine, is administered prophylactically to prevent the pneumococcal sepsis that sometimes occurs after splenectomy. Recombivax HB is a vaccine for hepatitis B. Attenuvax is a live, attenuated virus vaccine for immunization against measles (rubeola). Tetanus toxoid is administered to prevent tetanus resulting from trauma caused by an open wound.
Nursing process step: Planning
Cognitive level: Application

ENDOCRINE SYSTEM

CHAPTER 6

Endocrine System

1. Besides an elevated serum glucose level, which chemical study result is common in a patient with hyperosmolar nonketotic syndrome (HNKS)?
A. Elevated serum acetone level
B. Presence of serum ketone bodies
C. Serum alkalosis
D. Hypokalemia

CORRECT ANSWER—D. A patient with HNKS typically has an overall potassium deficit resulting from diuresis, which is secondary to hyperglycemia and hyperosmolarity because of the relative lack of insulin. Serum acetone and ketone bodies are characteristic of diabetic ketoacidosis. Serum alkalosis is not associated with HNKS, but lactic or renal metabolic acidosis may occur.
Nursing process step: Assessment
Cognitive level: Evaluation

2. A patient with hyperosmolar nonketotic syndrome (HNKS) is at risk for all of the following complications as the patient's condition worsens *except:*
A. Thromboemboli
B. Respiratory alkalosis
C. Renal impairment
D. Cerebrovascular accident

CORRECT ANSWER—B. Respiratory acidosis tends to occur secondary to decreased respiratory functioning as the patient's condition worsens. In a patient with HNKS, respiratory alkalosis may be noted initially as a compensatory mechanism. A patient with HNKS is more likely to have metabolic acidosis secondary to increased lactic acid or renal dysfunction. Increased blood viscosity caused by diuresis can lead to thromboemboli and cerebrovascular accident. Decreased blood flow to the kidneys secondary to volume depletion decreases the glomerular filtration rate and can cause renal impairment or failure.
Nursing process step: Planning
Cognitive level: Comprehension

3. Which intervention is appropriate for a patient with diabetic ketoacidosis?
A. Decrease the insulin I.V. infusion rate when the blood glucose level reaches 180 mg/dl
B. Switch from 0.9% sodium chloride solution to a glucose-containing fluid when the blood glucose level reaches 250 mg/dl
C. Administer insulin preparations subcutaneously when the blood glucose level reaches 200 mg/dl
D. Provide intermediate-acting insulin when the blood glucose level returns to 180 mg/dl

CORRECT ANSWER—**B.** The treatment of choice for a patient with diabetic ketoacidosis is I.V. insulin and 0.9% sodium chloride solution until the blood glucose level reaches 250 mg/dl. The fluid should then be changed to a glucose-containing solution to prevent hypoglycemia. After the blood glucose level reaches 250 mg/dl, insulin can be administered intravenously or subcutaneously. Only rapid-acting insulin preparations should be used until the patient is stabilized.
Nursing process step: Planning
Cognitive level: Application

4. Urinalysis findings for a patient with diabetic ketoacidosis are positive for proteinuria. Four days after the patient is admitted to the hospital, a repeat urinalysis also is positive for proteinuria. Why is this result of particular concern?
A. Proteinuria increases susceptibility to urinary tract infections
B. Proteinuria is an early sign of nephropathy
C. Protein stores are catabolized in the early stage of diabetic ketoacidosis
D. Proteinuria indicates the need for insulin reduction

CORRECT ANSWER—**B.** Proteinuria measured by urinalysis is an early sign of nephropathy. Microalbuminuria tests are now recommended for even earlier detection of diabetic nephropathy. Proteinuria is caused by damage to the glomerulus resulting from diabetes. Proteinuria is not associated with uncomplicated urinary tract infections, diabetic ketoacidosis, or insulin requirements.
Nursing process step: Assessment
Cognitive level: Analysis

5. All of the following interventions are appropriate for a patient with nephrogenic diabetes insipidus *except:*
A. Administering thiazide diuretics
B. Providing a low-sodium diet
C. Providing a low-protein diet
D. Administering desmopressin

CORRECT ANSWER—**D.** Desmopressin is used to treat patients with central diabetes insipidus. For patients with nephrogenic diabetes insipidus, treatment typically includes a low-sodium, low-protein diet and thiazide diuretics to induce volume depletion and improve sodium chloride and water reabsorption in the proximal tubules. This subsequently results in less volume delivered to the collecting ducts, which are lacking in antidiuretic hormone.
Nursing process step: Implementation
Cognitive level: Comprehension

Questions 6 to 8 refer to the following information:
A 69-year-old male patient is admitted to the cardiac care unit because of increased frequency of anginal events. His past medical history reveals recurrent peptic ulcer disease, which necessitated a Billroth II procedure approximately 2 months ago. He suffers from dumping syndrome despite dietary modifications.

---

6. Two hours after eating lunch, the patient appears pale. He also is irritable and complains of headache. Which nursing diagnosis is most appropriate?
A. High risk for injury related to central nervous system dysfunction
B. Knowledge deficit related to treatment for dumping syndrome
C. Decreased cardiac output related to impaired myocardial contractility
D. Altered tissue perfusion related to hypoglycemia

CORRECT ANSWER—D. Dumping syndrome, also known as gastrectomy syndrome, occurs soon after eating in patients who have undergone partial gastrectomy. The contents of the stomach empty too rapidly into the duodenum, resulting in hypoglycemia secondary to overcorrection of hyperglycemia with insulin release. Irritability and headache are signs of hypoglycemia. The other nursing diagnoses do not accurately reflect the patient's condition.
Nursing process step: Assessment
Cognitive level: Evaluation

7. Based on the patient's signs and symptoms, which nursing intervention is required?
A. Providing 50% glucose intravenously
B. Providing ½ cup of nondiet soda or orange juice
C. Administering glucagon intramuscularly
D. Providing a snack of peanut butter and crackers

CORRECT ANSWER—B. For a patient who can take carbohydrates by mouth, the best intervention for a hypoglycemic event is administration of a fast-acting carbohydrate, such as 4 to 6 ounces of fruit juice or nondiet soda. I.V. glucose or I.M. glucagon should be used only if the patient is unresponsive or cannot swallow. Peanut butter and crackers provide a protein supplement with complex carbohydrates and should be provided after the initial hypoglycemic event is effectively treated.
Nursing process step: Implementation
Cognitive level: Application

8. Which statement by the patient suggests he has effectively learned to cope with hypoglycemia secondary to dumping syndrome?
A. "I will monitor my blood glucose level 2 hours after I eat a meal."
B. "If I feel shaky and weak, I will drink a glass of orange juice."
C. "I will include fruit juices with each meal."
D. "If I feel weak and have palpitations, I will check my blood glucose level quickly."

CORRECT ANSWER—B. The patient can treat a hypoglycemic event with a fast-acting oral carbohydrate, such as orange juice. Routine postprandial serum glucose monitoring usually is not necessary for hypoglycemic conditions. A patient with dumping syndrome must avoid liquids and fast-acting carbohydrates during meals. Unless the patient also has diabetes mellitus, blood glucose monitoring for occasional episodes of hypoglycemia is not required.
Nursing process step: Evaluation
Cognitive level: Evaluation

9. A 66-year-old male is admitted to the intensive care unit with syndrome of inappropriate antidiuretic hormone (SIADH) resulting from pancreatic cancer. His serum sodium level on admission is 116 mEq/liter. He is lethargic and intermittently complains of headache, which he ranks as a 10 on a 10-point quantitative pain scale. Which nursing intervention is most appropriate for this patient?
A. Elevating the head of the bed more than 20 degrees
B. Administering a narcotic immediately, as ordered
C. Preparing the patient for a computed tomography scan
D. Administering a hypertonic solution

CORRECT ANSWER—**D.** Hyponatremia causes an osmotic gradient that pulls water from the intravascular space into the intracerebral cells, resulting in cerebral edema. Thus, the patient's assessment findings are caused by increased intracranial pressure. The severe hyponatremia experienced by this patient should be treated with I.V. replacement therapy with a hypertonic solution, such as 3% sodium chloride. Elevating the head of the bed no more than 20 degrees facilitates venous return to the heart and reduces secretion of antidiuretic hormone. Narcotics could interfere with ongoing neurologic assessments. Given the diagnosis, a computed tomography scan is not indicated at this time.
Nursing process step: Implementation
Cognitive level: Application

10. A diabetic patient should be closely monitored for the Somogyi effect. All of the following statements about this effect are true *except:*
A. The Somogyi effect is associated with undetected episodes of hypoglycemia during sleep
B. The Somogyi effect causes low early-morning blood glucose level and high postprandial blood glucose level
C. The Somogyi effect can be treated by increasing the insulin dosage
D. The Somogyi effect can be treated by decreasing the insulin dosage

CORRECT ANSWER—**C.** The Somogyi effect is associated with undetected episodes of hypoglycemia during sleep. A low early-morning blood glucose level and a high postprandial blood glucose level result from excess insulin and rebound hyperglycemia. Increasing the insulin dosage would worsen the condition. The treatment of choice is to counteract the Somogyi effect by reducing the insulin dosage.
Nursing process step: Implementation
Cognitive level: Comprehension

11. A diabetic patient is beginning intermediate-acting insulin therapy. When would a hypoglycemic event be most likely to occur in this patient?
A. At the peak of insulin activity
B. At the onset of insulin activity
C. At the end of insulin activity
D. Throughout the duration of insulin activity

CORRECT ANSWER—**A.** The peak of insulin activity is the period during which the insulin dose has its greatest effect; consequently, the patient is most likely to experience hypoglycemia at this time. However, the patient can become hypoglycemic at any point during therapy.
Nursing process step: Planning
Cognitive level: Analysis

12. A 72-year-old female has the following laboratory values: serum sodium (Na), 155 mEq/liter; serum potassium (K), 3.0 mEq/liter; blood urea nitrogen (BUN), 56 mg/dl; and serum glucose, 360 mg/dl. The nurse calculates that the patient's serum osmolarity is approximately:

A. 247 mOsm/liter

B. 180 mOsm/liter

C. 300 mOsm/liter

D. 356 mOsm/liter

CORRECT ANSWER—D. The formula for determining serum osmolarity is [2(Na + K)] + [BUN/2.8] + [serum glucose/18]. In a patient with hyperosmolar nonketotic syndrome, the serum osmolarity usually is greater than 350 mOsm/liter.

Nursing process step: Implementation

Cognitive level: Application

13. A 38-year-old male patient is admitted to the intensive care unit with a diagnosis of diabetic ketoacidosis. He also has cellulitis of the right forearm caused by I.V. drug abuse. The physician prescribes I.V. insulin. Which intervention is necessary to ensure safe delivery of the infusion?

A. Covering the delivery system with an occlusive wrapping to prevent insulin degradation

B. Flushing 50 ml of the I.V. insulin solution through the tubing to saturate insulin absorption sites

C. Mixing the insulin dose in a glass bottle to prevent leaching

D. Infusing insulin separately from phosphate supplements to prevent precipitate formation

CORRECT ANSWER—B. When added to I.V. solutions, insulin may be absorbed by the plastic container and tubing system. Flushing the system before connecting it to the patient saturates the container and tubing with insulin and ensures the patient will receive a consistent dosage. Insulin is not light-sensitive and can be mixed in plastic containers. Insulin does not form a precipitate with phosphate.

Nursing process step: Implementation

Cognitive level: Application

14. The physician prescribes demeclocycline for a patient with syndrome of inappropriate antidiuretic hormone (SIADH). This drug is given to:

A. Prevent seizure activity associated with hyponatremia

B. Inhibit the release of antidiuretic hormone

C. Prevent supraventricular rhythm disturbances

D. Interfere with the action of antidiuretic hormone at the renal tubules

CORRECT ANSWER—D. Demeclocycline, a tetracycline, causes nephrogenic diabetes insipidus by interfering with the action of antidiuretic hormone at the renal tubules, thereby allowing diuresis to occur. The drug has no effect on seizure activity or myocardial conduction, nor does it inhibit the release of antidiuretic hormone.

Nursing process step: Implementation

Cognitive level: Knowledge

15. Syndrome of inappropriate antidiuretic hormone (SIADH) is characterized by an increase in intravascular volume without peripheral edema. What is the physiologic basis for the absence of edema?

A. A concomitant increase in both intravascular and intracellular osmolarity occurs

B. Because urinary sodium is excreted despite the hyponatremic state, there is no difference in the osmotic gradient to cause movement of fluid into intercellular spaces

C. The increase in intravascular volume is insufficient to reflect third-space fluid shifts

D. The statement is not correct; SIADH does cause peripheral edema

CORRECT ANSWER—**B.** SIADH causes excessive fluid retention and hyponatremia. The hyponatremia is due to a dilutional effect and the loss of sodium via the renal tubules. The decreased serum osmolarity causes intracellular edema resulting from water being pulled into the cells; peripheral edema does not occur because the osmotic gradient does not encourage fluid shifts into the extracellular space. Intravascular osmolarity decreases, as reflected by a decrease in serum osmolarity to less than 275 mOsm/liter.
Nursing process step: Assessment
Cognitive level: Analysis

16. During fluid resuscitation and electrolyte replacement for a patient with diabetic ketoacidosis, the serum potassium level is a primary concern. All of the following statements about potassium are true *except*:

A. Potassium returns to the intracellular compartment via glucose

B. Potassium moves into the extracellular space in an acidotic state

C. Potassium loss in the renal tubules results from hyperglycemia, which promotes osmotic diuresis

D. Potassium-phosphorus supplements can be used to restore potassium and phosphate losses

CORRECT ANSWER—**A.** In a patient with diabetic ketoacidosis, the serum potassium level initially is elevated because of dehydration and metabolic acidosis. However, once fluids and insulin are administered, potassium begins moving into the intracellular compartments. This shifting is directly related to the administration of insulin, not glucose. The diuresis associated with hyperglycemia causes a profound loss of electrolytes, and the nurse must carefully assess for signs of hypokalemia as the glucose level is corrected. Although phosphorus replacement is controversial, simultaneous replacement of phosphorus and potassium can be accomplished with potassium-phosphorus supplements.
Nursing process step: Assessment
Cognitive level: Comprehension

17. Hypoglycemia can be triggered by certain drugs. Which drug should be avoided when treating a patient with a history of hypoglycemia?

A. Sulfisoxazole
B. Mannitol
C. Prednisone
D. Propranolol

CORRECT ANSWER—**A.** Sulfonamides, such as sulfisoxazole, are chemically related to oral hypoglycemic agents and may trigger hypoglycemia. Mannitol, an osmotic diuretic, does not cause hypoglycemia. Prednisone is a systemic glucocorticoid that alters carbohydrate metabolism; this can lead to increased glycogenesis and glycogenolysis by antagonizing the action of insulin. In some susceptible patients, prednisone can cause hyperglycemia and diabetes mellitus. Propranolol does not cause hypoglycemia but can mask its signs and symptoms.
Nursing process step: Planning
Cognitive level: Knowledge

18. A 38-year-old female is admitted to the intensive care unit with uncontrolled diabetes mellitus. She weighs 242 lb and has a medical history of peripheral vascular disease, diabetic ketoacidosis, coronary artery disease, and hypertension. Her blood glucose level has fluctuated from 102 mg/100 ml to 322 mg/100 ml, necessitating sliding-scale insulin for glucose coverage.

The patient had a 6-a.m. blood glucose level of 242 mg/100 ml, for which she received 8 units of Humulin regular insulin subcutaneously and 15 units of Humulin NPH insulin subcutaneously. At 8 a.m., she complains of palpitations and states, "I'm really hungry and weak. This diet isn't working and I need something to eat!" A stat fingerstick blood glucose test reveals a serum glucose level of 108 mg/100 ml. Which statement best describes the patient's condition?

A. A sudden drop in blood glucose, regardless of the final level reached, can trigger symptoms of hypoglycemia

B. The patient is attempting to obtain more food by manipulating the nursing staff

C. A consistently elevated blood glucose level causes palpitations and irritability

D. The patient's signs and symptoms result from the Somogyi effect

CORRECT ANSWER—A. Sudden, precipitous drops in the blood glucose level cause hypoglycemic symptoms regardless of the serum glucose endpoint. Palpitations, hunger, weakness, and irritability are symptoms of a hypoglycemic event. The Somogyi effect is related to rebound hyperglycemia resulting from undetected hypoglycemia.
Nursing process step: Assessment
Cognitive level: Application

19. Which dietary modification most commonly is recommended for a patient with hypoglycemia?
A. Increase simple sugar intake
B. Adhere to a low-carbohydrate, high-protein diet
C. Increase unsaturated fat intake
D. Increase vitamin supplements, particularly vitamin C

CORRECT ANSWER—B. A patient with hypoglycemia should follow a low-carbohydrate, high-protein diet and avoid simple sugars and fasting. Increased intake of unsaturated fats or vitamin supplements will not improve hypoglycemia.
Nursing process step: Implementation
Cognitive level: Analysis

20. A 44-year-old female with type I (insulin-dependent) diabetes mellitus is admitted to the intensive care unit with a diagnosis of diabetic ketoacidosis. Arterial blood gas analysis reveals a pH of 7.22. Which statement regarding the use of sodium bicarbonate therapy in the treatment of diabetic ketoacidosis is true?

A. Excessive amounts of bicarbonate can trigger hypokalemia

B. Bicarbonate therapy is recommended when the pH is greater than 7.2

C. Bicarbonate therapy is used to neutralize the release of free fatty acids

D. Bicarbonate therapy decreases the incidence of arrhythmias

CORRECT ANSWER—A. The use of sodium bicarbonate in nonemergencies is not recommended; rapid reversal of metabolic acidosis can cause severe hypokalemia and life-threatening arrhythmias. Sodium bicarbonate should be administered to patients with a pH of less than 7.1. Bicarbonate therapy has no effect on the release of free fatty acids; this release is stimulated by decreased insulin level.
Nursing process step: Implementation
Cognitive level: Comprehension

21. A 72-year-old male with non–insulin-dependent (type II) diabetes mellitus and cellulitis of the right foot is admitted to the hospital for hyperosmolar nonketotic syndrome (HNKS). His serum glucose level is 927 mg/dl and his serum osmolarity is 392 mOsm/liter. To control the blood glucose level, the patient will receive:

A. Short-acting insulin subcutaneously because glucose level decreases when fluid homeostasis is achieved

B. High-dosage insulin intravenously

C. Hourly insulin doses intramuscularly to gradually reduce the blood glucose level

D. Short-acting, low-dosage insulin intravenously

CORRECT ANSWER—D. Typically, an insulin protocol similar to that used for patients with diabetic ketoacidosis is prescribed for patients with HNKS because patients with either condition have similar insulin needs. Insulin should not be administered subcutaneously until the blood glucose level reaches approximately 250 mg/100 ml and stabilizes. High-dosage intravenous insulin can trigger a hypoglycemic event. Intramuscular administration of insulin is not the route of choice in managing HNKS.
Nursing process step: Implementation
Cognitive level: Analysis

Questions 22 and 23 refer to the following information:
A 64-year-old female patient is admitted to the intensive care unit with a diagnosis of diabetes insipidus resulting from a pituitary tumor. On admission, the patient is hypernatremic, with a serum sodium level of 152 mEq/liter. Her vital signs are temperature, 101.6° F (38.7° C); pulse, 124 beats/minute with sinus tachycardia; respirations, 22 breaths/minute; and blood pressure, 102/68 mm Hg.

22. The patient is lethargic and weak. Given her mental status, the physician orders I.V. fluids to replace the water deficit. Which statement regarding I.V. fluid volume replacement in a patient with diabetes insipidus is true?
A. The water deficit should be replaced quickly to prevent intravascular collapse leading to shock
B. The water deficit should be replaced gradually over 48 hours to prevent cerebral edema, seizures, and death
C. The water deficit should be corrected using a hypertonic saline solution to increase tubular water resorption
D. The water deficit should be replaced over a 24-hour period to support normal cardiac output

CORRECT ANSWER—B. If water is replaced too quickly, fluid shifts can move water from the intravascular space into the brain cells, resulting in cerebral edema, seizures, or death. The type of fluid used is determined by the patient's condition; however, oral or I.V. dextrose 5% in water commonly is used. An isotonic saline solution may be used initially to stabilize the patient's hemodynamic status.
Nursing process step: Implementation
Cognitive level: Application

23. The patient's diabetes insipidus results from a lack of which hormone?
A. Antidiuretic hormone
B. Corticotropin
C. Glucocorticoid hormones
D. Gonadotropin hormones

CORRECT ANSWER—A. Diabetes insipidus related to a pituitary dysfunction, such as a pituitary tumor, is caused by a deficiency of antidiuretic hormone. The lack of antidiuretic hormone in central diabetes insipidus also can be caused by head trauma, neurosurgery, cerebral injury, or infection. The other hormones listed are not associated with diabetes insipidus.
Nursing process step: Assessment
Cognitive level: Comprehension

24. All of the following are signs and symptoms of hyperosmolar nonketotic syndrome (HNKS) *except*:
A. Intracellular dehydration
B. Osmotic diuresis
C. Hyperglycemia
D. Fatty acid release

CORRECT ANSWER—D. For reasons not clearly understood, fatty acid release does not occur in HNKS. Patients with this condition probably have enough insulin to avoid lipolysis but not enough to prevent hyperglycemia. Intracellular dehydration and osmotic diuresis are other signs of HNKS.
Nursing process step: Assessment
Cognitive level: Comprehension

25. The serum glucose level in a patient with hyperosmolar nonketotic syndrome (HNKS) must be closely monitored. Which intervention is essential in the acute stage of HNKS?
A. Monitoring venous serum glucose level every hour
B. Monitoring venous serum glucose level every 30 minutes
C. Performing a fingerstick glucose test every hour
D. Collecting blood samples for glycosylated hemoglobin level testing every 4 hours

CORRECT ANSWER—C. In a patient with HNKS, a fingerstick test for glucose should be performed at least every hour. Venous serum glucose level is not necessary as long as fingerstick monitoring is possible. Glycosylated hemoglobin studies provide long-term data about the patient's average blood glucose level and are not appropriate for managing acute HNKS.
Nursing process step: Implementation
Cognitive level: Application

26. A goal of treatment for a patient with syndrome of inappropriate antidiuretic hormone (SIADH) is to achieve a normovolemic state. Improvement in the patient's condition would be indicated by all of the following assessment findings *except:*
A. Central venous pressure of 2 to 6 mm Hg
B. Orientation to person, place, and time
C. Urine specific gravity greater than 1.030
D. Intake approximating output plus insensible losses

CORRECT ANSWER—C. As a normovolemic state is attained, urine specific gravity should decrease to within the normal parameters of 1.010 to 1.025. The other options are evidence of improvement in the patient's fluid volume status.
Nursing process step: Evaluation
Cognitive level: Evaluation

27. Vasopressin is an aqueous preparation of purified antidiuretic hormone (ADH) infused intravenously for the short-term management of an ADH deficiency. Besides treating diabetes insipidus, vasopressin also may be prescribed to:
A. Provide a pressor effect for managing hypotension
B. Promote peristalsis in paralytic ileus
C. Decrease serum glucose level and increase insulin release
D. Control massive GI bleeding

CORRECT ANSWER—D. Because of its vasoconstricting effects, vasopressin is used to control massive GI bleeding, which often associated with esophageal varices. The drug is not recommended as a pressor agent because of its vasoconstricting effects on the myocardium and other body systems. Vasopressin does not reduce the glucose level nor does it promote peristalsis.
Nursing process step: Implementation
Cognitive level: Comprehension

28. All of the following stimulate the posterior pituitary gland to release antidiuretic hormone (ADH) *except:*
A. Hypercapnia via chemoreceptor stimulation
B. Hypovolemia via pressure-receptor stimulation
C. Hypotension via baroceptor stimulation
D. Hypothalamic osmoreceptor stimulation

CORRECT ANSWER—A. Hypercapnia does not trigger the release of ADH. Antidiuretic hormone is released in response to plasma osmolarity. Hypovolemia and hypotension also stimulate the release of ADH, which results in antidiuresis.
Nursing process step: Assessment
Cognitive level: Comprehension

29. A 42-year-old male patient with insulin-dependent diabetes mellitus is admitted to the intensive care unit after an episode of insulin shock. The nurse discusses appropriate interventions for controlling hypoglycemia at home with the patient and his wife. If the patient becomes groggy and lethargic, with an impaired ability to swallow, what should the wife do?

A. Immediately call emergency medical services
B. Provide orange juice or nondiet soda using a dropper
C. Place a teaspoon of honey between the gums and cheek
D. Provide hard candy and place the patient in high-Fowler's position

CORRECT ANSWER—C. The best initial response is to place honey or cake icing in the patient's buccal space. Providing oral fluids or food to a patient too lethargic to swallow increases the risk of aspiration. Typically, the patient improves rapidly once given a simple carbohydrate supplement, and emergency medical services usually are not needed.

Nursing process step: Implementation
Cognitive level: Application

Questions 30 and 31 refer to the following information:
A 39-year-old female patient is admitted to the hospital with a serum glucose level of 670 mg/dl. Serum electrolytes are potassium, 5.2 mEq/liter; sodium, 148 mEq/liter; and phosphate, 2.9 mg/dl. Arterial blood gas analysis shows a pH of 7.21.

---

30. Based on these findings, the nurse would expect treatment to begin with which I.V. solution?

A. 0.9% sodium chloride solution
B. Dextrose 5% in 0.45% sodium chloride solution
C. Lactated Ringer's solution
D. 0.9% sodium chloride solution with sodium bicarbonate

CORRECT ANSWER—A. Fluid resuscitation in a patient with diabetic ketoacidosis is initiated with 0.9% sodium chloride solution to replace fluid volume, sodium, and chloride. The acidosis will improve with insulin therapy and does not require sodium bicarbonate treatment. Although 0.45% sodium chloride solution is used for some patients, it should be free of dextrose in the early treatment of diabetic ketoacidosis. Once the blood glucose level reaches 250 mg/dl, dextrose 5% in 0.45% sodium chloride solution can be administered to prevent hypoglycemia, hypokalemia, and cerebral edema.

Nursing process step: Implementation
Cognitive level: Application

31. Once treatment has begun with I.V. fluids and low-dosage I.V. insulin, the nurse should closely watch for which serum abnormality?
A. Hypokalemia
B. Hyperphosphatemia
C. Hyponatremia
D. Metabolic alkalosis

CORRECT ANSWER—A. During acidosis, potassium shifts from the intracellular spaces to the extracellular spaces. As a result of hyperglycemia and its ensuing diuresis, potassium is lost, causing an overall total body deficit. As the acidotic state is corrected, potassium returns to the intracellular spaces. Profound hypokalemia is indicated by signs of cardiovascular collapse. Hyperphosphatemia, hyponatremia, and metabolic alkalosis are not concerns with standard fluid and insulin therapies.
Nursing process step: Evaluation
Cognitive level: Analysis

32. The nurse is caring for a diabetic patient with a nursing diagnosis of knowledge deficit related to lack of understanding of dietary measures recommended by the American Diabetes Association (ADA). Which statement by the patient indicates that he now understands the ADA diet?
A. "I should eat low-fat protein sources and use monounsaturated fats."
B. "My dietary calories should consist of 60% carbohydrates, 30% fats, and 20% protein."
C. "I should eat three meals a day and stop snacking."
D. "I should restrict my carbohydrate intake to prevent hyperglycemic episodes."

CORRECT ANSWER—B. The ADA recommends a diet in which 60% of the calories come from carbohydrates, 20% to 30% from fats, and 12% to 20% from proteins. Protein sources should be low in fat, and fat intake should be limited to polyunsaturated fats. Diabetic patients should eat three meals a day and an evening snack.
Nursing process step: Evaluation
Cognitive level: Synthesis

33. The classic signs and symptoms of hypoglycemia include:
A. Confusion, hypertension, and nausea
B. Headache, weakness, and irritability
C. Bradycardia, vomiting, and hypotension
D. Diplopia, restlessness, and tachypnea

CORRECT ANSWER—B. The classic signs and symptoms of hypoglycemia, which include headache, weakness, and irritability, result from stimulation of both the sympathetic and central nervous systems. Hypoglycemia tends to cause hypotension secondary to tachycardia. Tachypnea is not related to hypoglycemia.
Nursing process step: Assessment
Cognitive level: Evaluation

Questions 34 to 36 refer to the following information:

A 55-year-old female patient sustains a basilar skull fracture as a result of a forward fall and a blow to the frontal skull. Two days after the injury, the patient experiences a significant increase in thirst and frequent urination. A physical examination reveals sinus tachycardia of 102 beats/minute and blood pressure of 104/60 mm Hg. Her mucous membranes are dry. Blood pressure measurement reveals a systolic blood pressure decrease of 20 mm Hg from a supine to a standing position with an increase in the heart rate of 30 beats/minute, indicating orthostatic hypotension. The patient is diagnosed with diabetes insipidus related to cranial injury.

34. Primary laboratory findings in a patient with diabetes insipidus typically include:

A. Decreased urine osmolarity, increased urine specific gravity, and decreased serum osmolarity

B. Increased urine osmolarity, increased urine specific gravity, and increased serum osmolarity

C. Decreased urine osmolarity, increased serum osmolarity, and decreased urine specific gravity

D. Increased urine osmolarity, hypernatremia, and hypokalemia

CORRECT ANSWER—C. A patient with diabetes insipidus typically has polyuria in which the urine is dilute, with a specific gravity of less than 1.005 and an osmolarity of 200 mOsm/liter or less. Serum osmolarity is increased, but the degree of the increase depends on the patient's fluid intake.

Nursing process step: Assessment

Cognitive level: Comprehension

35. Which nursing intervention is appropriate for this patient?

A. Restricting fluid intake

B. Increasing sodium intake

C. Providing a high-potassium diet

D. Allowing unrestricted fluid intake

CORRECT ANSWER—D. Fluid intake should be encouraged in a patient with diabetes insipidus; this helps maintain a normovolemic state when urine output is increased. Water should be kept within reach of the patient, and an accurate intake and output record must be maintained. Sodium intake is restricted secondary to hypernatremia in patients with nephrogenic diabetes insipidus. An increased potassium intake is not required in diabetes insipidus.

Nursing process step: Planning

Cognitive level: Application

36. The physician orders drug therapy to control the diabetes insipidus. The nurse should question an order for which drug?

A. Oxytocin

B. Desmopressin acetate

C. Clofibrate

D. Hydrochlorothiazide

CORRECT ANSWER—A. Oxytocin is not used to treat diabetes insipidus. Desmopressin, an antidiuretic hormone (ADH) replacement agent, commonly is prescribed. Clofibrate may be prescribed because it stimulates the release of ADH from the posterior pituitary gland. Hydrochlorothiazide is a thiazide diuretic used to stimulate the kidneys' response to the loss of sodium and water by reabsorbing more water via mechanisms independent of ADH involvement.

Nursing process step: Implementation

Cognitive level: Analysis

37. Typical assessment findings in a patient with syndrome of inappropriate antidiuretic hormone (SIADH) include all of the following *except:*
A. Peripheral edema
B. Weight gain
C. Hyponatremia
D. Anorexia

CORRECT ANSWER—A. In patients with SIADH, weight gain without peripheral edema results from hyponatremia that is due to a concurrent loss of sodium and retained water. The hyponatremia is caused by dilutional effects, increased sodium secretion at the proximal tubules, and a decreased aldosterone level. Anorexia is a sign of hyponatremia.
Nursing process step: Assessment
Cognitive level: Comprehension

Questions 38 to 40 refer to the following information:
A 68-year-old female patient is admitted to the intensive care unit with a tentative diagnosis of hyperosmolar nonketotic syndrome (HNKS). Her medical history reveals that she has non–insulin-dependent diabetes mellitus that is being controlled with tolazamide, an oral hypoglycemia agent.

---

38. What is the most important laboratory test for confirming a diagnosis of hyperosmolar nonketotic syndrome (HNKS)?
A. Serum potassium level
B. Serum sodium level
C. Arterial blood gas values
D. Serum osmolarity

CORRECT ANSWER—D. Serum osmolarity is the most important test for confirming HNKS; it also is used to guide treatment strategies and determine evaluation criteria. A patient with HNKS typically has a serum osmolarity of over 350 mOsm/liter. Serum potassium, serum sodium, and arterial blood gas values also are measured, but they are not as important as serum osmolarity in confirming the diagnosis of HNKS. A patient with HNKS typically has hypernatremia and osmotic diuresis; arterial blood gas values reveal acidosis, and the potassium level is variable.
Nursing process step: Assessment
Cognitive level: Comprehension

39. The patient requires fluid resuscitation. Which statement about fluid replacement for a patient with hyperosmolar nonketotic syndrome (HNKS) is true?
  A. Administer 2 to 3 liters of I.V. fluid rapidly
  B. Administer 6 liters of I.V. fluid over the first 24 hours
  C. Administer a dextrose solution containing 0.9% sodium chloride
  D. Administer I.V. fluid slowly to prevent circulatory overload and collapse

CORRECT ANSWER—A. Regardless of the patient's medical history, rapid fluid resuscitation is critical for cardiovascular integrity. Profound intravascular depletion requires aggressive fluid replacement. A typical fluid resuscitation protocol is 6 liters of fluid over the first 12 hours, with more fluid to follow over the next 24 hours. Various fluids can be used, depending on the degree of hypovolemia. Commonly prescribed fluids include dextran (in cases of hypovolemic shock), isotonic 0.9% sodium chloride solution, and, once the patient is stabilized, hypotonic 0.45% sodium chloride solution.
Nursing process step: Planning
Cognitive level: Application

40. Once the patient is stabilized, the nurse develops a teaching plan to prepare the patient for eventual discharge and home management. Which statement indicates that the patient understands her condition and the preventive measures to control it?
  A. "I can avoid getting sick by not letting myself become dehydrated and by paying attention to my need to urinate, drink, or eat more than usual."
  B. "If I experience trembling, weakness, and headache, I should drink a glass of soda that contains sugar."
  C. "I will have to monitor my blood glucose level closely and notify the doctor if it is constantly elevated."
  D. "If I begin to feel especially hungry and thirsty, I will eat a snack high in carbohydrates."

CORRECT ANSWER—A. Inadequate fluid intake during hyperglycemic episodes often leads to hyperosmolar nonketotic syndrome HNKS. By recognizing the signs of hyperglycemia (polyuria, polydipsia, and polyphagia) and increasing her fluid intake, the patient may prevent HNKS. Drinking a glass of nondiet soda would be appropriate for hypoglycemia. A patient whose diabetes is controlled with oral hypoglycemic agents usually need not monitor the blood glucose level. A high-carbohydrate diet would exacerbate the patient's condition, particularly if her fluid intake was low.
Nursing process step: Evaluation
Cognitive level: Synthesis

41. A nursing diagnosis of risk for fluid volume excess related to aggressive fluid resuscitation is appropriate for a patient with diabetes insipidus who requires water replacement. When the nurse evaluates a patient's response to water replacement therapy, which signs would indicate that water intoxication has occurred?
  A. Confusion, weight gain, and seizures
  B. Lethargy, decreased urine output, and spasticity
  C. Flaccidity, restlessness, and disorientation
  D. Tetany, weight gain, and coma

CORRECT ANSWER—A. Classic signs of water intoxication include confusion and seizures, both of which are caused by cerebral edema, as well as weight gain. Spasticity, flaccidity, and tetany are unrelated to water intoxication.
Nursing process step: Evaluation
Cognitive level: Evaluation

42. When preparing a patient with insulin-dependent diabetes mellitus for discharge, the nurse should discuss the proper way to manage insulin needs. Which goal is appropriate for a patient with a nursing diagnosis of knowledge deficit related to lack of understanding of insulin therapy adjustment during periods of illness (such as those accompanied by nausea and vomiting)?

A. The patient will state that insulin should be withheld during periods of illness

B. The patient will state that doses of intermediate-acting insulin should be reduced during periods of illness

C. The patient will state that the usual insulin dosage schedule should be followed during periods of illness

D. The patient will state that serum glucose and urine ketone levels must be monitored during periods of illness to determine insulin requirements

CORRECT ANSWER—D. A patient with insulin-dependent diabetes mellitus should monitor serum glucose and urine ketone levels frequently during periods of illness because the physical stress associated with illness can increase insulin demand. The patient also should report any illnesses to the physician so that suitable dosage adjustments can be made. Insulin adjustments during illness should be based on glucose level, not the routine dosage schedule. Blood glucose control should be provided with short-acting insulin, especially if the patient is not eating due to nausea and vomiting. Adjustments in the insulin dosage should be discussed with the physician.
Nursing process step: Planning
Cognitive level: Evaluation

43. When administering regular Humulin insulin combined with intermediate-acting NPH insulin to a diabetic patient before breakfast, when should the nurse watch for a potential hypoglycemic reaction?

A. In the late morning
B. In the late afternoon
C. During the evening
D. At bedtime

CORRECT ANSWER—B. Although regular insulin peaks 2 to 3 hours after administration, the morning meal provides effective coverage. However, intermediate-acting NPH insulin peaks 6 to 8 hours after administration. Therefore, hypoglycemia or other evidence of the peak effects of morning NPH insulin would be seen in the late afternoon. This is why many insulin-dependent diabetic patients require an afternoon snack.
Nursing process step: Assessment
Cognitive level: Comprehension

44. Which fluid and electrolyte changes are common in a patient with syndrome of inappropriate antidiuretic hormone (SIADH)?

A. Decreased serum sodium, decreased plasma osmolarity, and increased urine sodium

B. Decreased urine volume, increased serum sodium, and increased urine sodium

C. Increased weight, increased serum sodium, and increased plasma osmolarity

D. Decreased weight, decreased serum sodium, and decreased plasma osmolarity

CORRECT ANSWER—A. Diagnostic test results in a patient with SIADH would include a decreased serum sodium level, decreased plasma osmolarity, increased urine osmolarity, and increased urine sodium level. Weight gain also occurs.
Nursing process step: Assessment
Cognitive level: Comprehension

Questions 45 and 46 refer to the following information:
A 57-year-old male patient who has diabetes mellitus and hypertension is admitted to the intensive care unit with a diagnosis of bronchogenic cancer occluding the right main bronchus and severe dyspnea requiring mechanical ventilation. He receives immediate radiation treatment, and his respiratory status subsequently improves. Two days after extubation, the patient is irritable and confused and has short-term memory deficits. He complains of headache. Serum studies are performed, and the patient is diagnosed with syndrome of inappropriate antidiuretic hormone (SIADH).

45. Which condition commonly is associated with SIADH?
   A. Diabetes mellitus
   B. Hypertension
   C. Myasthenia gravis
   D. Bronchogenic cancer

CORRECT ANSWER—D. Cancers of the lung are associated with SIADH. Stimulation of baroceptors in the lung caused by increased intrathoracic pressure triggers secretion of a physiologically active form of antidiuretic hormone. The other options are unrelated to SIADH.
Nursing process step: Assessment
Cognitive level: Knowledge

46. The patient has a nursing diagnosis of fluid volume excess related to electrolyte imbalance. Which signs and symptoms of hyponatremia should the nurse report immediately to the physician?
   A. Irritability and increased reflexes
   B. Diarrhea and swollen tongue
   C. Chvostek's sign and hyperreflexia
   D. Muscle weakness and lethargy

CORRECT ANSWER—D. Signs and symptoms of hyponatremia include muscle weakness and lethargy that can progress to stupor and coma. Additional signs and symptoms of hyponatremia include vomiting, abdominal pain, anxiety, lower extremity muscle cramping, and seizures. Irritability and increased reflexes are central nervous system signs of hypernatremia. Although diarrhea is a sign of hyponatremia, a swollen tongue indicates hypernatremia. Chvostek's sign and hyperreflexia may be seen in hypocalcemia.
Nursing process step: Implementation
Cognitive level: Analysis

47. A 62-year-old female patient is admitted to the intensive care unit with a diagnosis of pyelonephritis and possible septicemia. She has had five urinary tract infections over the past 2 years. During the nursing history interview, the patient expresses overwhelming fatigue from lack of sleep. She describes her urination pattern as "I seem to go all the time, even through the night." She notes that she has lost a few pounds over the last few days, although she drinks constantly. A serum laboratory panel reveals the following:
- sodium level, 152 mEq/liter
- osmolarity, 340 mOsm/liter
- glucose level, 125 mg/dl
- potassium level, 3.8 mEq/liter.

Based on the above information, which nursing diagnosis is most appropriate?

A. Fluid volume deficit related to inability to conserve water

B. Altered nutrition, less than body requirements, related to hypermetabolic state

C. Fluid volume deficit related to osmotic diuresis induced by hypernatremia

D. Altered nutrition, less than body requirements, related to catabolic effects of insulin deficiency

CORRECT ANSWER—A. The patient has signs and symptoms of diabetes insipidus, probably caused by failure of her renal tubules to respond to antidiuretic hormone as a consequence of the pyelonephritis. The hypernatremia is secondary to her water loss. Altered nutrition related to a hypermetabolic state or catabolic effect of insulin deficiency is an inappropriate nursing diagnosis for this patient.
Nursing process step: Assessment
Cognitive level: Application

48. Which nursing diagnosis is most appropriate for a patient with syndrome of inappropriate antidiuretic hormone (SIADH) and hyponatremia?

A. Risk for injury related to seizure activity

B. Impaired skin integrity related to peripheral edema

C. Fluid volume excess related to increased thyrotropin secretion

D. Impaired gas exchange related to pulmonary edema

CORRECT ANSWER—A. Patients with hyponatremia are at high risk for seizures. Nursing interventions should be aimed at safety and protection, including using padded side rails, administering supplemental oxygen, and keeping an oral airway readily available. Peripheral edema is not associated with SIADH. Thyrotropin is a hormone produced by the anterior pituitary gland; it has no role in SIADH. Pulmonary edema is a complication of hypernatremia and is not commonly seen in SIADH or hyponatremia.
Nursing process step: Planning
Cognitive level: Application

49. A 66-year-old male patient is recovering from a hypophysectomy for removal of a pituitary tumor. He is receiving desmopressin acetate nasal spray twice daily. When preparing the patient for discharge, the nurse should warn him about which adverse effects of desmopressin therapy?

A. Fatigue, sore throat, and fever
B. Weight gain and edema
C. Polyuria and polydipsia
D. Dizziness, palpitations, and lethargy

CORRECT ANSWER—B. Although adverse effects of desmopressin are uncommon, excessive fluid retention, as evidenced by weight gain and edema, may occur. The other signs and symptoms are not potential adverse effects of desmopressin therapy.
Nursing process step: Planning
Cognitive level: Knowledge

50. When caring for a patient with hyperosmolar nonketotic syndrome (HNKS), the nurse should assess for signs and symptoms of:

A. Lipolysis
B. Hyponatremia
C. Ketosis
D. Hypernatremia

CORRECT ANSWER—D. A patient with HNKS usually has concomitant hypernatremia resulting from the significant loss of water. The typical serum sodium level is 145 mEq/liter. Lipolysis and ketosis are hallmarks of diabetic ketoacidosis and are not seen in HNKS.
Nursing process step: Assessment
Cognitive level: Evaluation

51. The nurse prepares discharge instructions for a patient with chronic syndrome of inappropriate antidiuretic hormone (SIADH). Which statement indicates that the patient understands these instructions?

A. "I will check all food labels to make sure that I restrict my sodium intake."
B. "I will keep a log of my daily weight and call the physician if I gain 2 pounds or more in a day without changing my eating habits."
C. "I will check my pulse every morning and will contact my physician if it is irregular or rapid."
D. "I will measure my urine at home and check the specific gravity with a refractometer. If it begins to gradually rise, I will notify the physician."

CORRECT ANSWER—B. Daily weight is the most accurate means of monitoring hydration status at home. The patient should be encouraged to increase dietary intake of both sodium and potassium, particularly if diuretics are prescribed. Pulse checks and urine specific gravity measurements are unnecessary in a patient with chronic SIADH.
Nursing process step: Evaluation
Cognitive level: Synthesis

52. Which intervention is critical in managing a patient with chronic syndrome of inappropriate antidiuretic hormone (SIADH)?

A. Administering diuretics
B. Infusing a hypotonic sodium chloride replacement solution
C. Restricting fluid intake
D. Administering potassium supplements

CORRECT ANSWER—C. Fluid restriction is essential in treating chronic SIADH. Fluids typically are restricted to 800 to 1,000 ml/day. If diuretics are prescribed, sodium and potassium supplements may be needed. A hypertonic sodium chloride I.V. solution might be used in the acute phase of treatment if the patient is severely hyponatremic.
Nursing process step: Implementation
Cognitive level: Application

53. A 36-year-old female patient with a history of insulin-dependent diabetes mellitus is admitted to the critical care unit with a three-day history of nausea, vomiting, and abdominal pain. Her blood glucose level is 680 mg/dl. The interventions the nurse should first implement when treating this patient with diabetic ketoacidosis, *in order of importance,* are:

A. Monitor the patient's hemodynamic status and maintain a patent airway

B. Maintain a patent airway, and intervene to correct the patient's acidemia and hyperglycemia

C. Maintain a patent airway, and treat fluid volume excess and infection

D. Monitor the patient's fluid and electrolyte status, and maintain a patent airway

CORRECT ANSWER—**B.** The patient with diabetic ketoacidosis (DKA) is likely to have respiratory compromise related to the metabolic acidosis. Initially, maintaining a patent airway, monitoring the patient's respiratory pattern, and monitoring the patient's arterial blood gas analysis results will help determine if hypoxia or respiratory failure exists and if intubation is needed. Treatment for DKA is aimed at correcting the acidemia (decreased blood pH), hyperglycemia, and fluid volume deficits with rapid I.V. infusions of 0.9% sodium chloride solution. During the course of treatment, the nurse will need to monitor fluid and electrolyte status as well hemodynamic status to determine if any deficiencies exist and to evaluate the effectiveness of the treatment administered.

Nursing process step: Planning
Cognitive level: Analysis

HEMATOLOGIC AND IMMUNOLOGIC SYSTEMS

CHAPTER 7

Hematologic and Immunologic Systems

1. Reticulocytes are immature:
   A. Red blood cells
   B. Platelets
   C. Lymphocytes
   D. Monocytes

CORRECT ANSWER—**A.** All blood cells are made in the bone marrow and have several precursor cells that may be released from the marrow in times of stress or increased need, such as in anemia or hemorrhage. A slightly immature red blood cell is called a reticulocyte. Early platelets are called megakaryocytes. Mature white blood cells include granulocytes, lymphocytes, and monocytes. White blood cell precursors are called blasts and are identified with a prefix to match the cell type (for example, *lympho*blast or *mono*blast).
Nursing process step: Assessment
Cognitive level: Knowledge

2. Which assessment finding is indicative of early disseminated intravascular coagulation (DIC)?
   A. Acrocyanosis
   B. Hemoptysis
   C. Hematuria
   D. Hematochezia

CORRECT ANSWER—**A.** DIC is a secondary disorder that can occur with other serious conditions, such as septic shock, abruptio placentae, and massive tissue injury. Accelerated clotting mechanisms produce small clots that cause occlusion of the microcirculation. Acrocyanosis—a superficial bluish marking of the tissue in which cyanosis is clearly distal to the line and less apparent central to it—is evidence of localized microvascular clotting. Although bleeding is a common manifestation of DIC because of coagulation factor depletion and circulating anticoagulants, it signals that the clotting process has been in place for some time. Consequently, signs and symptoms of clotting (oliguria and cyanosis) occur earlier than signs of bleeding (hemoptysis, hematuria, and hematochezia).
Nursing process step: Assessment
Cognitive level: Evaluation

3. A patient experiencing acute rejection of the heart is prescribed lymphocyte immune globulin (also known as antithymocyte globulin, ATG). Nursing care during administration of this drug should include:

A. Administering concomitant fluids to maintain adequate hydration

B. Monitoring for hypotension and allergic reactions

C. Administering concomitant antiemetics

D. Monitoring the infusion site for signs of extravasation because drug is a vesicant

CORRECT ANSWER—B. Lymphocyte immune globulin is a protein product consisting of a complex of multiple antibodies that block T-lymphocyte function; it occasionally causes allergic or anaphylactic reactions. Symptoms of such reactions include fever, chills, rash, bronchospasm, and hypotension. The antibody is diluted in a large fluid volume, but hydration is not necessary during drug administration. Lymphocyte immune globulin is not a vesicant. However, it should be administered through an in-line filter over at least 4 hours to decrease the risks of infusing particulate matter and triggering hypersensitivity reactions. Concomitant administration of an antiemetic is not recommended unless the patient has a history of adverse GI symptoms with administration of this drug.
Nursing process step: Implementation
Cognitive level: Analysis

4. Infectious complications related to the immunosuppressant therapy used in transplant recipients include all of the following *except:*

A. Oral candidiasis (thrush)

B. Herpes zoster

C. Human immunodeficiency virus

D. Cytomegalovirus

CORRECT ANSWER—C. Immunosuppressant therapy can suppress the normal lymphocyte response, making patients prone to superinfection with fungus (such as *Candida*) and unable to resist opportunistic infections (such as tuberculosis or *Pneumocystis carinii* pneumonia) and viral infections (such as herpes zoster, herpes simplex, and cytomegalovirus). The human immunodeficiency virus is spread by direct inoculation via contact with contaminated blood or body fluids. A patient would not contract this infection as a result of immunosuppressant therapy.
Nursing process step: Planning
Cognitive level: Analysis

5. The patient most at risk for life-threatening coagulopathy is one who has just undergone surgery for:
   A. Ischemic stroke
   B. Uncomplicated aortic aneurysm repair
   C. Liver transplant
   D. Sickle cell crisis

CORRECT ANSWER—**C.** Patients at highest risk for coagulopathy are those with disorders of organs essential to the development of coagulation factors (such as the bone marrow, spleen, and liver) or with abnormalities of the actual coagulation factors. Consequently, patients who have received a liver transplant are at high risk for postoperative coagulopathy until the graft is fully functioning. Disorders that damage vessels or tissues (such as aortic aneurysm and ischemic stroke) and those that involve foreign bodies in the bloodstream (such as sickle cell crisis) can cause disseminated intravascular coagulation (DIC); however, DIC is a primary clotting disorder with bleeding as a secondary complication.
Nursing process step: Assessment
Cognitive level: Knowledge

6. A patient with chronic cirrhosis has bleeding around existing central line sites. Based on this finding, the nurse would assess the patient's:
   A. Bleeding time
   B. Factor VIII level
   C. Platelet autoantibody level
   D. Fibrinogen level

CORRECT ANSWER—**D.** The liver produces all coagulation factors except factor VIII. In a patient with known liver disease, coagulopathy is best diagnosed by assessing the coagulation factor levels. The fibrinogen level most accurately reflects coagulation factor levels because it is based on an absolute quantitative analysis of the amount of fibrinogen. The partial thromboplastin time (PTT) and prothrombin time (PT) are derived coagulation tests that reflect the amount of coagulation factors able to form a clot in the laboratory setting. Platelets are made in the bone marrow, and platelet problems are detected by monitoring the platelet count, bleeding time, and platelet autoantibody level.
Nursing process step: Assessment
Cognitive level: Analysis

7. All of the following local measures can be used to control skin, mucous membrane, and soft-tissue bleeding *except:*
  A. Absorbable gelatin sponge
  B. Topical thrombin
  C. Sandbags
  D. Xeroform

CORRECT ANSWER—**D.** Xeroform is a petrolatum-based antibacterial gauze that has no effect on coagulation. Local hemostatic agents control bleeding through a variety of mechanisms, ranging from pressure-induced clotting (sandbags) to forming a coagulant product (topical thrombin) when in contact with blood. An absorbable gelatin sponge is used as an adjunct to hemostasis in surgery; the sponge is saturated with normal 0.9% sodium chloride or thrombin and left in place after the bleeding is controlled.
Nursing process step: Implementation
Cognitive level: Knowledge

8. Which assessment finding is indicative of hepatic veno-occlusive disease after bone marrow transplantation?
  A. Weight gain and pulmonary crackles 20 to 40 days after transplantation
  B. Increased liver transaminase levels within 2 weeks after transplantation
  C. Right upper quadrant abdominal pain and increased bilirubin level 8 to 15 days after transplantation
  D. Fever, tender liver on palpation, and coagulopathy

CORRECT ANSWER—**C.** Hepatic veno-occlusive disease is the chemotherapeutic- or radiation-induced fibrous destruction of hepatic blood vessels that results in increased bilirubin without elevated transaminase levels. The most common presenting symptoms include right upper quadrant abdominal pain, weight gain, and ascites approximately 8 to 15 days after transplantation.
Nursing process step: Assessment
Cognitive level: Evaluation

9. If the physician orders I.V. co-trimoxazole for a patient with acquired immunodeficiency syndrome, the nurse would suspect that the patient has:
  A. Legionnaire's disease
  B. *Pneumocystis carinii* infection
  C. Candida septicemia
  D. Tuberculosis

CORRECT ANSWER—**B.** Co-trimoxazole is a broad-spectrum sulfonamide antibacterial effective against aerobic gram-negative bacteria, such as Enterobacteriaceae, and most gram-positive bacteria. It is also active against unusual and normally resistant organisms, such as *Nocardia asteroides* and *Pneumocystis carinii*. *Legionella* species are treated with erythromycin, and *Candida* species are managed with amphotericin or another antifungal agent. Tuberculosis is treated with antitubercular agents, such as isoniazid and rifampin.
Nursing process step: Evaluation
Cognitive level: Analysis

10. Which standard test initially is performed to crossmatch blood products?

A. Coombs' test
B. Erythrocyte sedimentation rate
C. Agglutination test
D. Hemoglobin antibody test

CORRECT ANSWER—C. The agglutination test is used to test ABO blood type and compatibility with possible donor blood. Coombs' test is used to detect minor antibodies when agglutination occurs despite ABO compatibility. Erythrocyte sedimentation rates can detect infection, especially in chronic inflammatory diseases, such as rheumatoid arthritis. A hemoblobin antibody test is necessary to confirm a blood incompatibility after a transfusion reaction occurs. Proof of incompatibility is the presence of hemoglobinuria, anti-A or anti-B antibodies in the serum, or low serum hemoglobin level.

Nursing process step: Implementation
Cognitive level: Knowledge

11. A 50-year-old leukemia patient is taking cyclosporine to prevent rejection 15 days after allogenic bone marrow transplantation. The patient's bone marrow is still aplastic with the following values: white blood cell count, $0.2/mm^3$; red blood cell count, $4.0/mm^3$; hematocrit, 30 %; hemoglobin level, 9.5 g/dl; and platelet count, $39,000/mm^3$. The patient complains of headache and blurred vision. Assessment findings reveal:

- temperature, 99.7° F (37.6° C)
- blood pressure, 200/96 mm Hg
- crackles in bases of lungs
- altered visual acuity
- normal pupillary response
- normal and equal arm and leg strength.

Which action should the nurse take?

A. Notify the physician because symptoms indicate impending intracranial bleeding with herniation
B. Notify the physician that the patient is exhibiting adverse effects of cyclosporine
C. Notify the physician that the patient is showing signs and symptoms of acute bone marrow rejection
D. Notify the physician so that the patient's renal function can be evaluated for complications of hemolytic-uremic syndrome

CORRECT ANSWER—B. Cyclosporine can cause neurologic adverse effects that are vague and difficult to define and often accompanied by hypertension, as in this example. The patient's neurologic symptoms are nonfocal, which reduces the possibility of herniation; however, because the platelet count is low, frequent neurologic assessments for focal deficits are indicated. Bone marrow rejection usually takes the form of graft-versus-host disease and manifests as skin rash, diarrhea, and hepatomegaly. Hemolytic-uremic syndrome is a late complication of bone marrow transplantation (occurring 50 days or more after the transplant) and causes hemolytic anemia and renal failure.

Nursing process step: Implementation
Cognitive level: Application

12. The most common cause of graft failure in renal transplantation is:
  A. Ischemic graft
  B. Rejection
  C. Surgical complications
  D. Infection

CORRECT ANSWER—**B.** Rejection is the most common cause of graft failure because human leukocyte antigen (HLA) tissue matching is difficult to perform and available immunosuppressant agents are not 100% effective. Hemorrhage is a surgical complication that could lead to hypoperfusion of the new kidney and a potentially ischemic graft. Infection is a significant complication of renal transplantation but does not necessarily lead to graft failure. The nurse should monitor for signs of infection, including wound drainage, poor wound healing, and leakage of urine.
Nursing process step: Assessment
Cognitive level: Comprehension

13. Patients with prolonged neutropenia (lasting more than 10 days) are at risk for which infection?
  A. Herpes simplex reactivation
  B. *Pneumocystis carinii* infection
  C. Oral candidal infection
  D. Tuberculosis

CORRECT ANSWER—**C.** A patient with prolonged neutropenia typically becomes susceptible to infection with opportunistic organisms or superinfection with normal or antibiotic-resistant flora. Because neutrophils combat bacteria, bacterial infections occur early in neutropenia; fungal infections resulting from normal flora occur after 7 to 14 days of neutropenia, and *Pneumocystis carinii* or other opportunistic infections occur after protracted periods of neutropenia. Prolonged neutropenia is not a specific risk factor for viral reactivation, although it may occur.
Nursing process step: Evaluation
Cognitive level: Evaluation

14. Risk factors for coagulopathy in patients who have undergone coronary artery bypass graft (CABG) surgery include all of the following *except:*

A. Longer time on bypass machine and large amount of blood replaced

B. Lower body temperature and insertion of postoperative intra-aortic balloon pump (IABP)

C. Preexisting biventricular failure and antiarrhythmic agent therapy

D. Number of vessels bypassed and administration of plasma expanders

CORRECT ANSWER—D. Patients undergoing CABG are likely to have numerous stressors that reduce the body's clotting ability; however, the number of vessels bypassed does not increase the risk for coagulopathy. Many patients undergo CABG surgery with hepatic congestion from preexisting heart disease, which can predispose them to a deficiency of coagulation factors. During the surgery itself, multiple red blood cell transfusions may be required to prime the perfusion circuit, and existing coagulation products are attracted to the device, thereby decreasing coagulation factors and increasing the chance of bleeding secondary to coagulopathy. In addition, anticoagulants are needed throughout the procedure. Patients are cooled during surgery, which reduces the quality of platelet function, and plasma expanders administered postoperatively have anticoagulant properties. The presence of an IABP induces thrombocytopenia in many patients. Many antiarrhythmic drugs cause adverse hematologic effects that could trigger coagulopathy.

Nursing process step: Assessment
Cognitive level: Comprehension

15. All of the following results are required before transplantation of solid organs *except:*

A. ABO compatibility

B. Human leukocyte antigen (HLA) matching

C. Positive mixed lymphocyte culture reaction

D. Negative test for antibodies to human immunodeficiency virus (HIV)

CORRECT ANSWER—C. A positive mixed lymphocyte culture reaction implies that the donor's and recipient's lymphocytes clumped when combined; this is a poor prognostic indicator for successful engraftment. ABO compatibility and HLA matching (or a close match) are essential to prevent graft rejection. Criteria that must be met for the patient to tolerate the necessary immunosuppressant therapy include absence of HIV infection, absence of active infections, and no history of metastasizing malignancies.

Nursing process step: Assessment
Cognitive level: Knowledge

16. The critical care nurse who believes a terminally ill patient's family may be amenable to donation of body organs should:
A. Discuss organ donation with the family
B. Have the physician discuss organ donation with the family as soon as possible to ensure adequate time to evaluate candidacy
C. Call the local or institutional transplant coordinator immediately to begin the evaluation process
D. Wait until the patient dies to call the local or institutional transplant coordinator

CORRECT ANSWER—C. Early evaluation of potential transplant candidates enhances the ability of practitioners to preserve organ function for possible transplantation. The nurse and physician should defer this process to transplant coordinators who are well trained in approaching families for permission to harvest organs. Family members should be reassured that they will not be responsible for costs incurred during the evaluation. It is preferable that immediate caregivers do not discuss the possibility of organ donation; family members may believe caregivers are anxious to hasten the patient's death in order to harvest organs for another patient.
Nursing process step: Implementation
Cognitive level: Application

17. Nursing care of a patient with disseminated intravascular coagulation (DIC) includes:
A. Frequently assessing peripheral pulses
B. Ensuring accurate coagulation tests through percutaneous venipuncture
C. Preventing fevers and enhancing body cooling
D. Using Trendelenburg's position to enhance blood flow to vital organs

CORRECT ANSWER—A. Patients with DIC have a primary clotting disorder of the microvasculature that leads to consumption of coagulation factors and thromboses throughout the body. Evaluation of a patient in the early phase of this disorder involves assessing for evidence of thromboses (such as ischemic stroke) and tissue ischemia (such as peripheral cyanosis and decreased pulses). Vasoconstriction and cool body temperatures can worsen DIC. Bleeding complications develop when injury occurs after the clotting system is compromised and coagulation factors are depleted. Tissue injury, such as from I.V. line insertions or venipunctures, and dependent injury, such as from dangling limbs or Trendelenburg's position, should be avoided when possible because they increase the risk of bleeding.
Nursing process step: Implementation
Cognitive level: Application

18. A patient is receiving corticosteroids to prevent rejection of a liver transplant. The physician is likely to prescribe which concomitant medication to counteract the adverse effects of corticosteroids?
- **A.** Diphenhydramine
- **B.** Cimetidine
- **C.** Colchicine
- **D.** Acetaminophen

CORRECT ANSWER—B. Corticosteroids have many systemic effects unrelated to the immunosuppressant actions of the drug. Because transplant patients require high-dosage or long-term corticosteroid therapy, the adverse effects of fluid retention, hypertension, hyperglycemia, emotional lability, and increased gastric acid secretion are common. Medications used to counteract the adverse effects of corticosteroids include insulin for hyperglycemia, diuretics for fluid retention and hypertension, and histamine$_2$ blockers, such as cimetidine, for increased gastric acid secretion. Diphenhydramine, colchicine, and acetaminophen are not used to counteract the adverse effects of corticosteroids.
Nursing process step: Planning
Cognitive level: Application

19. The nurse developing a plan of care for a patient with type A blood knows that the erythrocytes of a person with this blood type have A antigens on their surface. The nurse would not administer type B blood to this patient because the plasma of type A blood has:
- **A.** Anti-B antibodies
- **B.** Anti-B antigens
- **C.** Anti-A antibodies
- **D.** No antibodies

CORRECT ANSWER—A. The ABO blood typing system is based on identification of A and B antigens on the surface of red blood cells and circulating antibodies in the plasma, which are directed against antigens not present in the patient's blood. Therefore, a patient with A antigens would have anti-B antibodies in plasma. A patient with type O blood has no antigens on the red blood cells and antibodies against both A and B; consequently, this patient is considered a universal donor. A patient with AB blood has both antigens on the red blood cells and no antibodies in the plasma; such a patient is a universal recipient.
Nursing process step: Assessment
Cognitive level: Knowledge

20. Certain critical conditions, therapies, and medications can interfere with platelet functioning. The nurse should assess for signs of bleeding related to impaired platelet functioning in all of the following situations *except*:
   A. Severe infection and gentamicin use
   B. Leukemia and indomethacin use
   C. Hypothermia and dextran use
   D. Hyperalimentation and corticosteroid use

CORRECT ANSWER—D. Hyperalimentation and corticosteroids do not interfere with platelet functioning. However, in some conditions, such as leukemia or toxicity of certain drugs, platelet production is decreased or defective. In patients with cirrhosis of the liver and severe infection, increased destruction of platelets occurs outside the bone marrow. Patients who are hypothermic or have hypersplenism have a decreased number of circulating platelets secondary to sequestration or platelet loss. Many drugs can cause acquired thrombocytopenia by interfering with platelet functioning. These medications include volume expanders, such as dextran; antibiotics, such as gentamicin; and nonsteroidal anti-inflammatory drugs, such as indomethacin.
Nursing process step: Planning
Cognitive level: Analysis

21. A patient with congestive heart failure and hepatomegaly is admitted for open-heart surgery. There is no evidence of overt bleeding, but the following laboratory values are noted: hematocrit, 32%; hemoglobin, 11.4 g/dl; platelets, 154,000/mm^3; prothrombin time, 15 seconds (control, 10 seconds); partial thromboplastin time, 12.5 seconds (control, 11 seconds); fibrinogen, 170 mg/dl. Which blood product is required?
   A. Platelets
   B. Fresh frozen plasma
   C. Cryoprecipitate
   D. Red blood cells

CORRECT ANSWER—B. This patient has known hepatomegaly and is at high risk for coagulation factor deficiency. In addition, the abnormal prothrombin time and low-normal fibrinogen level suggest liver dysfunction. Given these clinical findings, the patient would require plasma, the blood product that replaces coagulation factors made in the liver. The nurse should monitor the patient's hematocrit because it is low; however, there are no signs of bleeding, and replacement therapy is not necessary. A normal platelet count is 200,000 to 300,000/mm^3; therefore, the patient's count is low, but a transfusion is not necessary at this point.
Nursing process step: Implementation
Cognitive level: Evaluation

22. What is the most common transfusion reaction?
A. Hemolytic reaction
B. Allergic reaction
C. Febrile reaction
D. Circulatory overload

CORRECT ANSWER—C. Because of minor genetic differences in the antigen/antibody makeup of individual patients, slight reactions to foreign proteins are common with all blood products. Reactions usually are febrile in nature. Typical allergic reactions, such as rash and itching, occur intermittently, and frank ABO (hemolytic) incompatibility is rare except when linked to human error in crossmatching. Circulatory overload is not a transfusion reaction, but a complication that can result from transfusion; signs and symptoms of circulatory overload include dyspnea, distended neck veins, chest pain, tachycardia, and crackles on auscultation.
Nursing process step: Evaluation
Cognitive level: Comprehension

23. Which statement about infection assessment in an immunocompromised patient is true?
A. Infections often are asymptomatic except for fever
B. Daily assessments usually reveal drainage in infected areas
C. Infections usually produce few symptoms, but cultures usually are positive
D. Systemic symptoms of infection, such as leukocytosis and myalgia, are pronounced

CORRECT ANSWER—A. The lack of an immune system response or an inflammatory response in immunocompromised individuals leads to few clinical symptoms of infection and often negative cultures despite systemic fever, possibly indicating infection. Fever, usually the low-grade type, commonly is the only sign of infection in an immunocompromised patient.
Nursing process step: Assessment
Cognitive level: Comprehension

24. A transplant patient receiving immunosuppressant therapy is most susceptible to which infection?
A. Herpes simplex reactivation
B. *Pneumocystis carinii* infection
C. *Candida albicans* infection
D. *Serratia* infection

CORRECT ANSWER—A. A patient on immunosuppressant medication to prevent graft rejection usually receives therapy directed against lymphoid function. Lymphocytes are most responsible for combating viral infection, making herpes simplex reactivation the most common infection in patients receiving immunosuppressants. The other infections may occur if immunosuppression is prolonged.
Nursing process step: Planning
Cognitive level: Knowledge

25. A patient with hemophilia is brought to the emergency department after injuring his knee playing soccer. The nurse should anticipate the need to administer:

A. Platelets
B. Fresh frozen plasma
C. Factor VIII concentrate
D. Red blood cells

CORRECT ANSWER—C. Hemophilia is a congenital deficiency of factor VIII or factor IX; a deficiency of factor IX is rare. When a patient with factor VIII deficiency is injured, coagulation initially occurs because of the existing platelets and bleeding is not immediately apparent. Because insufficient factor VIII is available to participate in the intrinsic coagulation pathway, bleeding occurs in areas in which factor VIII usually is prevalent, such as the joints, brain, kidneys, and oral mucous membranes. Immediate transfusion of factor VIII and repeated doses for 24 to 72 hours after injury can prevent bleeding. Factor VIII is available in two forms—blood bank formulations called cryoprecipitate and antihemophilic factor A (AHF) or concentrated factor VIII. Because hemophilia is caused by a deficiency or absence of factor VIII or factor IX, replacing these factors allows the coagulation cascade to occur. Administering fresh frozen plasma, red blood cells, or platelets would not correct the cause of the coagulopathy.
Nursing process step: Planning
Cognitive level: Analysis

26. Which nursing intervention is appropriate for a patient with cold agglutinin antibodies?

A. Administering blood according to institutional protocol
B. Administering packed red blood cells only
C. Administering blood warmed to body temperature
D. Administering blood through special filters

CORRECT ANSWER—C. The presence of nonspecific antibodies on the surface of red blood cells in certain diseases can cause agglutination (clumping) of red blood cells at temperatures below 39.2° F (4° C) and may cause hemolysis. The phenomenon does not occur at body temperature. Cold agglutinins are common in the elderly and after recent viral infection; they may be idiopathic. Warming the blood to body temperature prevents agglutination. Normal administration of blood does not include warming it. Administering packed red blood cells to a patient with cold agglutinin antibodies without warming the blood product can cause agglutination. Administering blood through special filters will not prevent agglutination.
Nursing process step: Implementation
Cognitive level: Application

27. A patient with acute myocardial infarction (MI) receives an I.V. bolus dose of tissue plasminogen activator (TPA), and an infusion of TPA is begun. Which of the following laboratory tests should be used to monitor the patient's response to treatment?
A. Platelet count
B. Thrombin time
C. Partial thromboplastin time
D. Fibrin split products

CORRECT ANSWER—B. TPA, a naturally occurring substance that accelerates clot breakdown, is administered to lyse existing clots in patients with MI, pulmonary embolism, or deep vein thrombosis. When TPA is administered, the patient is at high risk for excessive bleeding. A sensitive laboratory test is needed to detect the adequacy of treatment and assist in titrating the dosage to achieve therapeutic effects without bleeding. Thrombin time is a sensitive test that can detect small amounts of thrombin inhibitors in the blood. Platelet counts determine the number of platelets; they do not reveal any information about clotting. Partial thromboplastin time is not a sensitive test, and fibrin split products detect the presence of fibrin breakdown products.
Nursing process step: Evaluation
Cognitive level: Evaluation

28. What is the most common adverse effect of antibiotics used to treat gram-negative bacteria?
A. Oral ulcers
B. Platelet dysfunction
C. Oliguria and dysuria
D. Diarrhea

CORRECT ANSWER—D. Broad-spectrum antibiotics that destroy aerobic and anaerobic bacteria also destroy the normal flora of the GI tract that are responsible for absorbing water and certain nutrients, such as vitamin K. Destruction of normal flora commonly leads to diarrhea. Other less common adverse effects, such as oral stomatitis, platelet dysfunction, renal dysfunction, and liver dysfunction, are not caused by destruction of flora.
Nursing process step: Assessment
Cognitive level: Knowledge

29. Which nursing diagnosis is most appropriate for a patient with human immunodeficiency virus infection and cryptosporidiosis?
A. Risk for injury related to increased bleeding tendencies
B. Ineffective airway clearance related to loss of cough and gag reflex
C. Fluid volume excess related to heart failure
D. Fluid volume deficit related to diarrhea

CORRECT ANSWER—D. *Cryptosporidium* is a microbe that causes GI infection leading to diarrhea and fluid volume deficit (not fluid volume excess), abdominal discomfort, and nutritional or electrolyte imbalance. The patient is not at increased risk for bleeding tendencies or loss of protective reflexes.
Nursing process step: Assessment
Cognitive level: Comprehension

30. Which laboratory test is the first to become abnormal in a patient with disseminated intravascular coagulation (DIC)?
A. Platelet count
B. Fibrinogen level
C. Partial thromboplastin time (PTT)
D. Fibrin split products

CORRECT ANSWER—A. DIC is a disorder of accelerated and uncontrolled clotting triggered by normal clotting mechanisms (vessel injury, tissue injury, or presence of a foreign body in the bloodstream) but not checked by normal methods. The uncontrolled microvascular clotting uses platelets first for blood coagulation, followed by fibrinogen to make fibrin clots; ultimately, clots break down to create fibrin split products. Consequently, the platelet count decreases first, then the fibrinogen level decreases (after which PTT and the prothrombin time become prolonged), and, lastly, fibrin split products are detected as the clots lyse.
Nursing process step: Evaluation
Cognitive level: Evaluation

31. A trauma patient is bleeding profusely and receives massive blood transfusions. The nurse should assess for signs of transfusion reaction, including:
A. Hypocalcemia and hypercoagulability
B. Jaundice and alkalosis
C. Hyperkalemia and hyperammonemia
D. Hypothermia and hypermagnesemia

CORRECT ANSWER—C. Massive blood transfusions predispose patients to the adverse effects of stored preserved blood. Because banked blood is cold, it produces hypothermia. It also contains a significant number of dead or dying red blood cells, which increases the risk of hyperkalemia, hyperammonemia, increased blood urea nitrogen, and jaundice. Citrate, an acidic preservative used in banked blood, causes hypocalcemia by binding with serum calcium and causes acidosis because of the transfusion of a large volume of acidic fluid. Massive transfusions dilute existing coagulation factors, which causes coagulopathy in many patients unless coagulation factors are replaced simultaneously. The magnesium level is not affected by blood transfusions.
Nursing process step: Assessment
Cognitive level: Application

32. Aminocaproic acid is used to:
A. Prevent clotting
B. Prevent platelet formation
C. Prevent clot breakdown
D. Reduce by-products of clot breakdown in the blood

CORRECT ANSWER—C. Aminocaproic acid blocks the conversion of plasmin to plasminogen, which prevents the clot lysis process. Clots prevented from lysing remain at the site of injury. Aminocaproic acid is used to prevent bleeding in patients whose blood has already clotted.
Nursing process step: Implementation
Cognitive level: Knowledge

33. Close monitoring of bile drainage is required for a liver transplant patient in the immediate post-operative period. Which of the following is a reportable finding?
   A. Golden brown bile
   B. Light brown bile
   C. Dark, muddy brown bile
   D. Green bile

CORRECT ANSWER—C. Postoperative bile drainage from a T tube in a patient who has undergone liver transplantation normally is golden brown but may be light brown. As recovery continues, the bile may be greenish. Dark, muddy brown bile indicates potential ischemia or necrosis of the graft and should be reported.
Nursing process step: Assessment
Cognitive level: Evaluation

34. A patient recovering from a liver transplant is extubated on the third postoperative day; he is alert and follows all commands. The patient's laboratory findings at this time include a white blood cell count of 7,000/mm^3, normal coagulation studies, and a serum glucose level of 176 mg/dl. The patient is afebrile with normal vital signs. Two days later, the nurse notes the following on the patient's chart: normal blood pressure and heart rate, fever of 100.4° F (38° C), oriented but lethargic, slightly reddened incision site, and dark brown drainage from the T tube. Laboratory tests reveal normal hematocrit and hemoglobin values, a white blood cell count of 14,000/mm^3, slightly prolonged coagulation tests, and a serum glucose level of 100 mg/dl. Based on these findings, the nurse would:
   A. Do nothing because this postoperative course is normal
   B. Increase the patient's activity level because of possible pulmonary infection resulting from immobility
   C. Obtain a tissue sample of the wound for culture because the wound probably is the site of infection
   D. Notify the physician because the patient is exhibiting symptoms of possible organ rejection

CORRECT ANSWER—D. Fever, leukocytosis, mental status changes, abnormal coagulation tests, hypoglycemia, and brown bile drainage indicate graft ischemia and possible rejection, and the physician should be notified.
Nursing process step: Implementation
Cognitive level: Application

35. A 40-year-old male I.V. drug user has subacute bacterial endocarditis. Septicemia and disseminated intravascular coagulation develop, and the patient receives antibiotics and multiple blood transfusions. The physician decides that a pulmonary artery catheter and hemodialysis catheter must be inserted. The nurse assisting with these procedures will:

A. Administer red blood cells before catheter insertions

B. Wear gown, gloves, mask, and goggles

C. Wear gown, gloves, mask, and booties and treat all linens as contaminated

D. Wear gloves and goggles

CORRECT ANSWER—B. Patients at risk for human immunodeficiency virus (HIV) infection include I.V. drug users and those who engage in anal sex or have sexual partners who engage in anal sex. Thus, this patient is at risk for HIV, which is transmitted through direct contact with blood or body fluids. Nurses should protect themselves from exposure to all body fluids in daily practice and use particular caution during procedures that expose them to blood and semen. All mucous membranes should be protected from exposure, so gown, gloves, mask, and goggles should be worn for the catheter insertions, which will expose the nurse to the patient's blood.
Nursing process step: Implementation
Cognitive level: Application

36. The critical care nurse would be concerned about the risk of thrombocytopenia and plan to assess for signs of coagulopathy in a patient with:

A. An intra-aortic balloon pump who is receiving histamine blockers

B. Acute renal failure who is receiving heparin

C. Sepsis who is receiving dopamine

D. Immobility who has received excess red blood cell transfusions

CORRECT ANSWER—A. Several disorders and medications, including histamine blockers, reduce the number of circulating platelets by means of altered production, abnormal sequestration (as in the spleen), and accelerated destruction. Abnormal destruction also occurs when a patient has an indwelling device, such as an intra-aortic balloon pump, and in cases of hypermetabolism, as seen in sepsis. Heparin-induced thrombocytopenia is a possibility during heparin administration. Excess red blood cell transfusions can contribute to thrombocytopenia if antibodies develop from the transfusion. Acute renal failure, dopamine therapy, and immobility are not associated with thrombocytopenia.
Nursing process step: Planning
Cognitive level: Application

37. Which laboratory test is most specific for vitamin K-dependent factor depletion?

A. Platelet count

B. Prothrombin time (PT)

C. Partial thromboplastin time (PTT)

D. Fibrinogen level

CORRECT ANSWER—B. Vitamin K-dependent factors are used in the extrinsic coagulation pathway to form a fibrin clot. When these factors are not present, an extrinsic pathway deficiency can be detected. The extrinsic pathway is tested through the PT, and the intrinsic pathway is tested through the PTT; the final common pathway is tested via the fibrinogen level or thrombin time. Vitamin K is unrelated to the platelet count.
Nursing process step: Implementation
Cognitive level: Analysis

38. The risk of infection in an immunosuppressed patient can be decreased by:

A. Ensuring adequate sleep and immunoglobulin G (IgG) level

B. Providing progressive muscle relaxation therapy and a low-protein diet

C. Providing live plants and cut flowers and keeping doors closed

D. Using single-patient items and wearing a mask when providing care

CORRECT ANSWER—A. Immunosuppression and its infectious consequences can be decreased by various changes in nursing practice. Good hand washing is most essential, but adequate nutrition with a high-protein diet, rest, and stress reduction techniques, such as progressive muscle relaxation, also can enhance immunocompetence. The IgG level can be checked and, if found inadequate, intravenous IgG may be administered. Plants, fresh flowers, and standing water should be avoided because they harbor organisms. The benefits of wearing masks or implementing isolation procedures in immunosuppressed patients have not been conclusively proved.

Nursing process step: Implementation
Cognitive level: Application

39. Which diagnostic test would confirm a diagnosis of human immunodeficiency virus (HIV) infection?

A. Enzyme-linked immunosorbent assay

B. E rosette assay

C. Western blot assay

D. Immunofluorescence

CORRECT ANSWER—C. HIV infection is detected by analyzing the blood for antibodies to the virus. Antibodies occur approximately 2 to 12 weeks after exposure and denote infection. The enzyme-linked immunoabsorbent assay (ELISA) detects HIV antibody particles via immunofluorescence methods, but it can be inaccurate. A positive ELISA is followed by the Western blot assay, which involves electrophoresis of the antibody proteins. When used alone, the Western blot assay is not specific; when it is used in conjunction with ELISA, it is more than 98% accurate. The E rosette assay is used to count the number of T lymphocytes, but it is not used to confirm diagnosis of HIV infection. Immunofluorescence is used to detect infection in general, but not specifically HIV.

Nursing process step: Assessment
Cognitive level: Knowledge

40. A 49-year-old diabetic patient has been in the critical care unit for the past week recovering from diabetic ketoacidosis and cellulitis of the left leg. The patient has an undefined coagulopathy indicated by minor mucosal bleeding of the mouth, pink-tinged urine, and occult blood in the stools. When developing an assessment plan, the nurse should include:

A. Neurologic assessment every 2 to 4 hours
B. Heart sound assessment every 2 to 4 hours
C. GI assessment at least every 2 to 4 hours
D. Breath sound assessment every 2 to 4 hours

CORRECT ANSWER—**A.** Patients with minor or occult bleeding into body orifices, especially via the mucous membranes, may be exhibiting a problem with platelets, coagulation, or clot lysing. Regardless of the cause, morbidity and mortality in patients with coagulopathy are secondary to intracranial bleeding. This is especially likely with the type of capillary bleeding seen in this patient. Frequent neurologic assessments will detect abnormalities early. Assessments of other body systems, especially those beginning to show signs of bleeding (such as GI bleeding), also are important. However, other body systems may show few early sensitive indicators of bleeding and can be assessed less frequently when the bleeding is as vague and diffuse as that seen in this patient.
Nursing process step: Planning
Cognitive level: Application

41. The nurse would administer which type of plasma to a patient who has AB-negative blood?

A. O positive
B. A negative
C. B negative
D. AB positive

CORRECT ANSWER—**D.** Plasma administration does not require Rh compatibility, but it does require ABO matching. A patient with AB-negative blood has both A and B antibodies on the red blood cell surface and no antibodies in the plasma. The nurse must administer plasma that does not have antibodies that will destroy the patient's red blood cells. Therefore, only plasma of the AB blood type can be given.
Nursing process step: Implementation
Cognitive level: Application

42. Which of the following is an example of an altered barrier defense that directly predisposes a patient to infection?

A. Acidic urine
B. Injury to pulmonary cilia caused by smoking
C. Peripheral neuropathy of diabetes mellitus
D. Altered level of consciousness

CORRECT ANSWER—**B.** Infection can occur because of direct or indirect alterations in the barrier defense system, which consists of the external and internal coverings of the body (such as skin and mucous membranes), normal protective secretions (such as mucus and sweat), and special barrier properties (such as the acidity of the urine). The only example that directly alters one of these barriers is injury to pulmonary cilia from smoking. Acidic urine is normal, and neuropathies or altered consciousness indirectly predispose patients to barrier integrity problems.
Nursing process step: Assessment
Cognitive level: Knowledge

43. Nursing care for a patient receiving zidovudine (also known as azidothymidine, AZT) for human immunodeficiency virus (HIV) infection includes which intervention?

A. Administering zidovudine with milk or antacids

B. Checking pulse and blood pressure before zidovudine administration

C. Planning to treat drug-induced diarrhea

D. Evaluating central and peripheral neurologic function frequently

CORRECT ANSWER—D. Zidovudine is one of three currently available anti-HIV medications. The primary adverse effects of this drug are bone marrow suppression (especially of red and white blood cells), myalgia, and moderate neurologic symptoms (such as headache, tremors, and lowered seizure threshold). Other less common adverse effects include skin rash, altered taste sensation, and altered liver function. Dose-limiting toxicities include bone marrow suppression, renal dysfunction, and liver dysfunction. Zidovudine need not be administered with milk or antacids and does not cause diarrhea, but it does cause anorexia and nausea. The patient's pulse or blood pressure does not have to be checked before drug administration because zidovudine has no adverse cardiovascular effects.
Nursing process step: Implementation
Cognitive level: Application

44. A 23-year-old patient with chronic leukemia who underwent successful allogenic bone marrow transplantation 74 days ago has dyspnea, hypoxemia, and diffuse alveolar infiltrates on the X-ray film. This most likely reflects:

A. Acute graft-versus-host disease

B. Chronic rejection

C. Bronchiolitis fibrosa obliterans

D. Cytomegalovirus (CMV) pneumonia

CORRECT ANSWER—D. Late onset of pulmonary symptoms is likely to be a manifestation of chronic graft-versus-host disease (in the form of bronchiolitis fibrosa obliterans) or viral infection. The most common viral infection is CMV, although adenovirus and rhinovirus can occur. *Pneumocystis carinii* pneumonia also may occur, but it is not usually seen this late after transplantation. The acuteness of the symptoms and alveolar infiltrates are more compatible with CMV infection; bronchiolitis fibrosa obliterans would have a slower onset and symptoms related to pulmonary obstructive disease.
Nursing process step: Evaluation
Cognitive level: Evaluation

45. A patient who underwent kidney transplantation is most likely to receive which of the following medications to prevent rejection?
A. Interferon and methotrexate
B. Cyclosporine and hepatitis B vaccine
C. Cyclophosphamide and acetaminophen
D. Cyclosporine and azathioprine

CORRECT ANSWER—**D.** Immunosuppressant agents include corticosteroids; cyclosporine; certain antineoplastic agents given in smaller doses, such as methotrexate, cyclophosphamide, and azathioprine; and antibody products, such as lymphocyte immune globulin or muromonab-CD3. Interferon and hepatitis B vaccine enhance the immune response and would be detrimental for transplant patients. Acetaminophen is not indicated to prevent rejection and would be administered only if fever, ache, or headache occurs.
Nursing process step: Planning
Cognitive level: Application

46. A patient with easy bruising, gum bleeding, and difficulty achieving hemostasis after a sample of peripheral blood has been drawn is exhibiting a coagulation disorder of which etiology?
A. Break in vascular integrity
B. Platelet disorder
C. Malnutrition-induced coagulopathy
D. Excessive clot lysis

CORRECT ANSWER—**B.** Bleeding symptoms can be linked to the cause of the coagulopathy by observing the amount, vigorousness, location, and timing of the bleeding. Platelet problems manifest as skin, mucous membrane, and soft tissue bleeding, which is particularly prominent in dependent regions or those under pressure. Vascular hemorrhages are more massive and vigorous than coagulopathy induced by a platelet disorder and are associated with known injury. Excessive clot lysis can produce diffuse bleeding that is delayed in onset; the bleeding occurs when clots lyse, usually 24 to 72 hours after the event. Malnutrition-induced coagulopathy is associated with vitamin K deficiency and accompanied by abnormal bleeding tendencies and prolonged prothrombin time.
Nursing process step: Evaluation
Cognitive level: Evaluation

47. Patients who are the best candidates for pancreatic transplantation have which of the following?
A. Documented cardiovascular disease
B. Diabetes-induced renal disease
C. Diabetic neuropathies
D. Persistent infections related to diabetes

CORRECT ANSWER—**B.** Patients with diabetes mellitus who are eligible for pancreas transplant have refractory disease and at least one other severe complication of diabetes. Examples of acceptable disorders for transplant candidates include blindness, renal disease, and hypertension. Patients with coronary artery disease and active GI bleeding are excluded from transplantation because of the high surgical risk. Typical non-life-threatening problems of diabetes, such as infections, neuropathies, and foot disease, are not indications for transplantation.
Nursing process step: Assessment
Cognitive level: Evaluation

48. Third-degree heart block develops in a heart transplant patient with pacing wires on the second postoperative day and failure to capture is observed. The medication of choice to treat this problem is:

A. Atropine
B. Epinephrine
C. Phenylephrine
D. Isoproterenol

CORRECT ANSWER—D. A pure beta-adrenergic agonist, such as isoproterenol, would be used in a heart transplant patient. All sympathetic and parasympathetic fibers were severed in the transplanted heart during surgery; therefore, the heart will not respond to atropine. A patient with symptomatic bradycardia usually is treated with atropine, a pacemaker, and dopamine or epinephrine. Phenylephrine is an alpha-adrenergic agent primarily used to treat hypotension, especially hypotension secondary to spinal anesthesia.

Nursing process step: Implementation
Cognitive level: Application

49. The nurse caring for a patient with acquired immunodeficiency syndrome (AIDS) would implement appropriate measures to address which psychosocial problem most commonly reported among AIDS patients?

A. Denial
B. Anxiety about spreading the disease
C. Social isolation
D. Ineffective individual or family coping

CORRECT ANSWER—C. Patients with AIDS continue to be discriminated against by the general public and some health care providers. These patients are isolated from other patients, and, although universal precautions are required for all patient contacts, some special cleaning procedures are used for patients infected with human immunodeficiency virus. Other psychosocial reactions, such as denial and anxiety, occur according to individual situations, coping styles, and support systems.

Nursing process step: Implementation
Cognitive level: Application

50. A 49-year-old patient who underwent renal transplantation is readmitted to the intensive care unit (ICU) 7 days after the procedure for fevers and progressive renal failure. Assessment shows:
- blood pressure, 168/98 mm Hg
- temperature, 102.2° F (39° C)
- heart rate, 92 beats/minute with normal sinus rhythm
- respirations, 28 breaths/minute
- weight, 70 kg with a 2.5-kg weight gain over the last 2 days.

Previous intake and output were measured as intake of 3,250 ml and output of 1,800 ml. Blood chemistry levels drawn 3 hours before admission to the ICU include sodium, 134 mEq/liter; chloride, 97 mEq/liter; potassium, 5.3 mEq/liter; blood urea nitrogen (BUN), 56 mg/dl; glucose, 160 mg/dl; CO_2, 20 mmol/liter; and creatinine, 2.8 mg/dl. The patient is exhibiting symptoms of which type of transplant rejection?

A. Hyperacute rejection
B. Acute rejection
C. Accelerated rejection
D. Chronic rejection

CORRECT ANSWER—B. The patient is exhibiting symptoms of rejection, including hypertension, weight gain, low urine output, elevated creatinine level, and fever. The appearance of these symptoms 7 days after the procedure rules out hyperacute rejection, which occurs within minutes to hours of vascularization of the new kidney, and chronic rejection, which usually occurs 3 months after the transplant. Signs of acute rejection begin approximately 1 week after the procedure. These signs include return of previous organ failure symptoms, such as elevated BUN and serum creatinine levels, decreased urine output, and weight gain. Tenderness at the graft site, organ enlargement, and signs or symptoms of infection and tissue ischemia also suggest acute rejection. Accelerated rejection is thought to be a cellular response that occurs earlier than classic acute rejection and is diagnosed and treated in the same manner.
Nursing process step: Evaluation
Cognitive level: Comprehension

51. Nursing care of a patient receiving white blood cell (WBC) transfusions for profound sepsis with persistent neutropenia would include which intervention?
A. Checking vital signs at the beginning of, 30 minutes into, and at the end of the transfusion
B. Administering the blood product over 30 minutes to 1 hour
C. Premedicating the patient with acetaminophen, diphenhydramine, and steroids to prevent transfusion reactions
D. Agitating the bag gently every 15 minutes to prevent settling and rapid infusion of WBCs

CORRECT ANSWER—D. WBCs are administered only to seriously ill patients with sepsis whose WBC counts are unlikely to increase during the acute episode. WBCs contain many antigens and frequently cause severe reactions, including fever, chills, tremors, dyspnea, hypotension, and anaphylaxis. However, premedication to prevent such reactions is not routinely performed. Frequent vital signs assessments, such as every 15 to 30 minutes, during the infusion are recommended. WBCs are infused as a defined number of cells per minute, which is calculated by the blood bank before the product is sent to the nursing unit; they usually are infused over 3 to 6 hours. Because WBCs settle to the bottom of the bag and can infuse rapidly in succession, the bag must be agitated every 15 to 30 minutes to disperse the product. Because WBCs usually migrate to the site of infection, increased symptoms of infection may occur after transfusion.
Nursing process step: Implementation
Cognitive level: Application

52. Which of the following organ transplant procedures is the most successful in adults?
   A. Donor kidney transplantation
   B. Autologous bone marrow transplantation
   C. Cadaver liver transplantation
   D. Porcine pancreas transplantation

CORRECT ANSWER—**A.** The success of organ transplantation varies significantly and depends greatly on the general health of the recipient, the degree of tissue matching, and the physician's ability to perform the transplant with minimal tissue damage and maximal reconnection to the graft. Corneal transplants have the highest success rates in adults. The most successful organ transplant in an adult is a kidney transplant from a live donor; response rates are lower with cadaver kidneys. Variable response rates (from 20% to 60% for 5-year survival) are associated with liver, heart, pancreas, and bone marrow transplants. Allogenic, not autologous, bone marrow transplantation has a high success rate in children when such transplants are necessary for certain hematologic disorders.
Nursing process step: Assessment
Cognitive level: Comprehension

MULTISYSTEM REVIEW

CHAPTER 8

Multisystem Review

1. The nurse who suspects that a patient has disseminated intravascular coagulation (DIC) should assess all of the following *except:*
   A. I.V. and venipuncture sites
   B. Gastric output
   C. Intake and output
   D. Ability to ambulate with assistance

CORRECT ANSWER—D. A patient with suspected DIC must be protected from injury, and complete bed rest is indicated. If the patient is combative, he should be placed in a bed with padded side rails, and sedatives should be administered if necessary. All potential bleeding sites, including I.V. sites, GI tract, and genitourinary tract, must be monitored carefully for bleeding. In patients with acute DIC, intake and output must be monitored to assess fluid status and renal function.
Nursing process step: Assessment
Cognitive level: Application

2. All of the following are complications associated with septic shock *except:*
   A. Renal failure
   B. GI ulcers
   C. Septic arthritis
   D. Abnormal hepatic function

CORRECT ANSWER—C. Although it can lead to fatal septicemia, septic arthritis is not a complication of sepsis. This condition is caused by bacterial invasion of a joint; if untreated, septic arthritis eventually destroys the bone and cartilage. Renal failure, GI ulcers, abnormal hepatic function, heart failure, and disseminated intravascular coagulation are potential complications of sepsis.
Nursing process step: Evaluation
Cognitive level: Evaluation

3. Burn injuries are most commonly caused by:
   A. Chemicals
   B. Moist heat or steam
   C. Dry heat or fire
   D. Electricity

CORRECT ANSWER—C. Fire and sudden explosions of short duration (such as those caused by gasoline fumes or an electrical flash) are the most common causes of burn injury. Flash injury can cause inhalation injury because the superheated air can damage the larynx.
Nursing process step: Assessment
Cognitive level: Knowledge

Questions 4 to 8 refer to the following information:
A 26-year-old female patient with a psychiatric history is admitted to the intensive care unit after taking an overdose of lithium 1 hour ago. After establishing a patent airway, the physician orders gastric evacuation.

4. How should the nurse position the patient for gastric evacuation?
   A. Supine position, with the bed in reverse Trendelenburg's position
   B. Left lateral decubitus position, with the bed in Trendelenburg's position
   C. Left lateral decubitus position, with the bed in reverse Trendelenburg's position
   D. Right lateral decubitus position, with the bed in Trendelenburg's position

CORRECT ANSWER—B. The optimal patient position for gastric evacuation is left lateral decubitus, with the bed in Trendelenburg's position. This position confines the gastric contents to the left portion of the stomach, facilitates the evacuation of the ingested drug, and decreases the risk of aspiration.
Nursing process step: Implementation
Cognitive level: Comprehension

5. The nurse inserts a large-bore nasogastric (NG) tube into the oral cavity and begins to lavage. Which solution should be used for this procedure?
   A. 0.9% sodium chloride solution
   B. Tap water
   C. Sterile water
   D. Warm 0.9% sodium chloride solution

CORRECT ANSWER—B. After confirming placement of the NG tube, the nurse should use tap water for the lavage. The amount of drug evacuated with 0.9% sodium chloride solution would be no greater than that with tap water, and hypernatremia could result if the patient had underlying renal failure. Sterile water is of no benefit because the GI tract is not sterile.
Nursing process step: Implementation
Cognitive level: Comprehension

6. The nurse would continue gastric lavage and evacuation until:
   A. The aspirate is clear
   B. No further aspirate is evident
   C. At least 2 liters of water have been instilled and evacuated
   D. At least 5 liters of water have been instilled and evacuated

CORRECT ANSWER—D. Gastric lavage should continue until at least 5 liters of water have been instilled and evacuated, regardless of the clarity of the aspirate. This facilitates removal of the drug and prevents further drug absorption. Throughout the lavage, intake and output of the gastric contents should be equal. If the amounts are unequal, the nurse should stop the lavage and notify the physician. The patient is at risk for fluid volume excess or deficit, depending on the intake or output imbalance. Gastric lavage is contraindicated in any patient who lacks an intact gag reflex or secure airway.
Nursing process step: Assessment
Cognitive level: Comprehension

7. The patient does not respond to conventional treatment, and the physician is concerned about lithium toxicity. The nurse should continue to assess for all of the following signs and symptoms of lithium toxicity *except:*
A. Diarrhea
B. Polyuria
C. Oliguria
D. Muscle weakness

CORRECT ANSWER—C. Lithium toxicity is associated with lithium-induced diabetes insipidus syndrome, which causes polyuria and polydipsia. Other signs and symptoms of lithium toxicity include diarrhea, muscle weakness, nausea, vomiting, drowsiness, and ataxia.
Nursing process step: Assessment
Cognitive level: Evaluation

8. The patient requires hemodialysis. Which statement best explains the purpose of this treatment?
A. It helps improve kidney function
B. It removes extra water retained by the body because of the lithium
C. It removes lithium from the bloodstream
D. It removes lithium because the drug is poorly soluble in water

CORRECT ANSWER—C. Hemodialysis is indicated for drug overdose in which the patient has severe poisoning from a dialyzable drug and remains unstable despite conservative treatment. It is used to remove water-soluble drugs, such as lithium, that are not highly bound to plasma protein and to correct severe acid-base and electrolyte abnormalities. Hemodialysis temporarily assists the kidneys or acts as an external kidney; however, it does not improve kidney function. Lithium toxicity does not cause the body to retain extra water.
Nursing process step: Implementation
Cognitive level: Synthesis

9. Loss of circulating plasma volume occurs in burn injuries for all of the following reasons *except:*
A. Increased capillary permeability leads to escape of water, electrolytes, albumin, and protein into the interstitial and intracellular compartments
B. Increased basal metabolic rate leads to increased water loss via the respiratory system
C. Diuresis secondary to shifts in intravascular fluid further decreases intravascular volume
D. Insensible loss via the burn wound ranges from 90 to 350 ml/hour, further decreasing circulating plasma volume

CORRECT ANSWER—C. Diuresis does not occur in patients with burn wounds. Burn injuries trigger the release of antidiuretic hormone (ADH) in response to the hypovolemia; ADH decreases the production of urine by increasing water reabsorption by the renal tubules. Fluid volume is lost through increased capillary permeability, which begins when the injury occurs and extends to unburned tissue if the injury involves more than 30% of the body surface area. Insensible fluid loss through burn wounds and an increased basal metabolic rate contribute to the decreased circulating plasma volume.
Nursing process step: Assessment
Cognitive level: Comprehension

10. A 46-year-old female is admitted to the intensive care unit with crushing injuries to her pelvis and legs. After her cardiac and respiratory systems have been stabilized, the patient complains of slight shortness of breath on the second day. The nurse notes that a petechial rash has developed over the chest and axilla and notifies the physician. The nurse suspects the patient has:
A. Drug rash caused by prophylactic antibiotic therapy
B. Adult respiratory distress syndrome (ARDS)
C. Fat embolism
D. Complications from immobility

CORRECT ANSWER—C. Fat embolism is a complicated condition associated with long bone fractures and pelvic injuries. Fat emboli—fatty tissue that moves into the circulation and lodges in the pulmonary system—should be suspected in all trauma patients with crushing injuries. Signs and symptoms of fat embolism include petechial rash, respiratory problems, pulmonary edema, and central nervous system changes. Other minor clinical signs of fat embolism include tachycardia, pyrexia, retinal changes, decreased hemoglobin level, increased erythrocyte sedimentation rate, and thrombocytopenia. Although drugs can cause rashes, fat emboli are a more likely complication in this patient, especially with the associated shortness of breath. Trauma patients are at risk for ARDS, but this complication usually manifests as refractory hypoxemia, elevated pulmonary artery wedge pressure, and increased respiratory rate. Rashes are not associated with ARDS. Impaired skin integrity from immobility would cause a reddened area, not a rash, that progresses to open pressure ulcers.
Nursing process step: Assessment
Cognitive level: Evaluation

11. A patient in septic shock has a nursing diagnosis of fluid volume deficit related to distributional volume loss (resulting from a fluid shift to the interstitial space) and increased insensible loss with high fever. The nurse would plan all of the following interventions for a patient with this diagnosis *except:*
A. Assisting with insertion of hemodynamic monitoring devices
B. Instituting measures to control body temperature
C. Monitoring for signs of respiratory depression
D. Administering and monitoring prescribed fluid replacement therapy

CORRECT ANSWER—C. Although respiratory status should be monitored throughout all stages of septic shock, the nurse should assess specifically for tachypnea and crackles because these signs indicate fluid overload in the pulmonary system. Hemodynamic monitoring provides data about the effectiveness of fluid replacement; decreased mixed venous oxygenation indicates compromised tissue perfusion. Lowering the patient's high body temperature prevents an increased tissue metabolic rate, which can exacerbate tissue ischemia and hypoxia. Careful monitoring of fluid replacement therapy is necessary to prevent potential overtreatment and pulmonary congestion.
Nursing process step: Planning
Cognitive level: Analysis

12. The nurse caring for a patient with suspected sepsis should anticipate the need for a sputum culture, urine culture, and blood cultures from two separate sites because:
A. Identifying the causative organism may prevent the need for aminoglycosides
B. Determining the portal of entry and focus of infection is crucial to successful treatment
C. Culturing potential sources of infection can reveal the presence of endotoxins
D. Monitoring culture specimens can reveal abnormal prothrombin consumption

CORRECT ANSWER—B. To begin the most effective and prompt antibiotic treatment, the physician must know the specific organism and portal of entry. Because bacteremia can be transient, blood cultures from two separate sites should be obtained, but not via indwelling catheters, which can be colonized with bacteria not responsible for the septicemia. Because culture results typically are not available for at least 24 hours, any patient suspected of having sepsis will require two antibiotics, one of which is an aminoglycoside to expand the spectrum of antibacterial action. Endotoxins are released by causative microorganisms and trigger a variety of biochemical reactions that adversely affect the body, predisposing the patient to shock during sepsis; however, endotoxins are not obtained through culturing. Monitoring culture specimens provides information about the causative organism, not about abnormal prothrombin consumption, which also occurs with sepsis.
Nursing process step: Implementation
Cognitive level: Comprehension

13. The tissue layers involved in a burn injury are determined by the duration of contact with and the temperature of the burning agent. A partial-thickness burn affects which portions of the skin?
A. All of the epidermis and dermis
B. Epidermis and one-half to seven-eighths of the dermis
C. Epidermis and subcutaneous tissue
D. Dermis only

CORRECT ANSWER—B. A partial-thickness injury typically involves the epidermal layer and one-half to seven-eighths of the dermal layer of the skin; a partial-thickness burn wound is bright red to pink with glistening, serum-filled blisters. A full-thickness injury typically involves the epidermis, dermis, subcutaneous tissue, muscle, and bone; a full-thickness burn wound is snowy white, gray, or brown with a firm, leathery texture.
Nursing process step: Assessment
Cognitive level: Evaluation

Questions 14 to 18 refer to the following information:
A 22-year-old drug addict recently admitted for sharp substernal chest pain complains of a pounding heart. The nurse notes an increase in the patient's arterial blood pressure and sinus tachycardia of 144 beats/minute with premature ventricular contractions. On further questioning, the patient admits to recently ingesting cocaine.

---

14. The patient is at high risk for which complication related to cocaine use?
- **A.** Coronary artery spasm
- **B.** Bradyarrhythmias
- **C.** Neurobehavioral deficits
- **D.** Panic disorder

CORRECT ANSWER—A. Cardiac complications associated with cocaine use include coronary artery spasm, myocardial infarction, dilated cardiomyopathy, acute congestive heart failure, endocarditis, and sudden death. Tachyarrhythmias occur secondary to the blocked reuptake of norepinephrine, epinephrine, and dopamine, which results in an excess of these chemicals at postsynaptic receptor sites. Neurobehavioral deficits are common in neonates born to mothers who have used cocaine. Cocaine addicts often experience euphoria followed by depression as their craving for the drug increases; panic disorder is not associated with cocaine use.
Nursing process step: Planning
Cognitive level: Analysis

15. The nurse would expect the physician to treat the patient's hypertension and tachycardia with which drugs?
- **A.** Norepinephrine and lidocaine
- **B.** Nifedipine and lidocaine
- **C.** Nitroglycerin and esmolol
- **D.** Nifedipine and esmolol

CORRECT ANSWER—D. A vasodilator, such as nifedipine, would be used to treat the hypertension, and a beta-blocker, such as esmolol, would be used to lower the heart rate. The premature ventricular contractions may require treatment with the antiarrhythmic lidocaine; however, the question focuses only on the hypertension and tachycardia. Norepinephrine, an alpha-adrenergic blocker, is used in hypotensive emergencies, especially those that occur during spinal anesthesia. Nitroglycerin might be used for coronary vasospasm, but it is not the drug of choice for hypertension.
Nursing process step: Planning
Cognitive level: Analysis

16. The nurse assists with insertion of a pulmonary artery catheter to ensure better hemodynamic monitoring and management. The initial pressures readings include pulmonary artery wedge pressure, 19 mm Hg; central venous pressure, 16 mm Hg; and pulmonary artery pressure, 34/17 mm Hg. Cardiac output and systemic vascular resistance are 4.2 liters/minute and 1,359 dynes/second/cm^{-5}, respectively. The patient becomes increasingly tachypneic, and his ECG reading continues to show sinus tachycardia with a rate of 123 beats/minute. Based on these findings, the nurse suspects:

A. Endocarditis
B. Congestive heart failure
C. Myocardial ischemia
D. Myocardial infarction

CORRECT ANSWER—B. The catheter readings are indicative of a patient with congestive heart failure; the patient's filling pressures are high, and the heart is not working effectively (low cardiac output) against vasoconstricted arteries. Although all of the options are possible cardiac complications of cocaine use, the clinical signs and symptoms and pulmonary artery pressures indicate congestive heart failure.
Nursing process step: Assessment
Cognitive level: Evaluation

17. The ECG shows a 1-mm ST-segment elevation in the anteroseptal leads and a T-wave inversion in leads V$_3$ to V$_5$. The nurse would anticipate the physician ordering an infusion of which drug, keeping in mind the patient's drug history?

A. Lidocaine
B. Procainamide
C. Nitroglycerin
D. Digoxin

CORRECT ANSWER—C. Nitroglycerin dilates coronary arteries, which is necessary in a patient with ECG changes indicative of myocardial ischemia. Lidocaine, procainamide, and digoxin may be necessary at some point but are not used for coronary vasodilation.
Nursing process step: Planning
Cognitive level: Application

18. The nurse should monitor the patient's temperature and glucose level every 2 hours for the first 24 hours because:

A. Temperature and glucose level monitoring are part of the standard intensive care unit protocol
B. The patient is at risk for infection
C. The patient is at risk for hypoglycemia and hypothermia
D. The patient is at risk for hyperglycemia and hyperthermia, which are part of the "fight-or-flight" cocaine response

CORRECT ANSWER—D. The "fight-or-flight" response is triggered by cocaine use and the subsequent availability of excess epinephrine, norepinephrine, and dopamine at the postsynaptic receptor sites. Clinical signs of this response include hyperglycemia, hyperthermia, vasoconstriction, abrupt increase in arterial pressure, tachycardia, ventricular arrhythmias, and mydriasis. Any patient suspected of I.V. drug abuse is at risk for endocarditis and requires close monitoring; however, this would not include checking the glucose level every 2 hours. No standard protocol for glucose monitoring exists in the intensive care unit, unless the patient is receiving an I.V. insulin drip.
Nursing process step: Evaluation
Cognitive level: Analysis

19. The nurse who suspects fat embolism in a trauma patient would initiate which action?
  A. Restricting fluid intake
  B. Administering oxygen as ordered
  C. Helping the patient from the bed to a chair
  D. Monitoring nutritional intake

CORRECT ANSWER—B. Treatment of suspected fat embolism includes immobilization of the long bone fracture, oxygen therapy, early intubation, and mechanical ventilation with positive end-expiratory pressure, as needed, to open collapsed alveoli and prevent further collapse as well as blood and fluid replacement therapy to supply the dilated heart with adequate venous return. Right-sided heart dilation results from the increased work of breathing secondary to blockage of the pulmonary vessels. Immobilization of the long bone fracture requires bed rest. Monitoring of nutritional intake is required in a trauma patient because of increased caloric needs, not fat embolism.
Nursing process step: Planning
Cognitive level: Application

Questions 20 to 22 refer to the following information:
A 64-year-old male patient with chronic obstructive pulmonary disease (COPD) is admitted to the intensive care unit for unilateral lung transplantation. Postoperatively, a mediastinal shift develops and the patient is reintubated with a double-lumen tube to treat the hypoxia. His arterial blood gas values after intubation include pH, 7.31; partial pressure of oxygen in arterial blood (PaO_2), 66 mm Hg; partial pressure of carbon dioxide in arterial blood ($PaCO_2$), 48 mm Hg; and HCO_3^-, 24 mEq/liter. The ventilator to the newly transplanted lung is set at assist-control mode with a respiratory rate of 12 breaths/minute; tidal volume, 1,000 cc; positive end-expiratory pressure, 5 cm H_2O; and fraction of inspired oxygen (FIO_2), 0.8. The ventilator to the native lung is set on a continuous positive airway pressure mode with a fraction of inspired oxygen of 0.5.

---

20. How would the nurse interpret the arterial blood gas values?
  A. Metabolic acidosis with hypoxia
  B. Respiratory acidosis with hypoxia
  C. Metabolic alkalosis with hypoxia
  D. Uncompensated respiratory acidosis with hypoxia

CORRECT ANSWER—D. The patient clearly is hypoxic, with a PaO_2 of 66 mm Hg. Uncompensated respiratory acidosis is indicated by the high $PaCO_2$ level and normal HCO_3^- level. The patient clearly is acidotic with a pH below 7.35. Metabolic acidosis would be evident if the HCO_3^- is less than 22 mEq/liter. If the patient were able to compensate for his respiratory acidosis, then he would increase his respiratory rate to rid his body of excess carbon dioxide and to bring his pH into the normal range.
Nursing process step: Evaluation
Cognitive level: Application

21. A double-lumen tube is being used to treat the patient's hypoxia because:
A. Patients with COPD still experience complications associated with the remaining emphysematous lung after unilateral lung transplantation
B. Oxygen can be infused directly into each lung field
C. A mediastinal shift has occurred secondary to the native lung, which can now be deflated passively
D. It facilitates removal of increased secretions

CORRECT ANSWER—C. The native emphysematous lung with overdistended alveoli continues to trap air and cause a mediastinal shift onto the new lung, decreasing oxygen flow to that lung. A double-lumen endotracheal tube allows the native lung to be passively deflated with the patient on a continuous positive airway pressure mode, thereby increasing oxygen flow to the new lung. Although it is true that patients with COPD still experience complications associated with the remaining lung, the double-lumen tube is used to correct the complication described in option C. Double-lumen tubes do not allow for more direct oxygen administration or removal of increased secretions.
Nursing process step: Implementation
Cognitive level: Comprehension

22. To decrease the risk of hypoxia, the nurse should place the patient in which position?
A. With the head of the bed elevated 30 degrees
B. In a side-lying position, with the head of the bed elevated 30 degrees
C. In reverse Trendelenburg's position
D. In a side-lying position on the native lung, with the head of the bed elevated 30 degrees

CORRECT ANSWER—D. Most patients who undergo unilateral lung transplantation benefit from lying on the native lung with the new lung facing upward. This position helps decrease edema resulting from lung transplantation and encourages ventilation perfusion of the new lung, which should increase the patient's PaO_2 level. The other positions would not be as beneficial for this patient.
Nursing process step: Implementation
Cognitive level: Analysis

23. The nurse is caring for a patient whose burn wounds are being treated with an open-exposure dressing. The nurse would anticipate performing all of the following interventions *except:*
A. Checking the patient's temperature every 2 hours
B. Changing linens frequently
C. Assessing the wound for signs of infection
D. Promoting self-care by encouraging the patient to apply a topical antibiotic to the wound

CORRECT ANSWER—D. Open-exposure dressings allow the wound to be visually inspected and may suppress bacterial growth through the drying effect of air. However, a patient with open wounds is susceptible to increased heat and insensible water loss and requires frequent temperature checks, particularly during the early acute stages. Strict isolation and frequent linen changes are indicated, especially if the wound is draining copiously. The patient must avoid direct or indirect contamination, which would occur if a topical antibiotic was applied to the wound.
Nursing process step: Planning
Cognitive level: Application

24. The nurse must distinguish among bacteremia, septicemia, and septic shock to appropriately assess, implement, and evaluate patient care. Which of the following statements is most accurate?
A. Bacteremia is the presence of bacteria in the blood as evidenced by a positive blood culture
B. Septicemia, or blood infection, is diagnosed solely through the clinical findings of fever, chills, and a high white blood cell count; the causative organism is unknown
C. Septic shock is a type of shock that occurs secondary to hypovolemia and cardiac failure
D. Cold sepsis is hypothermia related to endotoxin release that occurs after blood is contaminated with *Escherichia coli*

CORRECT ANSWER—A. Bacteremia is the presence of bacteria in the blood as evidenced by a positive blood culture. Septicemia is a systemic infection in which pathogens are present in the circulating bloodstream, having spread from an infection in any part of the body. A patient with septicemia exhibits signs and symptoms characteristic of infection. Septicemia is diagnosed by a blood culture and treated aggressively with antibiotics and fluids to prevent septic shock. Septic shock usually is preceded by signs of severe infection. It is treated by identifying the causative organism and providing aggressive therapy with fluids, antibiotics, and vasopressors to maintain hemodynamic stability. The release of endotoxins leads to peripheral vasodilation, decreased blood pressure, increased respiratory rate, and confusion; it eventually can lead to organ failure and death. Cold sepsis is not a medical diagnosis.
Nursing process step: Evaluation
Cognitive level: Comprehension

25. All of the following statements about systemic inflammatory response syndrome (also known as sepsis syndrome) are true *except:*
A. Cytokines, such as interleukins 1, 2, 6, and 8, are released
B. Tumor necrosis factor is released
C. Gram-positive bacteria are the exogenous cause in 90% of the cases in which the causative organism is identified
D. Approximately 400,000 to 500,000 cases are reported in the United States each year

CORRECT ANSWER—C. In approximately two-thirds of cases of sepsis syndrome with known etiology, the causative organisms are gram-negative bacteria; only 20% to 25% of cases are caused by gram-positive bacteria. All of the other statements are true. Sepsis syndrome consists of a systemic inflammatory response generally initiated by an exogenous source, mainly bacterial endotoxins stimulating an endogenous host response, that triggers the release of cytokines, tumor necrosis factor, and other proinflammatory mediators. In several clinical trials, the mortality rate for sepsis syndrome averaged 40%.
Nursing process step: Assessment
Cognitive level: Comprehension

26. What is the most common portal of entry for microorganisms associated with sepsis syndrome?
A. Skin
B. GI tract
C. Respiratory tract
D. Urinary tract

CORRECT ANSWER—D. Although microorganisms that cause sepsis syndrome can enter through the skin, GI tract, or respiratory tract, the most common portal of entry is the urinary tract via urinary catheters, suprapubic tubes, and cystoscopic examination.
Nursing process step: Assessment
Cognitive level: Knowledge

27. Nursing interventions for a patient with a thermal injury include all of the following *except:*
A. Lavaging with 2 to 3 liters of 0.9% sodium chloride solution if the eyes are affected
B. Obtaining as much information as possible about the burning agent
C. Applying ice to the burn wound
D. Removing all of the patient's clothing and jewelry

CORRECT ANSWER—C. Ice should never be applied to a burn wound caused by a thermal source because it constricts blood vessels and can damage surrounding tissues. Halting the burning process, removing clothing and jewelry (which can retain heat and increase the depth of injury), decreasing the degree of corneal ulceration, and obtaining information about the causative agent are appropriate interventions for a patient whose skin integrity is compromised by thermal injuries.
Nursing process step: Implementation
Cognitive level: Application

28. What is the primary nursing intervention in the emergency management of a patient with a thermal injury?
A. Instituting the ABCs of trauma resuscitation
B. Stabilizing the patient and controlling hemorrhage associated with the injury
C. Halting the burning process
D. Covering the wound with clean sheets to prevent further contamination

CORRECT ANSWER—C. The burning process must be stopped and the wound cooled to decrease the depth and extent of the injury before the ABCs (airway, breathing, and circulation) of resuscitation are initiated. Afterward, the nurse must stabilize the patient and control any hemorrhage resulting from the associated injury. Treatment for hypovolemic shock should be instituted within the first few minutes and continued with close monitoring of hemodynamic pressures. Preventing further wound contamination is necessary but not the immediate priority.
Nursing process step: Implementation
Cognitive level: Application

29. A patient with third-degree burns on both legs will have a nursing diagnosis of risk for altered peripheral perfusion related to:
A. Circumferential eschar
B. Fat emboli
C. Infection
D. Femoral artery occlusion

CORRECT ANSWER—A. As edema develops with circumferential burns, eschar forms a tight, constricting band and compromises circulation to the extremity distal to the circumferential site. Pain in the extremities is a useful indicator of increasing pressure and decreasing circulation. The patient's limbs should be elevated to decrease edema and promote venous return. A patient with third-degree burns is not at increased risk for fat emboli unless he also has long bone or pelvic fractures. Infection does not alter peripheral perfusion. Burns to the legs are not associated with femoral artery occlusion.
Nursing process step: Implementation
Cognitive level: Analysis

Questions 30 to 34 refer to the following information:
A 22-year-old male near-drowning victim is admitted to the intensive care unit (ICU). Having regained consciousness in the emergency department, the patient is transported to the ICU with a 0.5 Venturi mask and an intravenous line infusing dextrose 5% in 0.45% sodium chloride solution at 125 ml/hour.

30. Twenty-four hours after admission to the ICU, the patient suddenly develops signs and symptoms that alarm the nurse, who notifies the anesthesiologist. Which of the following assessment findings would prompt this action?
A. Arterial blood gas values of pH, 7.34; PaO_2, 91 mm Hg; and $PaCO_2$, 42 mm Hg
B. Pink, frothy sputum and a respiratory rate of 44 breaths/minute
C. Increasing confusion
D. Bilateral rales of the lower lobes

CORRECT ANSWER—B. All of the options are possible signs and symptoms of impending pulmonary insufficiency, and the need for elective mechanical ventilation must be evaluated. A patient with a respiratory rate of 44 breaths/minute and pink, frothy sputum has serious symptoms of impending respiratory failure despite his ability to maintain an adequate pH, PaO_2, and $PaCO_2$. A change in mental status could be secondary to both hypoxia and increasing cerebral edema.
Nursing process step: Assessment
Cognitive level: Analysis

31. After the nurse and anesthesiologist collaborate to treat the patient medically and avoid intubation, the patient experiences bronchospasm. What would the nurse administer in this situation?
A. Bronchodilator and antibiotics
B. Antibiotics, phenytoin, and oxygen
C. Epinephrine, steroids, and aminophylline
D. Epinephrine and oxygen

CORRECT ANSWER—C. Bronchospasm commonly is treated with a beta-adrenergic drug, such as epinephrine or isoproterenol, that causes bronchodilation. Aminophylline also is used to dilate the bronchi, and steroids are administered to decrease inflammation. Although antibiotics may be ordered, they typically are administered to combat potential or known infection. The patient already is receiving oxygen.
Nursing process step: Implementation
Cognitive level: Analysis

32. The nurse obtains a copy of the patient's most recent arterial blood gas values. Which interpretation is correct?

A. The results are pH, 7.26; PaO_2, 82 mm Hg; $PaCO_2$, 30 mm Hg; and HCO_3^-, 16 mm Hg; the patient has respiratory acidosis with metabolic compensation and requires immediate intubation

B. The results are pH, 7.34; PaO_2, 63 mm Hg; and $PaCO_2$, 45 mm Hg; the patient is working hard to breath but maintaining normal blood gas levels

C. The results are pH, 7.20; PaO_2, 42 mm Hg; and $PaCO_2$, 55 mm Hg; the patient has severe metabolic acidosis and requires immediate intubation

D. The results are pH, 7.26; PaO_2, 50 mm Hg; and $PaCO_2$, 50 mm Hg; the patient has respiratory acidosis with hypoxia and requires immediate intubation

CORRECT ANSWER—D. A patient recovering from a near-drowning accident typically experiences combined alveolar and interstitial pulmonary edema, which alters surfactant production and damages alveolar capillary membranes. Even an awake and alert patient can suffer from hypoxia unresponsive to oxygen therapy. Severe pulmonary edema can occur up to 24 hours after a near-drowning event. As the patient's oxygenation efforts fail, the $PaCO_2$ level begins to increase and respiratory acidosis occurs. In this situation, the body is not oxygenating adequately, and the patient requires immediate intubation and mechanical ventilation to maintain a patent airway and to prevent respiratory arrest. A patient with a pH of 7.26, PaO_2 of 82 mm Hg, $PaCO_2$ of 30 mm Hg, and HCO_3^- of 16 mm Hg (as in option A) has uncompensated metabolic acidosis and requires intubation. A PaO_2 of 63 mm Hg (option B) is abnormal. A patient with the readings listed in option C probably has acidosis from a respiratory source; although the base excess and bicarbonate level are not given, the patient probably would be intubated.
Nursing process step: Assessment
Cognitive level: Analysis

33. A nursing diagnosis for this patient would be at increased risk for impaired gas exchange related to all of the following *except:*

A. Accumulated secretions
B. Aspiration of foreign material
C. Bronchospasm
D. Decreased cardiac output

CORRECT ANSWER—D. The patient is at increased risk for impaired gas exchange related to hypoxia, pulmonary edema, hypercapnia, changes in level of consciousness, aspiration of foreign material, bronchospasm, and accumulated secretions. A patient with decreased cardiac output is at risk for insufficient oxygen at the tissue level; the appropriate nursing diagnosis in this case would be altered pulmonary tissue perfusion related to decreased cardiac output.
Nursing process step: Planning
Cognitive level: Analysis

34. Because altered cerebral tissue perfusion can result from asphyxiation, which nursing action is necessary for this patient?

A. Suctioning frequently to avoid increased peak inspiratory pressures

B. Assisting with intubation and hyperventilation to decrease $PaCO_2$ blood level

C. Assessing neurologic status at least every 8 hours during the first 24 hours

D. Notifying the psychiatric resident on call if the patient becomes increasingly restless and combative

CORRECT ANSWER—B. A patient suffering from asphyxia after a near-drowning accident is highly susceptible to hypoperfusion and cerebral hypoxia produced by brain tissue acidosis and neural cell damage. Cellular edema occurs along with potentially devastating increases in intracranial pressure (ICP), which typically develop during the first 24 hours. To prevent increased ICP, the patient should be mechanically hyperventilated to decrease $PaCO_2$ and ICP levels by vasoconstricting arterioles. Although suctioning should be performed as needed, it should be used judiciously because it increases ICP. Neurologic status should be assessed every 2 hours; any changes, including behavioral changes, may indicate altered cerebral tissue perfusion or increasing ICP and should be reported to the physician or medical resident.
Nursing process step: Implementation
Cognitive level: Application

35. A patient in the advanced stages of septic shock may have disseminated intravascular coagulation (DIC), which is indicated by which of the following laboratory findings?

A. Increased white blood cell count and increased coagulation factors

B. Increased fibrin split products, decreased fibrinogen, and thrombocytopenia

C. Decreased coagulation factors and metabolic alkalosis

D. Decreased white blood cell count and increased hemoglobin

CORRECT ANSWER—B. DIC is associated with septic shock; it causes clotting in the microcirculation and bleeding from larger vessels. The endotoxins produced by the microorganism causing the septic shock damage endothelial cells, which activates factor XII and the intrinsic coagulation pathway. As a result, fibrin clots form in the microcirculation. Fibrin formation and vascular wall damage promote the aggregation of platelets, which are directly damaged by endotoxins. The end result clinically is decreased tissue perfusion because of clot formation in the microcirculation with resultant lactic acidosis, cellular death, and organ death. From a laboratory perspective, the result is thrombocytopenia, decreased circulating coagulation factors, and activation of the fibrinolytic system, which is indicated by increased fibrin split products and decreased fibrinogen. If the blood loss is significant, hemoglobin may be low.
Nursing process step: Assessment
Cognitive level: Evaluation

36. Patients with septic shock may have severe blood dyscrasia, such as thrombocytopenia resulting from microembolization of platelets. A patient with thrombocytopenia should not be given which drug?
  A. Phytonadione (vitamin K)
  B. Ferrous sulfate
  C. Aspirin
  D. Nifedipine

CORRECT ANSWER—C. Aspirin impedes clotting by preventing platelet aggregation; it should not be given to a patient with preexisting thrombocytopenia, which commonly occurs as a complication of disseminated intravascular coagulopathy during sepsis. Vitamin K promotes hepatic formation of active prothrombin and is administered to patients with hypoprothrombinemia secondary to vitamin K malabsorption or vitamin K deficiency. Ferrous sulfate provides elemental iron, which is necessary for hemoglobin formation in patients with iron deficiency. Nifedipine, an antianginal drug, does not cause blood dyscrasia.
Nursing process step: Planning
Cognitive level: Analysis

Questions 37 and 38 refer to the following information:
A patient admitted to the intensive care unit because of a phenobarbital overdose is given activated charcoal 1 g/kg body weight.

37. The nurse carefully evaluates the effectiveness of therapy and observes for potential complications. Which of the following is *not* a potential complication of activated charcoal treatment?
  A. Bowel obstruction
  B. Pulmonary aspiration
  C. Vomiting
  D. Diarrhea

CORRECT ANSWER—D. Diarrhea can result from the accompanying laxative agent, not as a complication of activated charcoal therapy. Bowel obstruction can occur if the activated charcoal is not administered with a laxative. Fatal pulmonary aspiration is possible if activated charcoal is administered to a patient who lacks an intact gag reflex or protected airway. Nausea, vomiting, black stools, and constipation are potential adverse GI effects of activated charcoal treatment. Vomiting can be prevented by administering activated charcoal with a laxative over at least 30 minutes (via nasogastric tube or intermittent oral doses).
Nursing process step: Evaluation
Cognitive level: Comprehension

38. Which of the following would be administered with activated charcoal?
A. Calcium chloride
B. 70% sorbitol
C. Diazepam
D. Oxygen

CORRECT ANSWER—B. Magnesium sulfate, magnesium citrate, and 70% sorbitol are effective laxatives administered with activated charcoal to enhance its elimination. Concomitant administration of a laxative significantly decreases the GI transit time of activated charcoal, which causes constipation. If activated charcoal remains in the GI system, bowel obstruction may occur. Calcium chloride is not a laxative. Diazepam would not be administered to a patient suffering from an overdose of a barbiturate, such as phenobarbital. Oxygen therapy is not required with activated charcoal treatment, although the patient may receive oxygen, depending on his level of respiratory depression.
Nursing process step: Implementation
Cognitive level: Application

39. The severity of a burn injury is influenced by the:
A. Depth, size, and location of the injury and the patient's age
B. Patient's medical history, gender, and associated trauma
C. Depth and location of the injury and the causative burning agent
D. Depth, size, and location of the injury and the patient's gender

CORRECT ANSWER—A. The severity of a burn injury is related to the depth, size, and location of the injury, the associated trauma, and the patient's age and medical history. The severity of a burn injury is not influenced by a patient's gender or the burning agent.
Nursing process step: Assessment
Cognitive level: Comprehension

40. Which complication should the nurse anticipate in a patient with a burn injury and which primary intervention should be initiated to prevent it?

A. Sepsis associated with the burn wound, which can be prevented by providing daily aseptic wound care

B. Inhalation injury associated with carbon monoxide poisoning, which can be prevented by maintaining a patent airway

C. Renal failure associated with hypovolemia, which can be prevented by administering lactated Ringer's solution and potassium supplements as ordered

D. Neurovascular compromise related to inelastic eschar formation over wounds, which can be prevented by evaluating pulses in the burned extremity every 15 minutes and keeping the extremity in a dependent position

CORRECT ANSWER—B. Carbon monoxide poisoning is the most immediate cause of death associated with burns. Smoke or chemical inhalation injury causes sudden loss of bronchial cilia, decreased alveolar surfactant, atelectasis, mucosal edema, and wheezing. Maintaining a patent airway is imperative, and the patient may require mechanical ventilation, humidified oxygen, bronchodilators, and vigorous pulmonary toilet to prevent pulmonary infection. Sepsis, acute tubular necrosis secondary to hypovolemia and release of myoglobin, and neurovascular compromise are life-threatening complications of thermal injury. However, the interventions for these complications would include meticulous, aseptic wound care; administration of lactated Ringer's solution and careful evaluation for hyperkalemia associated with cellular trauma and release of potassium into the extracellular fluid; frequent evaluation of pulses in the extremities; and maintenance of the affected extremity in an elevated position to promote venous return and decrease edema.

Nursing process step: Implementation
Cognitive level: Application

Questions 41 to 43 refer to the following information:
A 33-year-old mother of two children is admitted to the intensive care unit (ICU) after arriving at the emergency department with a fever of 103° F (39.4° C), respiratory rate of 38 breaths/minute, blood pressure of 92/50 mm Hg, and increasing lethargy and confusion. She has no previous medical or surgical history. Her husband reports that the patient had been experiencing increasing back pain and urinary frequency over the past 5 days that was unrelieved by nonsteroidal anti-inflammatory drugs.

41. Based on the patient's signs and symptoms, which actions should the nurse take first?

A. Orienting the patient and family to the ICU and obtaining a more detailed description of recent signs and symptoms

B. Administering a broad-spectrum antibiotic, then collecting urine, blood, and sputum specimens

C. Inserting an indwelling urinary (Foley) catheter; obtaining baseline vital signs; and collecting urine, blood, and sputum specimens

D. Reassessing vital signs; inserting an indwelling urinary catheter; obtaining urine, blood, and sputum specimens for immediate culturing; and preparing the patient for invasive monitoring

CORRECT ANSWER—D. In this situation, the patient's vital signs should be reassessed to determine hemodynamic stability. Monitoring fluid intake and output and electrolyte levels as well as collecting specimens are important; in many cases, they are done simultaneously in the ICU. However, specimens must be obtained before antibiotics are given, although the patient probably would receive a broad-spectrum antibiotic well before culture results are available. Other actions aim to reduce fever and the metabolic rate. Obtaining a detailed history is less important than establishing hemodynamic and pulmonary stability, which typically are monitored using invasive means, such as a pulmonary catheter. An indwelling urinary catheter used to monitor urine output would not be inserted before vital signs assessment was performed.

Nursing process step: Implementation
Cognitive level: Analysis

42. A Swan-Ganz catheter is inserted, and the patient's initial pressures include systolic pulmonary artery pressure, 13 mm Hg; diastolic pulmonary artery pressure, 5 mm Hg; pulmonary artery wedge pressure, 4 mm Hg; and central venous pressure, 3 mm Hg. Other findings include blood pressure, 86/52 mm Hg; heart rate, 112 beats/minute; cardiac output (CO), 7.5 liters/minute; and systemic vascular resistance (SVR), 435 dynes/second/cm^{-5}. The nurse should suspect which condition and implement which immediate action?

A. Renal calculi, which requires obtaining a urine specimen

B. Early septic shock related to urinary tract infection, which requires administration of fluids, antibiotics, and vasopressors as ordered

C. Septic shock, which requires helping family members understand the seriousness of the condition and letting them visit the patient while she is still somewhat responsive

D. Septicemia, which requires obtaining an arterial blood gas (ABG) sample and administering vasopressors as ordered to maintain adequate blood pressure and organ perfusion

CORRECT ANSWER—B. The patient's CO and SVR, along with her clinical signs and symptoms, indicate early septic shock, probably resulting from a urinary tract infection that has remained untreated. The patient is dehydrated and has very low filling pressures; fluid therapy is required to maintain an adequate blood pressure. The fever and probable release of endotoxins from the causative microorganism have left the patient peripherally vasodilated; vasoactive medications will be needed if fluids do not sustain her blood pressure. Fluids must be administered before vasoactive drugs because of the low filling pressures. Respiratory and cardiovascular status also must be evaluated. Because of the increasing lethargy, the nurse should prepare the patient for mechanical ventilation if indicated. The psychosocial needs of the family must be addressed but do not take precedence over emergency patient care. Renal calculi is accompanied by pain, nausea, vomiting, and, sometimes, fever, anuria, and hematuria; the patient does not exhibit these symptoms, except for pain. She will require an ABG analysis; however, fluids must be administered prior to vasoconstrictor therapy.

Nursing process step: Implementation
Cognitive level: Analysis

43. The patient is intubated and, despite aggressive fluid and antibiotic therapy, requires norepinephrine and a renal dose of dopamine to maintain blood pressure and organ perfusion. What is the appropriate dosage of dopamine and its mechanism of action?
A. At 1 to 8 mcg/kg/minute, dopamine promotes renal dilation without vasoconstriction
B. At 0.5 to 2 mcg/kg/minute, dopamine promotes vasodilation by acting primarily on the dopaminergic receptors
C. At 2 to 10 mcg/kg/minute, dopamine provides necessary cardiac stimulation and renal dilation
D. At 10 mcg/kg/minute, dopamine dilates only the renal vasculature

CORRECT ANSWER—B. At low dosages of 0.5 to 2 mcg/kg/minute, dopamine acts on the dopaminergic receptors in the renal, mesenteric, coronary, and intracerebral vascular beds to cause vasodilation. At low dosages, dopamine also can cause cardiac stimulation, but this therapeutic effect is not necessary for this patient. At dosages ranging from 5 to 8 mcg/kg/minute, dopamine will cause increased peripheral vasoconstriction, which is not considered a therapeutic effect for this patient. At dosages greater than 10 mcg/kg/minute, alpha-adrenergic stimulation occurs and causes vasoconstriction.
Nursing process step: Implementation
Cognitive level: Comprehension

44. The cellular response resulting from thermal injury includes all of the following *except:*
A. Disseminated intravascular coagulation (DIC) secondary to decreased platelet and fibrinogen levels
B. Converging of neutrophils in the injured area with phagocytosis of bacteria
C. Decreased number of circulating monocytes and increased number of macrophages attacking foreign material and digesting debris
D. Red blood cell destruction at the site of injury and partial red blood cell destruction at the wound periphery

CORRECT ANSWER—C. The cellular response to thermal injury includes an increased number of circulating monocytes that convert to macrophages in the tissues and begin the repair process by attacking and digesting wound debris and transporting it from the wound site. Neutrophils converge on the area of injury and phagocytosis of bacteria occurs. Initially, the inflammatory response triggers vasoconstriction and fibrin clot formation. Fibrinogen and platelet levels subsequently decrease, predisposing the patient to DIC. Interference with cellular enzyme processes leads to red blood cell destruction.
Nursing process step: Assessment
Cognitive level: Comprehension

Questions 45 to 47 refer to the following information:
A 50-year-old male patient involved in a motor vehicle accident is admitted to the intensive care unit after being intubated and initially stabilized in the emergency department. He has multiple fractured ribs and fractures of both femurs. A peritoneal tap is negative, but a chest X-ray film reveals a small pneumothorax on the left side.

---

45. The patient is connected to a mechanical ventilator set on assist-control mode. The nurse becomes concerned after noting that the patient's peak inspiratory pressure has increased and he is breathing at more than 10 respirations above the ventilator rate. The patient's oxygen saturation level as measured by pulse oximetry has fallen from 95% to 88%, and he has diminished breath sounds on the left side. The patient points to his left chest and indicates he is in pain. After notifying the physician, the nurse would take what primary action?

A. Preparing for needle aspiration and chest tube insertion

B. Obtaining a blood sample for arterial blood gas analysis

C. Ordering a chest X-ray film

D. Assessing for continued chest pain

CORRECT ANSWER—A. The patient's pneumothorax probably has expanded to the point at which his left lung collapsed, and he should be prepared for needle aspiration and possible chest tube insertion. Other signs and symptoms of lung collapse include tachycardia, cessation of chest wall movement on the affected side, palpation of subcutaneous air, sudden sharp chest pain, hypotension, and anxiety. Although arterial blood gas analysis and chest X-ray results would be helpful, the patient requires immediate intervention to prevent further deterioration of his condition. An assessment of continued chest pain may be appropriate after immediate interventions have been performed.
Nursing process step: Implementation
Cognitive level: Application

46. After the chest tube is inserted and connected to suction, the patient begins to improve. After 30 minutes, the nurse reassesses vital signs, which include blood pressure, 110/74 mm Hg; heart rate, 106 beats/minute with sinus tachycardia; respirations, 24 breaths/minute; and core temperature, 96° F (35.6° C). Ventilator settings are FIO_2, 0.7; synchronized intermittent mandatory ventilation (SIMV), 12 breaths/minute; tidal volume, 850 cc; positive end-expiratory pressure, 5 cm H_2O; and pressure support, 12 cm H_2O. Arterial blood gas values include PaO_2, 71 mm Hg; $PaCO_2$, 26 mm Hg; and pH, 7.46. Which nursing action to increase available oxygen at the tissue level is appropriate at this time?

A. Increase SIMV to 15 breaths/minute

B. Increase tidal volume to 950 cc

C. Place the patient on a hypothermia unit

D. Place the patient on a hyperthermia unit

CORRECT ANSWER—D. The hypoxia can be corrected by treating the patient's hypothermia and respiratory alkalosis, both of which move the oxyhemoglobin-dissociation curve to the left and increase the affinity of hemoglobin for oxygen. Increasing SIMV and tidal volume would further contribute to the low $PaCO_2$ and respiratory alkalosis.
Nursing process step: Implementation
Cognitive level: Evaluation

47. The patient suddenly experiences arrhythmias and full cardiopulmonary arrest. The initial arterial blood gas reading obtained after the cardiac arrest has occurred reveals respiratory acidosis with $PaCO_2$, 78 mm Hg; PaO_2, 32 mm Hg; pH, 7.27; and HCO_3^-, 21 mEq/liter. The acidosis should not be treated with sodium bicarbonate because the:

A. Acidosis causes a shift to the right on the oxyhemoglobin curve

B. $PaCO_2$ level is 78 mm Hg

C. PaO_2 level is 32 mm Hg

D. Patient is at risk for hypernatremia

CORRECT ANSWER—A. A shift to the right on the oxyhemoglobin-dissociation curve can be caused by acidosis, increased metabolic functions (fever), and hypoxia, which increases the level of 2,3-diphosphoglycerate. A shift to the right decreases the affinity of hemoglobin for oxygen and results in the release of oxygen to the tissues, which is necessary when tissue perfusion is decreased or absent, as occurs in patients suffering cardiopulmonary arrest. Administration of sodium bicarbonate will cause an increase in the sodium level; however, this is not the reason to avoid this therapy. Although sodium bicarbonate does affect acid-base balance, treatment of the $PaCO_2$ and PaO_2 levels requires different interventions.
Nursing process step: Planning
Cognitive level: Comprehension

48. A patient's metabolic status must be monitored throughout all stages of septic shock. Which acid-base imbalances typically occur during the early stage and late stage of septic shock, respectively?

A. Respiratory acidosis and respiratory alkalosis

B. Respiratory acidosis and metabolic acidosis

C. Metabolic alkalosis and metabolic acidosis

D. Respiratory alkalosis and metabolic acidosis

CORRECT ANSWER—D. Respiratory alkalosis is evident during the early stage of septic shock secondary to compensatory hyperventilation. In the late stage of septic shock, decreased tissue perfusion and metabolic acidosis occur.
Nursing process step: Evaluation
Cognitive level: Evaluation

49. A male patient who attempted suicide with an overdose of acetaminophen is assessed by the admitting nurse in the intensive care unit. In the emergency department, the patient was alert but not oriented to place. The patient now appears confused and unable to follow commands. He is normothermic, with a stable heart rate, blood pressure, and respiratory rate. The nurse's initial action should be to:

A. Notify the physician of the change in level of consciousness and institute seizure precautions

B. Obtain a blood specimen to check liver function

C. Administer atropine

D. Administer succimer

CORRECT ANSWER—A. The most common complications of poisoning and drug overdose are central nervous system depression and coma. Other complications include seizures, alterations in blood pressure, arrhythmias, and tissue damage. Although the patient's vital signs and respiratory rate are stable, the nurse should anticipate a further decrease in level of consciousness and take necessary measures to protect the patient's airway. Acetaminophen can cause severe hepatotoxicity and liver function will need to be checked; however, this action is not yet a priority. The antidote for acetaminophen poisoning is acetylcysteine, a dispositional antagonist that hastens detoxification of acetaminophen. Atropine and succimer are the antidotes for anticholinesterase poisoning and lead poisoning, respectively.
Nursing process step: Implementation
Cognitive level: Analysis

50. A 32-year-old male with chronic renal failure is admitted to the intensive care unit with bilateral infiltrates of the lungs. His first arterial blood gas readings reveal pH, 7.24; $PaCO_2$, 40 mm Hg; PaO_2, 64 mm Hg; and HCO_3^-, 13 mEq/liter. His respiratory rate is 22 breaths/minute. What is the patient's acid-base status?
A. Uncompensated respiratory alkalosis with hypoxia
B. Uncompensated respiratory acidosis with hypoxia
C. Uncompensated respiratory acidosis with mixed metabolic alkalosis
D. Uncompensated metabolic acidosis with hypoxia

CORRECT ANSWER—**D.** The patient is acidotic, with a pH of 7.24. The normal $PaCO_2$ and low HCO_3^- indicate a metabolic problem not compensated by the increased respiratory rate or acidosis. The patient may require mechanical ventilation because of the low PaO_2 level and known pulmonary infiltrates.
Nursing process step: Evaluation
Cognitive level: Evaluation

51. A patient with sepsis is being treated with a cooling blanket for a fever of 103° F (39.4° C). How often and by which route should the patient's temperature be checked?
A. Every hour via a rectal temperature
B. Every 2 hours via a rectal temperature
C. Every hour via a core temperature
D. Every 4 hours via a core temperature

CORRECT ANSWER—**C.** Unless a continuous monitoring system is available, the best method of evaluating the patient's fever is by taking a core temperature reading. Regardless of how the temperature is measured, a reading is necessary at least every hour to prevent hypothermia, which can lead to chills, shivering, and increased myocardial consumption at a time when the patient needs all of the available cardiac reserve.
Nursing process step: Implementation
Cognitive level: Application

52. What is the most important, immediate goal of therapy for a patient with a burn injury?
A. Maintaining fluid, electrolyte, and acid-base balance
B. Planning for rehabilitation and discharge
C. Providing emotional support to the patient and family
D. Preserving full range of motion of all affected joints

CORRECT ANSWER—**A.** Although all of the goals are important, the most immediate and life-sustaining goal is to maintain fluid, electrolyte, and acid-base balance. This helps prevent potentially life-threatening complications, including burn shock, disseminated intravascular coagulation, respiratory failure, cardiac failure, and acute tubular necrosis.
Nursing process step: Planning
Cognitive level: Application

53. A patient with an electrical burn injury must be carefully assessed because electrical burns cause:
A. More severe pain than other types of burns and large doses of analgesics will be required
B. Significant internal destruction that is difficult to detect
C. Severe electrolyte disturbances
D. Wounds that require immediate attention to prevent continued damage by the electrical current

CORRECT ANSWER—**B.** The internal destruction along the pathway of the electrical current usually is greater than the surface burn might indicate; consequently, special monitoring is needed to evaluate the body systems affected by an electrical burn. An electrical current damages tissue as it passes through the body; the current also can cause flash burns and surface thermal burns from heat or flames. Loss of muscle contraction and reflex control, changes in level of consciousness, and respiratory paralysis occur with the initial electrical shock. Hyperventilation may follow, and lethal arrhythmias are common even with the smallest electrical shock. The pain associated with a burn is related to the degree of injury, which is determined by the size and depth of the burn. The pain from electrical burns is not necessarily more severe than that caused by thermal or other burn injuries. The first priority of treatment is to stop the burning process and institute advanced cardiac life support (ACLS) measures. However, continued damage from the electrical current does not occur. Electrolyte disturbances can occur with all types of burns; they are not necessarily more severe with electrical burns but do require close monitoring.
Nursing process step: Assessment
Cognitive level: Comprehension

54. A patient with burn injuries develops acute renal failure and requires hemodialysis. The nurse notes a prolonged QT interval on the ECG and observes localized seizure activity. Which electrolyte disturbance would cause these symptoms?
A. Hypokalemia
B. Hypernatremia
C. Hypocalcemia
D. Hypophosphatemia

CORRECT ANSWER—**C.** A patient with a burn injury is at risk for acute renal failure secondary to inadequate fluid resuscitation and the release of myoglobin and hemoglobin. Acute renal failure predisposes the patient to hypocalcemia because the kidneys cannot convert vitamin D to the usable form necessary to facilitate calcium absorption from the intestinal tract. Hypocalcemia causes signs and symptoms of nervous system irritability, including seizure activity, cramps, tetany, and positive Trousseau's and Chvostek's signs. A prolonged QT interval, bronchospasm, and stridor also may occur. Seizure activity and muscle twitching are associated with hyponatremia. Other electrolyte abnormalities that may occur in a patient with a burn injury are hyperkalemia and hyperphosphatemia.
Nursing process step: Evaluation
Cognitive level: Evaluation

55. All of the following can cause upper airway obstruction *except:*
A. Tumor
B. Thickened secretions
C. Thrombus
D. Edema of the epiglottis

CORRECT ANSWER—C. Upper airway obstruction interrupts airflow to the lungs and can be caused by tumors, vocal cord paralysis, edema of the epiglottis or larynx (resulting from tonsillitis), infection of the oral or pharyngeal area, thickened secretions, tongue positioning or swelling, foreign body aspiration, laryngeal or tracheal trauma, and anaphylaxis. A thrombus will cause an obstruction in the pulmonary vasculature and, subsequently, ventilation-perfusion mismatch.
Nursing process step: Assessment
Cognitive level: Comprehension

56. A patient suffering from a drug overdose is treated in the emergency department and transferred to the intensive care unit. The nurse asks the patient and his spouse about the specific drug ingested and the reason for taking the drug. The nurse also would question the patient about all of the following *except:*
A. Patient's weight
B. Patient's height
C. Whether vomiting occurred after ingestion
D. Concurrent use of medication, alcohol, or illicit drugs

CORRECT ANSWER—B. To develop an effective plan of care, the nurse must gather essential facts about the patient and the circumstances surrounding the overdose. In this situation, the patient's height is not relevant. Questioning should focus on the patient's medical history and the route and time of drug ingestion.
Nursing process step: Assessment
Cognitive level: Synthesis

57. During the initial assessment of a patient with a burn injury, the nurse would be concerned if the:
A. Lactated Ringer's solution was being infused at a rate of 175 ml/hour
B. ECG showed atrial fibrillation with 110 beats/minute
C. Urine was tea-colored and output was less than 30 ml/hour
D. Wound was blistering and was very painful

CORRECT ANSWER—C. Tea-colored urine in less than adequate amounts (that is, less than 30 ml/hour) is caused by the release of myoglobin into the bloodstream resulting from muscle damage, which is especially common in patients with electrical burn injuries. These proteins can precipitate in the renal tubules, causing tubular necrosis and renal shutdown. Patients with burns require aggressive fluid resuscitation at high flow rates, such as 175 ml/hour. A controlled atrial fibrillation with a ventricular rate of 110 beats/minute should be reported and monitored. However, because the ventricular rate is controlled, the nurse need not treat it as an emergency. Burn injuries are painful and can be expected to blister, especially if the patient has partial-thickness injuries.
Nursing process step: Assessment
Cognitive level: Evaluation

58. Before applying the topical antibiotic mafenide to a burn wound, the nurse should tell the patient that:

A. Mafenide absorption is increased by using only a light dressing

B. Mafenide is applied once a day

C. Mafenide causes pain on application and analgesics will be administered before it is applied

D. Mafenide penetrates eschar and is applied every 3 hours

CORRECT ANSWER—C. Mafenide is a topical antibiotic with broad-spectrum coverage that rapidly and deeply penetrates the wound. It is applied three or four times daily, and the wound is left open, exposed to air. However, mafenide inhibits wound healing and causes pain on application; the patient will require analgesics before the antibiotic is applied. Adverse effects of mafenide include pulmonary toxicity, metabolic acidosis, and hypersensitivity.

Nursing process step: Implementation
Cognitive level: Synthesis

59. The venous oxygen saturation (SvO_2) level of a patient with sepsis must be monitored throughout the course of the illness to identify possible threats to oxygen delivery and consumption. A high SvO_2 level probably would be secondary to:

A. Decreased respiratory rate

B. Increased cardiac output

C. Increased hemoglobin level

D. Decreased oxygen extraction at the tissue level

CORRECT ANSWER—D. A patient with sepsis has an imbalance between systemic oxygen supply and demand. During treatment, the increased level of oxygen consumption requires increased systemic blood flow and oxygen delivery because the increased metabolic rate and circulatory abnormalities impair the tissues' ability to maximally extract oxygen. A decreased respiratory rate could lower the SvO_2 level if the oxygen supply to the tissues is decreased. Increased cardiac output and increased hemoglobin level probably would raise the SvO_2 level, a desirable outcome in this situation. However, in a patient with sepsis, the initial increase in SvO_2 is secondary to the primary metabolic failure, shifts in the oxyhemoglobin-dissociation curve, and circulatory abnormalities.

Nursing process step: Assessment
Cognitive level: Analysis

60. The hypovolemia that occurs after a burn injury involving more than 20% of the body surface area produces splanchnic vasoconstriction with reflex ileus. Which nursing intervention would help treat this condition?

A. Checking gastric pH every 2 hours

B. Administering antacids to neutralize gastric secretions

C. Collecting stool specimens for guaiac testing

D. Inserting a nasogastric (NG) tube and suctioning the patient

CORRECT ANSWER—D. Although all of the interventions would be helpful, only insertion of an NG tube and suctioning would treat the reflux ileus. Other GI responses to a burn injury include abdominal distention, regurgitation, malabsorption, ulcers, and hyperacidity leading to Curling's ulcer. Therefore, the nurse should monitor the patient's gastric pH, administer antacids, and order a guaiac test on all drainage.

Nursing process step: Implementation
Cognitive level: Application

61. A patient in septic shock requires frequent skin assessments because:
A. Peripheral edema can lead to blistering
B. Immobility and decreased tissue perfusion can impair skin integrity
C. Skin rash may develop
D. Pruritus accompanying septicemia can lead to scratching and bleeding

CORRECT ANSWER—**B.** The skin of a patient with septic shock should be assessed frequently for signs of breakdown or pressure ulcers stemming from immobility and decreased tissue perfusion. The nurse should institute appropriate measures to prevent tissue breakdown, including using a low-air-loss mattress, turning the patient every 2 hours, performing passive range-of-motion exercises, and teaching the patient to shift position frequently if possible. A skin rash with subsequent pruritus may develop, possibly secondary to a reaction to antibiotic treatment. However, neither rashes nor peripheral edema are characteristic of septic shock.
Nursing process step: Assessment
Cognitive level: Comprehension

62. A female patient severely burned in a car fire is brought to the intensive care unit and stabilized. When she awakens, the patient asks about her husband, who was killed in the accident. How should the nurse respond?
A. Explain that the patient should focus on her own problems now
B. Answer the question honestly and allow the patient to grieve
C. Change the subject until the chaplain arrives
D. Tell the patient her husband was taken to another hospital for treatment

CORRECT ANSWER—**B.** In many situations involving burn injuries, other persons may have been injured or killed. The nurse caring for a burn victim who asks about a loved one should understand that the patient is ready to hear an immediate answer, even if the news is tragic. The nurse should always answer truthfully and never lie to the patient or avoid the subject once it comes up; doing so will only increase the patient's anxiety. However, explanations should be brief to allow the patient to begin grieving.
Nursing process step: Implementation
Cognitive level: Synthesis

63. The mother of a patient admitted to the intensive care unit after a drug overdose cannot identify the capsules her son ingested. She gives the nurse one of the capsules, which she found near the patient's body. What would be the nurse's initial action in this situation?
A. Report the incident to the physician
B. Call the regional poison control center
C. Compare the imprinted letters or numbers on the capsule with the Identadex
D. Send the capsule to the laboratory for analysis

CORRECT ANSWER—**C.** The first step is to attempt to identify the drug by comparing letters or numbers with the Identadex or Poisindex. Either the nurse or the physician can assume responsibility for identifying the drug; therefore, reporting the incident to the physician is unnecessary. Staff members at the regional poison control center can provide helpful information and act as consultants to the health care team; however, this would require some time. Laboratory analysis is the most time-consuming step, and the information may arrive too late to be useful.
Nursing process step: Implementation
Cognitive level: Comprehension

64. After a frank discussion involving the health care team and the family of a patient in the late stage of septic shock, the nurse overhears a family member say to relatives, "Mom has a little blood infection but otherwise is doing really well." Based on this comment, the nurse should realize that the family:

A. Is in a crisis and is coping by denying the gravity of the situation

B. Has a good understanding of the prognosis and degree of care the patient is receiving

C. Is angry and unable to accept the truth about their mother

D. Needs further education about septic shock

CORRECT ANSWER—A. Although the family members will need further education about septic shock and its potentially grave complications, they are evidently under a great deal of stress because of the potential loss of a loved one and probably are incapable of handling such news at this time. No evidence indicates that the family members are angry; rather, they seem to be denying the reality of the situation. The family will require psychosocial services, possibly from a psychiatric nurse liaison or chaplain, to help them cope with the situation.

Nursing process step: Analysis
Cognitive level: Synthesis

65. After emergency treatment is administered to a patient suffering a drug overdose, the nurse should focus on:

A. Decreasing GI absorption of the toxic substance

B. Decreasing systemic absorption of the toxic substance

C. Arranging for psychiatric evaluation and counseling

D. Obtaining a history and clinical assessment

CORRECT ANSWER—D. The nurse should obtain as much information as possible from the patient or family members regarding the drug and how it was ingested to better control the drug toxicity. Decreasing GI and systemic absorption and arranging for psychiatric evaluation and counseling should follow the clinical assessment and history taking, which provide data necessary for appropriate treatment.

Nursing process step: Assessment
Cognitive level: Application

SAMPLE TEST

Questions

1. A female patient is admitted to the intensive care unit while the operating room is prepared for her emergency aneurysm repair. The patient's blood pressure is 219/130 mm Hg. Which of the following I.V. antihypertensive medications would the nurse expect to administer in this situation?
   A. Hydralazine hydrochloride (Apresoline)
   B. Methyldopa (Aldomet)
   C. Nitroprusside sodium (Nipride)
   D. Enalapril (Vasotec)

2. When changing the dressing of a patient with a burn injury, the nurse should:
   A. Use maximum-absorption bandages to ensure that all drainage is absorbed
   B. Use elastic bandages on dependent areas to limit edema and bleeding and to facilitate grafting
   C. Wrap the extremities proximally to distally to promote venous return
   D. Use strict aseptic technique when removing the bandages

3. The nurse should plan to monitor for which complication that occurs routinely after splenectomy?
   A. Leukopenia
   B. Leukocytosis
   C. Thrombocytopenia
   D. Thrombocytosis

Questions 4 to 5 refer to the following information: An 82-year-old female patient is admitted to the hospital complaining of severe, colicky abdominal pain in the periumbilical area. She has bloody diarrhea and, on assessment, exhibits rebound abdominal tenderness. Her assessment findings include blood pressure, 88/52 mm Hg; white blood cell count, 14,000/mm^3; heart rate, 118 beats/minute and irregular; respirations, 32 breaths/minute; and temperature, 101.2° F (38.4° C).

4. Based on the assessment data, the nurse suspects that the patient most likely has:
   A. Bowel obstruction
   B. Acute appendicitis
   C. Occlusion of the superior mesenteric artery
   D. Crohn's disease

5. Which treatment would the nurse anticipate for this patient?
   A. Permanent ileostomy
   B. Embolectomy and possible bowel resection
   C. Miller-Abbott tube insertion
   D. Appendectomy

6. The initial goals of treatment for a patient with bowel infarction include:
   A. Relieving pain
   B. Maintaining skin integrity
   C. Providing adequate nutrition
   D. Maintaining fluid and electrolyte balance

7. Which treatment most effectively lowers the potassium level in a patient with hyperkalemia?
   A. Glucose and insulin therapy
   B. Sodium bicarbonate therapy
   C. Sodium polystyrene sulfonate (Kayexalate) therapy
   D. Hemodialysis

8. Which pathogen for pneumonia is associated with the highest mortality rate in the elderly?
   A. *Streptococcus pneumoniae*
   B. *Klebsiella*
   C. *Staphylococcus aureus*
   D. *Legionella*

9. A chest tube connected to a multiple-chamber drainage system is inserted in a patient with an acute pneumothorax. The nurse would expect to see bubbling in which chambers of the drainage system?
   A. First drainage collection chamber and water-seal chamber
   B. First and second drainage collection chambers
   C. Water-seal chamber and suction-control chamber
   D. Suction-control chamber and second drainage collection chamber

10. Two hours after eating dinner, a 55-year-old female patient is admitted to the emergency department for evaluation of acute abdomen. The patient has severe epigastric pain, nausea, and a fever of 102.6° F (39.2° C). After ruling out a gynecologic disorder, the surgeon performs an exploratory laparotomy for suspected ruptured appendix. The nurse caring for the patient after surgery knows that she is at increased risk for:
    A. Adenovirus pneumonia
    B. Fungal pneumonia
    C. *Pseudomonas* pneumonia
    D. Aspiration pneumonia

11. During the acute phase of myocardial infarction, which ECG change is most common?
    A. Significant Q waves
    B. Widened QRS complex
    C. ST-segment elevation
    D. ST-segment depression

12. A patient with acute heart failure is receiving digoxin. The nurse becomes concerned with which of the following assessment data, as it represents an electrolyte imbalance which could potentiate digoxin toxicity?
    A. Skeletal muscle weakness, numbness and tingling, and abdominal cramps
    B. Depressed ST segments, hyporeflexia, and decreased peristalsis
    C. Carpopedal spasm, perioral paresthesia, and muscle cramps
    D. Bradycardia, diminished sensorium, and respiratory depression

13. Primary ECG findings for a patient with Wolff-Parkinson-White syndrome include:
    A. Widened QRS complex and inverted P wave
    B. Prolonged PR interval and delta wave
    C. Prolonged PR interval and widened QRS complex
    D. Shortened PR interval and delta wave

14. During the early postoperative assessment of a patient who underwent abdominal aortic aneurysm repair, the nurse should observe for foul-smelling, watery stools because:
    A. Patients with diarrhea can easily become dehydrated
    B. Aortic rupture reduces mesenteric artery blood flow and can cause bowel ischemia
    C. Oral feedings cannot begin until the patient has a normal bowel movement
    D. These symptoms may indicate GI bleeding

Questions 15 to 17 refer to the following information:
A 64-year-old male patient underwent coronary artery bypass graft surgery 3 weeks ago. He had an uneventful postoperative recovery and was discharged on the fifth postoperative day. He has returned to the hospital with a persistent fever of 101.2° F (38.4° C) and positional chest pain; he has an elevated erythrocyte sedimentation rate and a white blood cell count of 11,200/mm^3 with normal differential. His vital signs are stable, and his wounds are healing well.

15. Based on these findings, the nurse suspects that the patient has:
A. Pneumonia
B. Mediastinitis
C. Dressler syndrome
D. Influenza

16. Which medication would the nurse expect to administer to this patient?
A. Acetaminophen
B. Ibuprofen
C. Antibiotics
D. Propoxyphene hydrochloride

17. Which patient-teaching information would the nurse include in the patient's plan of care?
A. Dressler syndrome is a chronic condition that can be well controlled with anti-inflammatory agents
B. Dressler syndrome is a self-limiting inflammatory process that will resolve with or without treatment
C. Positioning, heat, and upper-extremity exercises will be used to alleviate pain
D. If the pain does not resolve, the ibuprofen dosage will be doubled

18. A 49-year-old female patient appeared in good health until 5 days ago when she experienced an explosive headache while mowing the lawn. Arteriography revealed a small aneurysm of the middle cerebral artery, with a grade II hemorrhage. After clipping of the aneurysm, the patient had mild left hemiparesis but no other deficits. Five days after surgery, she is difficult to arouse, confused, and disoriented with left hemiplegia. A computed tomography scan rules out rebleeding and hydrocephalus. Hypervolemic hemodilution with moderate hypertension is used to overcome vasospasm. This treatment should include:
A. Assessing neurologic status frequently, monitoring for increased pulmonary artery pressure and cardiac output, and administering diuretics
B. Assessing neurologic status frequently and monitoring for increased blood pressure, pulmonary artery wedge pressure increase to between 14 and 17 mm Hg, cardiac output increase to between 7 and 8 liters/minute, and hematocrit drop to less than 30%
C. Assessing neurologic status frequently, darkening the room, and monitoring hourly urine output for decreased volume
D. Assessing neurologic status frequently and monitoring for increased blood pressure and hemoglobin increase to more than 30 g/dl

19. The physician prescribes corticosteroids for a patient with a pelvic fracture for prophylaxis against the complications of hypoxia and fat emboli in the pulmonary vasculature. The nurse understands that this controversial treatment has its risks and benefits. Assuming the availability of all of the following studies, which blood study results should be evaluated to monitor for risks associated with steroid use?
A. partial pressure of oxygen in arterial blood (PaO$_2$) levels
B. Blood cultures
C. White blood cell counts
D. Intracranial pressure readings

20. The most common electrolyte disturbance in a renal transplant patient in the acute postoperative phase is:
A. Hyponatremia
B. Hypernatremia
C. Hypokalemia
D. Hypermagnesemia

21. When ranitidine is given to a patient with peptic ulcer disease, it acts by:
A. Neutralizing gastric pH
B. Preventing gastric acid secretion via inhibition of histamine action
C. Inhibiting basal and stimulated gastric acid secretion
D. Blocking histamine₂ antagonists

22. Which sign or symptom is not indicative of renal injury?
A. Costovertebral angle tenderness
B. Hematuria
C. Pyuria
D. Flank pain

23. Which statement about inverse ratio ventilation is correct?
A. Flow rate is decreased and respiratory rate is increased
B. Minute ventilation is increased and tidal volume is decreased
C. Inspiratory time is increased and expiratory time is decreased
D. Pressure support is initiated and expiratory time is increased

24. A patient is prescribed diltiazem hydrochloride after an extensive workup because the patient complained of which of the following symptoms?
A. "My heart is racing."
B. "My feet are swollen."
C. "I have a crushing pain in my chest."
D. "I feel hungry and have been sweating a lot."

25. For a patient in hypertensive crisis who had a recent cerebrovascular accident resulting from thrombosis, the blood pressure should be lowered to:
A. Normal
B. 160 to 180 mm Hg systolic
C. 100 to 110 mm Hg diastolic
D. Both B and C

26. The nurse caring for a patient in cardiogenic shock is asked by a family member about the patient's chances of survival. The nurse would need to be as consistent as the physician in answering the family member's question and should tell him that, despite recent advances in medical technology, the mortality rate for cardiogenic shock remains at:
A. 80%
B. 50%
C. 30%
D. 10%

27. The nurse would expect to administer all of the following drugs during the acute phase of aortic dissection *except:*
A. Propranolol (Inderal)
B. Nitroprusside sodium (Nipride)
C. Diltiazem (Cardizem)
D. Trimethaphan camsylate (Arfonad)

28. A 44-year-old male is diagnosed with diabetic ketoacidosis. His initial laboratory data include pH, 7.2; potassium, 3.8 mEq/liter; and sodium, 149 mEq/liter. Despite the patient's metabolic acidosis, the physician does not order sodium bicarbonate therapy. The rationale for not using sodium bicarbonate to treat the acid-base imbalance is best described by which statement?
A. Metabolic acidosis provides the necessary stimulus to breathe
B. Sodium bicarbonate therapy is not warranted for a pH above 6.8
C. Sodium bicarbonate therapy can reverse acidosis too quickly, thereby causing severe hypokalemia
D. Indiscriminate use of sodium bicarbonate therapy can cause hyperkalemia

29. The nurse caring for a patient whose blood glucose level is 67 mg/dl would expect to note which findings during the physical examination?
A. Bradycardia and lethargy
B. Tachycardia and diaphoresis
C. Bradycardia and seizures
D. Tachycardia and lassitude

Questions 30 and 31 refer to the following information:
A 29-year-old female patient involved in a bicycle accident sustained a right femur fracture and blunt abdominal trauma with splenic rupture. After splenectomy, she is transferred to the intensive care unit and is in stable condition. Her femur fracture will be stabilized in a few days.

---

30. The patient complains of severe pain in her right leg. Distal pulses cannot be obtained by Doppler ultrasonography, and the nurse notes that the patient's right foot is considerably cooler than the left. The nurse's next step would be to:
A. Notify the physician and prepare for emergency angiography
B. Administer analgesics and monitor the neurovascular status of the patient's right leg
C. Apply warm compresses and elevate the patient's right leg
D. Apply cold compresses and place the patient's right leg in a dependent position

31. A small laceration of the deep femoral artery is found. After emergency surgery, the patient is admitted to the critical care unit. The nurse prioritizes the evaluation of this patient's injuries as follows:
A. Monitoring hemodynamic status, neurovascular status of the right leg, and urine output
B. Monitoring respiratory status, urine output, and neurologic status
C. Monitoring hemodynamic status, neurovascular status of the right leg, and respiratory status
D. Monitoring hemodynamic status, neurovascular status of the right leg, and neurologic status

32. The nurse is caring for a patient recently prescribed procainamide. What changes in rhythm would indicate an adverse reaction to this medication?
A. Prolonged PR interval
B. Prolonged QT interval
C. ST-segment elevation
D. ST-segment depression

33. When planning the care of a patient with syndrome of inappropriate antidiuretic hormone (SIADH), the nurse formulates a nursing diagnosis of fluid volume excess related to increased serum antidiuretic hormone and renal sodium excretion. The nurse would plan to restrict the patient's total fluid intake, including fluids required with medications, to how many milliliters in a 24-hour period?
A. 240 ml
B. 500 ml
C. 1,000 ml
D. 1,500 ml

34. After a thermal injury occurs, all body systems are affected. Which statement about the ensuing effect on the cardiac system is true?
A. Cardiac output is decreased if the injury affects more than 50% of the total body surface area
B. Drugs with both vasoconstrictive and positive inotropic properties are needed to support the cardiac system
C. Fluid restriction is necessary to avoid increasing the workload of the heart
D. Although arrhythmias are uncommon, careful ECG monitoring is necessary

35. A "shift to the left" in the white blood cell count usually indicates:
A. Pernicious anemia or hepatic disease
B. Viral infection
C. Allergy
D. Bacterial infection

36. Which of the following laboratory values is consistent with fulminant hepatic failure?
A. Increased albumin
B. Decreased serum bilirubin
C. Increased serum glucose
D. Increased blood urea nitrogen

37. A 40-year-old patient involved in a motor vehicle accident is admitted to the intensive care unit for observation of a questionable splenic injury. The nurse ensures that serial abdominal examinations, serial hematocrit testing, and continuous blood pressure monitoring are performed. Which type of tube should be inserted in this patient?
A. Jejunostomy tube
B. Nasogastric tube
C. Dobhoff feeding tube
D. Cecostomy tube

38. Proper chest tube placement for a patient with a right hemothorax would be at the:
A. Right second intercostal space
B. Left fourth intercostal space
C. Right eighth intercostal space
D. Left ninth intercostal space

39. What is the lowest range of negative pressure acceptable for weaning a patient from a ventilator?
A. -10 to -15 cm H_2O
B. -20 to -25 cm H_2O
C. -30 to -40 cm H_2O
D. -35 to -40 cm H_2O

Question 40 refers to the following laboratory information:

Serial enzyme	Creatine kinase (CK)	Creatine kinase-MB (CK-MB)	Lactate dehydrogenase (LD)
Normal level	32 to 150 U/liter	4% to 6%	140 to 280 U/liter
8 a.m.	280 U/liter	6%	160 U/liter
4 p.m.	200 U/liter	4%	154 U/liter
12 a.m.	160 U/liter	3%	148 U/liter
8 a.m. next day	70 U/liter	0%	136 U/liter

40. These serial enzyme results indicate that:
A. Acute myocardial infarction has occurred
B. Skeletal muscle damage may have occurred
C. Liver damage may have occurred
D. No information can be obtained from these enzyme results

41. Atrial fibrillation can be medically treated with:
A. Digoxin
B. Amrinone
C. Dobutamine
D. Captopril

42. Autonomic dysreflexia is more common with lesions at the T7 level or above. This medical emergency is characterized by:
A. Vasodilation and hypotension
B. Severe orthostatic hypotension and loss of sympathetic nervous system function
C. Extreme hypertension, bounding headache, and profuse sweating
D. Arrhythmias and severe chest pain

Questions 43 to 46 refer to the following information:
A 27-year-old male patient is admitted to the intensive care unit with head trauma, blunt abdominal injuries, and bilateral femur fractures after a motor vehicle accident. At admission, the patient has purposeful response to painful stimuli, blood pressure of 90/56 mm Hg, pulse rate of 122 beats/minute and regular, and respiratory rate of 24 breaths/minute. Laboratory data include serum sodium, 146 mEq/liter; blood urea nitrogen, 33 mg/dl; hemoglobin, 14.5 g/dl; and serum alcohol level, 0.2 mg/dl.

43. During the initial assessment, the nurse notes that the patient's urine output is 300 ml/hour. Based on this finding, the nurse should implement interventions to treat which disorder?
A. High-output renal failure
B. Diabetes insipidus
C. Syndrome of inappropriate antidiuretic hormone (SIADH)
D. Hypervolemia

44. Which intervention would the nurse include in the patient's plan of care?
A. Limiting I.V. fluids to prevent hypervolemia
B. Preparing for pulmonary artery catheterization to monitor central venous pressure
C. Providing unlimited oral fluids to replace urine loss
D. Monitoring urine output hourly

45. Which medication would most likely be administered to this patient?
A. Furosemide (Lasix)
B. Ethacrynic acid (Edecrin)
C. Vasopressin (Pitressin)
D. Potassium chloride

46. Which other possible cause of volume depletion should the nurse consider when caring for this patient?
A. Temporary decrease in antidiuretic hormone secretion resulting from the effects of alcohol
B. Blood loss secondary to blunt abdominal trauma
C. Diuretic abuse
D. Fluid extravasation resulting from bilateral femur fractures

47. A bullet wound places a patient at high risk for embolization if:
A. The patient is active after being injured
B. The bullet enters the groin area
C. The exit wound or bullet cannot be located
D. The bullet enters the chest

48. The nurse might administer which of the following medications to a patient with chronic atrial fibrillation?
A. Digoxin, warfarin, and verapamil
B. Digoxin, hydralazine, and verapamil
C. Warfarin, hydralazine, and diltiazem
D. Warfarin, verapamil, and diltiazem

49. Negative nitrogen balance can contribute to skin breakdown, poor wound healing, and lack of energy for rehabilitation exercises in patients with spinal cord injuries. Negative nitrogen balance can be prevented by:
A. Administering medications to stimulate GI peristalsis
B. Providing early parenteral and later enteral nutritional support
C. Decreasing caloric intake and increasing nitrogen and protein intake
D. Encouraging early mobilization and administering frequent nutritional supplements

50. The nurse caring for a patient with acute anterior wall myocardial infarction notes the following rhythm:

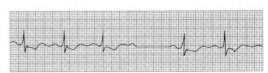

The patient is asymptomatic with this rhythm. Which treatment is most appropriate?
A. Dopamine I.V. infusion
B. Temporary atrioventricular sequential pacing
C. Intra-aortic balloon pump counterpulsation therapy
D. Monitoring for progression of the block

51. To prevent hepatic encephalopathy in a patient with liver disease, the nurse would administer all of the following *except*:
A. Oxygen based on arterial blood gas levels
B. Stool softeners
C. Potassium chloride based on serum potassium level
D. Sedatives to treat agitation

52. What is the best indicator of renal failure?
A. Blood urea nitrogen level
B. Serum potassium level
C. Serum creatinine level
D. Urine creatinine level

53. A patient who recently ingested a toxic dose of a caustic agent is stabilized in the emergency department, then transported to the intensive care unit for further evaluation and treatment. The greatest amount of information about the patient's immediate condition would be obtained by:
  A. Examining an abdominal X-ray film
  B. Administering syrup of ipecac
  C. Evaluating blood level of the toxic substance
  D. Administering oxygen

54. A patient with a burn injury would be given enteral tube feedings despite his ability to receive oral nourishment because:
  A. Negative nitrogen balance must be maintained
  B. Patients undernourished before the injury require greater than normal nutritional intake
  C. Patients with burn injuries require additional calories, and protein mass must be maintained to ensure survival
  D. Patients with burn injuries require up to 8,000 calories daily

55. A patient whose spinal cord is compressed by a tumor initially will exhibit:
  A. Root pain and segmental sensory or motor changes
  B. Anterior cord syndrome
  C. Paralysis below the lesion
  D. Brown-Séquard syndrome

Questions 56 to 59 refer to the following information:
A 52-year-old male patient has a long cardiac history, including three previous myocardial infarctions and two coronary artery bypass procedures. He is admitted to the critical care unit with congestive heart failure and ischemic cardiomyopathy. An echocardiogram reveals an ejection fraction of 15%. A pulmonary artery catheter is inserted on admission.

56. Which finding would be unusual in this patient?
  A. S_3 gallop
  B. S_4 gallop
  C. Pulmonary crackles
  D. Jugular vein distention

57. Which diagnostic test would the patient most likely undergo?
  A. Treadmill exercise test
  B. Endomyocardial biopsy
  C. Electrophysiology studies
  D. Cardiac catheterization

58. The patient is prescribed a regimen of nitroglycerin, nitroprusside, and dobutamine I.V. infusions as well as I.V. digoxin once daily. The nurse observes that the patient's pulmonary artery wedge pressure has decreased to 4 mm Hg and the systolic blood pressure to 82 mm Hg. Which therapeutic measure would the nurse initiate?
  A. Increase the dobutamine infusion rate
  B. Rapidly infuse fluids while decreasing the dobutamine infusion rate
  C. Increase the nitroprusside infusion rate and decrease the nitroglycerin infusion rate
  D. Temporarily decrease the nitroprusside infusion rate while cautiously infusing fluid

59. The patient's urine output is decreasing and his serum creatinine level has increased to 2.4 mg/dl. Which nursing intervention is most appropriate?
  A. Adding a dopamine I.V. infusion at a rate of 10 to 15 mcg/kg/minute
  B. Monitoring serum levels of medications excreted via the kidneys
  C. Cautiously infusing I.V. fluid challenges
  D. Infusing furosemide

60. Hepatomegaly, peripheral edema, and jugular vein distention are clinical signs of:
  A. Right-sided heart failure
  B. Left-sided heart failure
  C. Compensated heart failure
  D. Acute heart failure

61. A 57-year-old male with unstable angina is admitted to the critical care unit and immediately tells the nurse he is experiencing a crushing sensation in his chest. Two sublingual nitroglycerin tablets do not relieve the discomfort, and the patient says the pain is worsening. What is the most likely cause of this unrelieved pain?
A. Unstable angina
B. Acute myocardial infarction
C. Congestive heart failure
D. Ventricular septal defect

62. A male patient has the following rhythm:

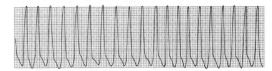

During the initial assessment, the patient has a blood pressure of 62/40 mm Hg. The patient also complains of dizziness. The nurse would interpret this rhythm as:
A. Asystole
B. Pulseless ventricular tachycardia
C. Ventricular tachycardia with a pulse
D. Ventricular fibrillation

63. The clinical manifestations of endocarditis result from all of the following pathophysiologic mechanisms *except:*
A. Generalized infection
B. Valvular destruction
C. Embolism
D. Dyspnea

64. The nurse would assess for which of the following symptoms that are indicative of the most likely embolic complication resulting from tricuspid valve vegetation?
A. Shortness of breath and hypoxia
B. Decreased level of consciousness and right-sided paralysis
C. Cold, mottled left arm without pulses
D. Urine output of less than 30 ml/hour for 4 hours

65. Which is a typical profile of a person at risk for hyperosmolar nonketotic syndrome (HNKS)?
A. Obese diabetic patient whose diabetes is well controlled with oral hypoglycemic agents
B. Elderly patient with inadequately treated type II diabetes mellitus
C. Patient with transiently elevated blood glucose levels who is receiving steroid therapy
D. Elderly patient with type I diabetes mellitus

66. A 66-year-old female patient is admitted to the intensive care unit after her daughter found her unresponsive on the kitchen floor. The patient has a rapid respiratory rate of 30 breaths/minute, blood pressure of 88/42 mm Hg, and heart rate of 152 beats/minute with sinus tachycardia. The daughter tells the nurse that the patient has diabetes and uses Orinase. The patient also has coronary artery disease and congestive heart failure. The physician diagnoses hyperosmolar nonketotic syndrome (HNKS) coma. After a GI assessment is performed, which intervention would be required for this patient?
A. Gastric lavage
B. Gastric intubation
C. Intestinal intubation
D. Enema or laxative therapy

67. The nurse ensures that a patient with an ischemic lower extremity secondary to atherosclerosis is adequately hydrated because:
A. Fluid sequesters in the affected extremity
B. Dehydration is a leading cause of thrombosis formation
C. Renal failure secondary to myoglobinuria may occur
D. Tissue ischemia releases lactic acid, which acts systemically as an osmotic diuretic

68. When assessing the abdomen, the nurse would follow which sequence?
A. Inspection, percussion, palpation, and auscultation
B. Auscultation, percussion, palpation, and inspection
C. Palpation, percussion, inspection, and auscultation
D. Inspection, auscultation, percussion, and palpation

69. Tension pneumothorax is a potential complication of mechanical ventilation in an asthmatic patient. Which findings are most consistent with a diagnosis of tension pneumothorax?
A. Distended neck veins, decreased breath sounds on the affected side, and tracheal deviation toward the affected side
B. Distended neck veins, absent breath sounds on the affected side, and tracheal deviation toward the unaffected side
C. Flat neck veins, absent breath sounds on the affected side, and tracheal deviation toward the affected side
D. Flat neck veins, decreased breath sounds on the affected side, and tracheal deviation toward the unaffected side

70. An immunocompromised patient with active tuberculosis is placed in respiratory isolation. When can the isolation be safely discontinued?
A. When the patient is discharged from the hospital
B. After 1 week of treatment with antitubercular agents
C. After 4 weeks of treatment with antitubercular agents
D. After sputum smears are negative for 3 consecutive days

71. Which of the following patients is not at risk for hyperkalemia caused by excessive cellular destruction and potassium release?
A. 21-year-old patient with crush trauma
B. 45-year-old patient with third-degree burns
C. 60-year-old patient with cardiac failure
D. 72-year-old patient with acute acidosis

72. A patient with hemorrhagic pancreatitis develops ecchymosis along both flanks. This finding is known as:
A. Cullen's sign
B. Turner's sign
C. Homan's sign
D. Kernig's sign

73. Which nursing intervention would be inappropriate for a patient with acute pancreatitis?
A. Administering histamine$_2$-receptor antagonists
B. Aspirating gastric secretions via nasogastric tube suctioning
C. Providing nothing by mouth except ice chips
D. Limiting physical activity

74. Common malignancies in patients with acquired immunodeficiency syndrome (AIDS) include:
A. Lymphoma
B. Gastric carcinoma
C. Spinal neoplasm
D. Malignant melanoma

75. Induced emesis to evacuate gastric contents is recommended for which of the following patients?
A. Alert 49-year-old man with an intact gag reflex who is suspected of recently ingesting a noncaustic substance
B. 17-year-old boy who ingested an unknown substance and is having a seizure
C. 8-month-old infant who ingested a toxic dose of a noncaustic substance
D. 35-year-old woman who ingested an overdose of tricyclic antidepressants

76. Which medication would best assist a patient with a failing heart in the acute phase of congestive heart failure?
A. Dobutamine (Dobutrex)
B. Diltiazem (Cardizem)
C. Propranolol (Inderal)
D. Digoxin (Lanoxin)

77. Which bedside measurement is best for assessing cardiac function?
A. Cardiac output
B. Right atrial pressure
C. Cardiac index
D. Pulmonary capillary wedge pressure

78. A 30-year-old male patient with pneumocystic pneumonia is admitted to the intensive care unit. He is allergic to bacitracin, so pentamidine and I.V. corticosteroids are started. Which changes best indicate that the patient is experiencing adverse reactions to pentamidine?
A. Decreased white blood cell count, hypertension, and hypoglycemia
B. Decreased sodium level, increased prothrombin time, and hypertension
C. Increased white blood cell count, hypotension, and hyperglycemia
D. Low platelet count, hypotension, and hypoglycemia

Questions 79 to 81 refer to the following information:
Attempts to wean a 54-year-old female patient from mechanical ventilation have been unsuccessful. The physician decides to perform a tracheostomy and mechanically ventilate the patient via a #8 Shiley tracheostomy tube. Twenty-four hours later, weaning is tried again. The patient's vital signs include temperature, 102.2° F (39° C); heart rate, 146 beats/minute; blood pressure, 156/92 mm Hg; and respirations, 10 breaths/minute. The patient is not assisting the ventilator.

79. Which of the patient's vital signs is the primary contraindication to weaning?
A. Temperature
B. Heart rate
C. Blood pressure
D. Respiratory rate and not assisting the ventilator

80. The physician replaces the endotracheal tube with a tracheostomy tube because it will decrease which of the following?
A. Compliance
B. Resistance
C. Elasticity
D. Functional residual capacity

81. The patient is prescribed antibiotics and all attempts to wean her are halted. After she is afebrile for 48 hours, weaning is attempted again. The nurse caring for this patient should discuss nutritional status and requirements with the nutrition support nurse because adequate levels of which electrolytes must be maintained for successful weaning?
A. Potassium, sodium, and chloride
B. Magnesium, sodium, and chloride
C. Magnesium, phosphate, and potassium
D. Magnesium, phosphate, and calcium

82. Which data would indicate that treatment of hypernatremia was effective?
A. Serum sodium level of 144 mEq/liter and serum osmolarity of 300 mOsm/liter
B. Serum sodium level of 148 mEq/liter and serum osmolarity of 310 mOsm/liter
C. Serum sodium level of 145 mEq/liter and serum osmolarity of 295 mOsm/liter
D. Serum sodium level of 140 mEq/liter and serum osmolarity of 300 mOsm/liter

83. A patient with acute pancreatitis should be monitored closely for all of the following potential complications *except:*
A. Pneumonia
B. Hepatitis
C. Pulmonary emboli
D. Pulmonary edema

84. Common, potentially life-threatening complications of allogenic bone marrow transplantation within the first 30 days after the procedure include all of the following *except:*

A. Hemolytic-uremic syndrome and acute graft-versus-host disease

B. Idiopathic hyperammonemia and gram-negative sepsis

C. Pulmonary hemorrhage and aplastic anemia

D. Cytomegalovirus pneumonia and thrombocytosis

85. The nurse is caring for a 90-kg male patient recently intubated for the third time for respiratory failure and heavily sedated after the intubation. The patient's arterial blood gas results are base excess, +5; HCO_3^-, 32 mm Hg; pH, 7.39; partial pressure of carbon dioxide in arterial blood ($PaCO_2$), 52 mm Hg; and PaO_2, 60 mm Hg. The patient is on synchronized intermittent mandatory ventilation (SIMV) at 8 breaths/minute, with a tidal volume of 800 ml, positive end-expiratory pressure of 7.5 cm H_2O, and fraction of inspired oxygen (FIO_2) of .50. Based on these findings, the nurse should:

A. Administer bicarbonate to decrease lactic acid production

B. Check for causes of hyperventilation

C. Check for causes of hypoventilation

D. Administer additional oxygen

86. What is the most important nursing goal for a patient in septic shock?

A. Promoting adequate tissue perfusion and supporting ventilation, oxygenation, and hemodynamic stability

B. Maintaining accurate intake and output records and optimizing nutritional support

C. Preventing skin and soft tissue breakdown

D. Promoting comfort and providing psychosocial support to the patient and family

87. A 30-year-old male is brought to the emergency department suffering from photophobia, blurred vision, and nuchal rigidity. During the evaluation, he suffers a tonic-clonic seizure. A computed tomography scan reveals a large arteriovenous (AV) malformation in the frontal region with subarachnoid hemorrhage. The patient undergoes embolization of the vessels connected to the AV malformation, resection of the malformation, and removal of a hematoma created by the hemorrhage. After surgery, the patient is taken to the intensive care unit, where he is alert, oriented, and extubated with no focal deficits. Postoperative care for this patient would include:

A. Hyperventilating the patient to reduce intracranial pressure

B. Increasing systolic blood pressure to between 150 and 160 mm Hg via dopamine administration to overcome vascular spasm

C. Elevating the head of the bed 15 to 30 degrees, maintaining the neck in straight alignment, and keeping systolic blood pressure between 90 and 100 mm Hg via nitroprusside administration

D. Administering mannitol and furosemide to reduce circulating blood volume

88. A 52-year-old male admitted to the intensive care unit with a tentative diagnosis of diabetes insipidus is scheduled for a water deprivation test. Which nursing intervention is a priority during this test?

A. Providing adequate I.V. support to maintain a urine output of more than 20 ml/hour

B. Encouraging oral fluid intake only and maintaining accurate intake and output records

C. Providing emotional support and closely monitoring for signs and symptoms of intravascular collapse

D. Closely monitoring for signs and symptoms of fluid volume overload

Questions 89 and 90 refer to the following information:
A 66-year-old male patient is admitted to the intensive care unit with acute arterial occlusion of the right popliteal artery documented by arterial Doppler ultrasonography. He is in intense pain while the nurse prepares him for emergency angiography.

89. The nurse would expect to encounter which findings when assessing the patient's pulses in the right leg?
  A. Absent femoral, popliteal, anterior tibial, and pedal pulses
  B. Palpable femoral pulse and absent popliteal, anterior tibial, and pedal pulses
  C. Palpable femoral, popliteal, and posterior tibial pulses and absent pedal pulse
  D. Palpable femoral, popliteal, and pedal pulses and absent posterior tibial pulse

90. The patient has a large thrombus in the popliteal artery and receives an intra-arterial infusion of urokinase. Which medication would be administered concomitantly with urokinase?
  A. I.V. heparin
  B. Subcutaneous heparin
  C. Dipyridamole
  D. Warfarin sodium

91. The left ventricle of a patient with hypertrophic cardiomyopathy typically is:
  A. Uniformly enlarged and distended
  B. Stiff and noncompliant
  C. Abnormally shaped, with a disproportionately hypertrophied ventricular septum
  D. Rigid, with thin walls and a low ejection fraction

92. Which diagnostic procedure is used to identify an abdominal aortic aneurysm?
  A. Computed tomography scan of the chest
  B. Cardiac catheterization
  C. Abdominal ultrasonography
  D. Echocardiography

Questions 93 and 94 refer to the following information:
An 80-kg male patient with adult respiratory distress syndrome is mechanically ventilated at the following ventilator settings: FIO_2, 1.00; assist-control ventilation, 10 breaths/minute; tidal volume, 800 ml; and positive end-expiratory pressure (PEEP), 5 cm H_2O. The patient received a sedative and a neuromuscular blocker. His peak inspiratory pressure is 35 cm H_2O, and arterial blood gas readings are as follows: $PaCO_2$, 48 mm Hg; PaO_2, 55 mm Hg; and pH, 7.36.

93. The nurse would take which action next?
  A. Increase tidal volume to 1,100 ml
  B. Increase PEEP to 7.5 cm H_2O
  C. Monitor the patient's acid-base balance
  D. Administer a diuretic

94. The patient is started on broad-spectrum antibiotics, and his ventilator settings are changed to: FIO_2, 1.00; positive end-expiratory pressure (PEEP), 10 cm H_2O; tidal volume, 700 ml; and assist-control mode, 10 breaths/minute. The following arterial blood gas readings are obtained 30 minutes later: pH, 7.34; $PaCO_2$, 43 mm Hg; PaO_2, 110 mm Hg; and HCO_3^-, 24 mEq/liter. The nurse would anticipate which additional change in the ventilator settings?
  A. Decrease in FIO_2
  B. Decrease in tidal volume
  C. Decrease in respiratory rate
  D. Decrease in PEEP

95. The critical care nurse would obtain which laboratory test results to monitor the effects of heparin therapy?
  A. Partial thromboplastin time and prothrombin time
  B. Partial thromboplastin time and platelet count
  C. Prothrombin time and platelet count
  D. Fibrinogen and platelet counts

96. Which nursing intervention is appropriate for a patient with a Minnesota tube?
A. Inflate the esophageal balloon to 20 to 40 mm Hg and release it periodically to prevent necrosis
B. Inflate the gastric balloon to 20 to 40 mm Hg and apply traction
C. Deflate the esophageal balloon after decompressing the gastric balloon to evaluate the status of bleeding varices
D. Inflate the gastric balloon with 100 cc of air and frequently check for high pressures in the balloon

97. Which finding indicates that warfarin sodium therapy is effective?
A. Prothrombin time between 16 and 22 seconds
B. Partial thromboplastin time between 45 and 75 seconds
C. Fibrinogen count less than 50 mg/dl
D. Platelet count less than 100,000/mm^3

98. Succimer is a heavy-metal chelating agent used to treat:
A. Paint chip ingestion
B. Iron tablet overdose
C. Aspirin overdose
D. Excess ingestion of vitamin C

99. A 44-year-old male with a history of insulin-dependent diabetes mellitus is admitted to the intensive care unit. During the past 3 days, he has experienced rhinitis, productive cough, and low-grade fever. He now exhibits Kussmaul's respirations. Which statement about Kussmaul's respirations is true?
A. Kussmaul's respirations result from a central nervous system response to hyperglycemia
B. Kussmaul's respirations occur as a result of chemoreceptors detecting metabolic acidosis and triggering deep, rapid breathing as a compensatory mechanism
C. Kussmaul's respirations are a sign of respiratory acidosis
D. Kussmaul's respirations occur as a result of certain baroreceptors, which are located in the aortic arch, triggering the medulla to increase the rate and depth of breathing in response to hypovolemia

100. What is the most valuable nursing assessment tool in a patient with cardiac contusion?
A. Serum cardiac enzyme studies
B. Grade of anginal-type pain
C. Serial ECGs
D. Evaluation of tachycardic response

101. Cerebral perfusion pressure, a measure of blood flow to the brain, is defined as the pressure at which brain cells are perfused and must be at least 50 mm Hg. Cerebral perfusion pressure can be increased by:
A. Increased mean arterial pressure (MAP) or decreased intracranial pressure (ICP)
B. Decreased MAP or increased ICP
C. Increased MAP and increased ICP
D. Decreased MAP and decreased ICP

Questions 102 and 103 refer to the following information:
A 75-year-old male patient with chronic obstructive pulmonary disease and a history of atrial fibrillation is brought to the emergency department with right-sided weakness and expressive dysphasia. His pupils are equal and reactive to light.

102. This situation indicates a probable embolus in the:
A. Left frontal lobe
B. Right frontal lobe
C. Left temporal lobe
D. Right parietal lobe

103. To reduce the risk of future emboli, the patient might receive:
A. Digoxin to control atrial fibrillation
B. Sequential compression devices for the lower legs
C. Low-dose heparin in the hospital and oral warfarin sodium after discharge
D. Dextran to reduce platelet cohesiveness

104. The nurse is caring for a recently admitted trauma patient who has developed adult respiratory distress syndrome. The patient's arterial blood gas levels are as follows: $PaCO_2$, 35 mm Hg; PaO_2, 73 mm Hg; and pH, 7.37. The nurse maintains normal body temperature in this patient because hypothermia has what effect on the oxyhemoglobin dissociation curve?
A. Shift to the left, with red blood cells releasing oxygen
B. Shift to the right, with red blood cells releasing oxygen
C. Shift to the left, with red blood cells retaining oxygen
D. Shift to the right, with red blood cells retaining oxygen

105. A 34-year-old patient who underwent a liver transplant 12 hours ago is most likely to receive:
A. Continuous platelet transfusion
B. Continuous insulin infusion
C. Continuous furosemide infusion
D. Continuous or intermittent antiemetic therapy

106. A 36-year-old female patient arrives in the emergency department with tachypnea and dyspnea. The woman's companion relates the client's history of asthma and reports that she does not have any allergies. The patient's status continues to deteriorate. To treat this woman, the nurse would expect to administer which of the following medications?
A. Inhaled beta$_2$-agonist
B. I.V. corticosteroid
C. Subcutaneous epinephrine
D. I.V. aminophylline

107. The most important reason for monitoring the blood pressure of a patient suffering an acute exacerbation of asthma is to evaluate the:
A. Hemodynamic effects of hyperinflation
B. Cardiovascular effects of dehydration
C. Hypertensive effects of aminophylline
D. Hypertensive effects of diuretics

108. The fluid status of a patient with congestive heart failure is best monitored by inserting which of the following?
A. Indwelling urinary (Foley) catheter
B. Radial arterial I.V. line
C. Pulmonary artery catheter
D. Intra-aortic balloon pump

109. When asystole is suspected, the nurse should:
A. Administer lidocaine and defibrillate the patient
B. Obtain a 12-lead ECG
C. Begin an isoproterenol I.V. infusion
D. Checking the results of two ECG leads to confirm asystole

110. Negative inspiratory force evaluates:
A. How deep a breath a patient can take
B. How effectively a patient can move a volume of air sufficient to maintain adequate ventilation
C. Negative pressure within the airways
D. Negative pressure within the trachea

111. The nurse caring for a patient in acute respiratory failure plans to obtain an arterial blood gas sample when the oxygen saturation, as measured by pulse oximetry, drops to 90%. This oxygen saturation level correlates with a PaO_2 of approximately:
A. 90 mm Hg
B. 80 mm Hg
C. 70 mm Hg
D. 60 mm Hg

112. A 37-year-old male trauma patient with a flail chest is receiving morphine for severe pain. He has the following arterial blood gas readings: pH, 7.28; $PaCO_2$, 65 mm Hg; PaO_2, 58 mm Hg; and HCO_3^-, 20 mEq/liter. After notifying the physician, the nurse would:
A. Obtain a chest X-ray film
B. Intubate and ventilate the patient
C. Discontinue the morphine
D. Continue to monitor the patient

113. A 39-year-old patient with a resolving hemothorax is scheduled for sclerotherapy. The nurse who assists during this procedure must turn the patient frequently to:
A. Facilitate emptying of the cavity after sclerosis is completed
B. Enhance absorption of the sclerosing agent
C. Enhance distribution of medication across the pleura
D. Ensure that the procedure is minimally painful for the patient

114. Which position best promotes oxygenation in a patient with pneumonia of the left lung?
A. Left lateral decubitus position
B. Right lateral decubitus position
C. Prone position
D. Supine position

115. Which assessment findings would most likely be heard over an area of pulmonary consolidation?
A. Wheezes and decreased fremitus
B. Bronchial breath sounds and egophony
C. Crackles and absent breath sounds
D. Rhonchi and friction rub

116. When caring for a patient in prerenal failure, the nurse would do all of the following *except*:
A. Administer fluid replacements to restore body fluid balance
B. Administer dobutamine
C. Administer diuretics
D. Administer low-dosage dopamine

117. A patient with esophagitis is admitted with upper GI bleeding and hypotension. A total of 10 units of blood are administered over a 6-hour period. Later the patient is hemodynamically stable (blood pressure, 126/80 mm Hg; hematocrit, 32%) but is still losing about 150 ml of blood per shift. The physician orders the administration of various blood products. Which would the nurse give first?
A. Platelets
B. Fresh frozen plasma
C. Packed red blood cells
D. Cryoprecipitate

118. Patients receiving immunosuppressant therapy should be taught about all of the following points *except:*
A. The need to monitor weight because weight loss is common in patients taking immunosuppressants
B. The need to immediately report fever, commonly the only sign of infection, to the physician
C. The need for follow-up visits to monitor the degree of immunosuppression
D. The fact that inflammatory and immune responses are reduced by immunosuppressant therapy

119. The Rule of Nines can be used to determine fluid resuscitation requirements in a patient with a burn injury. This method commonly is used because:
A. It is quick and convenient, dividing the body into nine sections
B. It is accurate in both children and adults
C. It uses the palm of the hand, which represents 15% of the total body surface area
D. It allows for age- and gender-related differences in body size

120. The nurse checks on a 45-year-old female patient with insulin-dependent diabetes mellitus and finds her lying on the bed, pale, obtunded, and diaphoretic. Her heart rate is 136 beats/minute. What action should the nurse take first?
A. Administer a rapid I.V. bolus of 0.9% sodium chloride solution
B. Administer an I.V. bolus of insulin
C. Administer an I.V. bolus of 50% dextrose solution
D. Administer an I.V. bolus of mannitol

121. The nurse cannot rely on the central venous pressure reading to guide fluid replacement in a patient in hypovolemic shock when the patient has:
A. Chronic renal failure
B. Hypovolemia secondary to third-space fluid shifts
C. Pulmonary disease
D. Head trauma

122. The nurse would initiate progressive activity in a patient with cardiac contusion:
A. As soon as associated injuries allow
B. When ECG changes stabilize
C. As soon as possible to prevent deconditioning
D. When the patient expresses interest in increasing activity

123. A female is admitted to the hospital with a fever of 102° F (38.8° C) of unknown origin. Her white blood cell count is elevated, yet all X-ray films and cultures are negative. The patient has been on the medical-surgical unit for 4 days. An emergency computed tomography scan of the brain shows a parameningeal abscess. If the abscess irritates the meninges, what symptoms are likely to occur?
A. Decreased level of consciousness
B. Respiratory acidosis and hypotension
C. Status epilepticus and photophobia
D. Nuchal rigidity, headache, and irritability

124. A 34-year-old male patient diagnosed with acquired immunodeficiency syndrome 2 years ago has been taking zidovudine. He is admitted to the intensive care unit after experiencing a tonic-clonic seizure that lasted 1 minute. He is confused, lethargic, and weak on the right side. A computed tomography scan shows multiple abscess lesions in both hemispheres and a large lesion in the left frontal lobe that is causing increased intracranial pressure. What treatment would this patient receive?
A. Antibiotics for the opportunistic infection
B. Diuretics to reduce the swelling
C. Craniotomy to drain the large lesion and to obtain a culture of the infected area
D. Supportive care for a terminal illness

125. A 53-year-old male hemodialysis patient with a history of chronic obstructive pulmonary disease (COPD), coronary artery disease, chronic renal failure, and diabetes mellitus has an exacerbation of COPD and is admitted to the intensive care unit. On the patient's second day in the unit, hemodialysis is initiated. The patient experiences hypotension and chest pain after 1 hour on dialysis. His ECG shows ST-segment elevation in the inferior leads that resolves when the flow of the dialysis machine is slowed and 5% albumin is administered. What is the most likely explanation for the patient's symptoms?
A. Hypovolemia exacerbated by hemodialysis
B. Coronary artery disease exacerbated by blood volume loss
C. Pericarditis affecting cardiac output
D. Pulmonary embolus resulting from catheter insertion

Questions 126 and 127 refer to the following information:
A seemingly healthy 30-year-old male is admitted to the intensive care unit after fainting at work. A nasogastric tube, which is draining frank blood, was inserted in the emergency department. Endoscopic examination reveals multiple esophageal varices.

126. The most effective way to stop the bleeding in this patient is to:
A. Insert a quadruple-lumen Minnesota tube
B. Perform injection sclerotherapy
C. Administer I.V. vasopressin
D. Surgically decompress portal hypertension

127. After a few days, the patient is stable and transferred from the intensive care unit. When reviewing the transfer orders, the nurse would expect the physician to prescribe which of the following medications to lower portal pressure?
A. Vasopressin
B. Propranolol
C. Vitamin K
D. Furosemide

128. All of the following nursing interventions are appropriate for resolving high airway pressure during mechanical ventilation *except:*
A. Increasing pressure within the endotracheal cuff
B. Administering bronchodilator nebulizations
C. Suctioning the endotracheal tube
D. Humidifying the ventilator circuitry

129. All of the following are causes of open pneumothorax *except:*
A. Knife wound to the left upper thoracic cavity
B. Bullet wound to the right middle thoracic cavity
C. Fracture of the sternum and third to fifth ribs resulting from cardiopulmonary resuscitation
D. Entry-and-exit bullet wound in the right upper lobe of the lung

130. Successful chest tube therapy in a patient with a pneumothorax is evidenced by:
A. Chest tube drainage of less than 100 ml per shift
B. PaO_2 greater than 80 mm Hg on 35% oxygen delivered via face mask
C. Equal chest expansion
D. Bubbling in the water-seal chamber

131. The nurse is caring for a patient with severe chronic obstructive pulmonary disease. A normal finding on this patient's ECG would be:
A. Large amplitude in all leads with right-axis deviation
B. Small amplitude in all leads with right-axis deviation
C. Large amplitude in all leads with left-axis deviation
D. Small amplitude in all leads with left-axis deviation

132. When assessing a 62-year-old male patient admitted with a diagnosis of acute myocardial infarction, the nurse auscultates an S_4 gallop. Which statement about an S_4 gallop is false?
A. It is common in persons with healthy hearts
B. It usually is related to a pathologic process
C. It cannot be detected in patients with atrial fibrillation
D. It commonly is referred to as an atrial gallop

133. Thrombolytic therapy is most successful when administered:
A. Up to 6 hours after the initial insult
B. 6 to 12 hours after the initial insult
C. 12 to 18 hours after the initial insult
D. Up to 24 hours after the initial insult

134. A patient who suffered complete heart block after an anterior wall infarction receives a temporary pacemaker. The following rhythm develops:

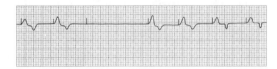

The nurse would respond by initiating which pacemaker action?
A. Changing the pacing mode from paced to fixed (asynchronous)
B. Increasing the output
C. Decreasing the output
D. Increasing the paced rate

135. Clinical signs and symptoms of cardiogenic shock include:
A. Normal urine output, tachycardia, and systolic blood pressure 90 mm Hg or lower
B. Urine output of less than 30 ml/hour
C. Tachypnea, tachycardia, and cardiac output of 5 to 8 liters/minute
D. Tachypnea, tachycardia, and cardiac index of 3.5 to 5 liters/minute/m^2

136. Signs of a basilar skull fracture include all of the following *except:*
A. Raccoon eyes
B. Otorrhea
C. Unequal pupils
D. Rhinorrhea

137. All of the following nursing diagnoses are appropriate for a patient with encephalitis *except:*
A. Risk of injury related to increased intracranial pressure
B. Ineffective airway clearance related to increased accumulation of secretions or decreased level of consciousness
C. Pain related to meningeal irritation
D. Hypothermia related to decreased body metabolism

138. A vision-impaired female accidentally ingests a large dose of salicylates and is brought to the medical intensive care unit after being intubated for marked respiratory alkalosis. In addition to changes in level of consciousness, which finding would indicate that the patient is suffering from complications of salicylate toxicity?
A. Constipation
B. Bleeding
C. Hyperglycemia
D. Infection

139. Clotting is triggered by all of the following factors *except:*
A. Vessel injury
B. Tissue injury
C. Vasodilation
D. Foreign body in the bloodstream

140. A 33-year-old female patient is admitted to the hospital by her general practitioner after complaining of headache, blurred vision, anxiety, and abdominal pain occurring with exercise and with heavy lifting; her blood pressure also is markedly elevated. Upon admission to the hospital, the patient's blood pressure is 170/110 mm Hg. The physician orders a 24-hour urine collection for total free catecholamines and vanillylmandelic acid as well as a computed tomography scan of the abdomen. Based on the assessment findings and the tests ordered, the nurse realizes that the patient is being evaluated for which condition?
A. Appendicitis
B. Pancreatitis
C. Pheochromocytoma
D. Crohn's disease

141. A patient is at increased risk for complete heart block and requires temporary pacemaker back-up if which of the following rhythms occurs?
A. First-degree heart block
B. Second-degree atrioventricular block, Mobitz type I
C. Second-degree atrioventricular block, Mobitz type II
D. Sinus bradycardia

142. A 28-year-old patient suffers an epidural hematoma after falling off a fence. As soon as the diagnosis is made, the nurse would prepare for:
A. Emergency surgery
B. Surgery in the morning, with intracranial pressure monitoring overnight
C. Lumbar puncture to detect an associated subarachnoid hemorrhage
D. Careful monitoring of intracranial pressure and neurologic assessments, with surgery being unlikely

143. Ranitidine can affect anticonvulsants by:
A. Increasing metabolism of the anticonvulsant
B. Decreasing metabolism of the anticonvulsant
C. Decreasing the potassium level, thus lowering the seizure threshold
D. Increasing the potassium level, thus raising the seizure threshold

144. To prevent injury during a seizure, the nurse must remember to:
- A. Restrain the patient
- B. Insert an oral airway
- C. Protect the patient's head
- D. Intubate the patient

145. A patient with second- and third-degree burns over 25% of his body is admitted to the intensive care unit. The nurse expects that this patient will have:
- A. Major burns in which the skin blisters and is black and leathery
- B. Burns in which the skin is deeply charred and damage extends through the subcutaneous tissue to the muscle and bone
- C. Burns damaging the epidermis, causing erythema and pain
- D. Burns that cause only minimal pain because nerve endings have been damaged

146. All of the following statements about hypokalemia are true *except*:
- A. Hypokalemia predisposes a patient to digitalis toxicity despite normal digoxin level
- B. Loop diuretics can cause profound electrolyte disturbances, including hypokalemia
- C. Hypokalemia can be reversed by correcting alkalosis
- D. Hypokalemia depresses myocardial function

147. To evaluate the pulmonary and cardiac structures of a patient with thoracic trauma, the nurse would obtain which chest X-ray film view?
- A. Supine anteroposterior
- B. Left lateral
- C. Upright
- D. Right lateral

Questions 148 to 150 refer to the following information:

A 32-year-old male patient with acute respiratory distress syndrome is on mechanical ventilation and has been in the intensive care unit for 3 days. Repeated attempts to decrease his FIO_2 to .50 or less have failed. The physician orders a positive end-expiratory pressure (PEEP) of 10 cm H_2O.

148. Lowering the patient's FIO_2 to .50 or less will:
- A. Decrease barotrauma
- B. Facilitate mechanical ventilation
- C. Decrease oxygen toxicity
- D. Increase PaO_2

149. What is the primary hemodynamic effect of this level of PEEP?
- A. Increased cardiac output
- B. Increased heart rate
- C. Increased pulmonary circulation
- D. Decreased pulmonary circulation

150. Fifteen minutes after PEEP has been set at 10 cm H_2O, the nurse notes that the patient has an increased heart rate, decreased blood pressure, and distant right-sided breath sounds. The ventilator high-pressure alarm sounds with each ventilator cycle. The nurse suspects that the patient has:
- A. Tension pneumothorax
- B. Ruptured pulmonary artery
- C. Cardiac tamponade
- D. Esophageal tear

151. Which of the following are signs and symptoms of the late stage of septic shock?
- A. Warm skin, decreased level of consciousness, and tachycardia
- B. Cold and clammy skin, decreased cardiac output, decreased urine output, and tachycardia
- C. Chills, metabolic acidosis, and normal urine output
- D. Decreased central venous pressure, anxiety, and normal urine output

152. The nurse would expect to administer which of the following during the initial stage of septic shock?
  A. Oxygen and nitroprusside
  B. Norepinephrine and dobutamine
  C. Oxygen and dopamine
  D. Oxygen and procainamide

153. Positive Kernig's and Brudzinski's signs often are seen in patients with:
  A. Meningeal irritation resulting from subarachnoid hemorrhage or meningitis
  B. Cerebral thrombosis
  C. Viral encephalitis
  D. Status epilepticus

154. A 67-year-old patient is admitted to the surgical intensive care unit after aneurysm repair. During surgery, the patient received multiple blood transfusions, including fresh frozen plasma and platelets. Which complication might result from the multiple blood products administered in the operating room?
  A. Transfusion reaction
  B. Hepatitis
  C. Hypervolemia
  D. Adult respiratory distress syndrome

155. A dopamine I.V. infusion at a rate of 11 mcg/kg/minute will:
  A. Increase renal blood flow
  B. Decrease renal blood flow
  C. Cause mild tachycardia
  D. Increase pulmonary capillary wedge pressure

156. The nurse's first priority when treating a patient in cardiogenic shock is to:
  A. Administer I.V. fluids and vasoactive drugs
  B. Assess level of consciousness
  C. Insert an intra-aortic balloon pump
  D. Insert a transvenous pacing wire

157. The nurse caring for a patient with heart disease should:
  A. Restrict all visitors
  B. Allow unlimited visitation
  C. Assess the patient before all visits
  D. Establish individual visiting guidelines

158. A 29-year-old female is admitted to the intensive care unit with progressive hypoxia of unknown origin. Her medical history includes a recent upper respiratory tract infection treated with antibiotics. Her pulmonary status has deteriorated to the point at which she requires full mechanical ventilation and paralysis to maximally lower oxygen demands. Despite aggressive efforts, extracorporeal membrane oxygenation (ECMO) is needed to treat her severe hypoxia. Which independent nursing intervention is necessary with this treatment?
  A. Adjusting the flow of ECMO based on the patient's condition
  B. Adjusting the rate of ECMO based on the patient's condition
  C. Monitoring the patient's condition through daily chest X-ray films
  D. Monitoring for bleeding, infection, and complications related to immobility

159. Which antidote would be administered to a person suffering from carbon monoxide poisoning?
  A. Calcium
  B. Sodium bicarbonate
  C. Oxygen
  D. Naloxone

160. An 82-year-old male with pneumococcal pneumonia is admitted to the intensive care unit. What atypical signs and symptoms of infection are common in elderly patients?
  A. Mental status changes and normal temperature
  B. Increased respiratory rate and low sodium level
  C. Normal white blood cell count and tachycardia
  D. Normal chest X-ray film and low albumin level

161. A 74-year-old male patient is being fed via continuous tube feedings when the nurse notes a change in his tracheal secretions from clear to creamy tan in color. The nurse aggressively suctions the tracheostomy tube to clear secretions and notifies the physician of the possibility of aspiration. Because the patient was not in respiratory distress, the nurse and physician decide to monitor this patient's respiratory status closely every 15 minutes for how many hours?
A. 2 to 4 hours after aspiration
B. 4 to 8 hours after aspiration
C. 10 to 12 hours after aspiration
D. 12 to 24 hours after aspiration

162. An intoxicated patient has aspirated small food particles. One sign of aspiration is:
A. Decreased $PaCO_2$
B. Increased compliance
C. Bloody suction material within 6 hours after aspiration
D. Decreased intrapulmonary shunting

163. A Denver shunt is used to treat:
A. Esophageal varices
B. Ascites
C. Hepatic encephalopathy
D. Hepatorenal syndrome

164. In the early stage of septic shock, a patient typically has:
A. High systemic vascular resistance and high cardiac output
B. Low systemic vascular resistance and high cardiac output
C. Low systemic vascular resistance and low cardiac output
D. High systemic vascular resistance and low cardiac output

165. The nurse auscultates a new, high-pitched decrescendo diastolic murmur over the second right intercostal space in a patient with blunt chest trauma. What does this murmur indicate?
A. Aortic valve regurgitation
B. Mitral valve regurgitation
C. Ventricular septal defect
D. Aortic dissection

166. The critical care nurse is aware that atherosclerotic changes usually originate:
A. At arterial bifurcations because laminar flow becomes turbulent at points of arterial branching
B. In the media of the artery because smooth-muscle cells are necessary for lipid changes
C. Along the uncurved portions of the artery because atherosclerotic plaques cannot proliferate when surrounded by turbulent flow
D. Independent of the anatomic site of the artery

167. The most useful, noninvasive diagnostic tool for assessing valvular disease is:
A. Cardiac catheterization
B. ECG
C. Echocardiography
D. Chest X-ray film

168. In a patient with acute left-sided heart failure and severe hemodynamic compromise, which of the following would best assist the failing left ventricle?
A. Diuretic therapy
B. Semi-Fowler's position
C. Intra-aortic balloon pump therapy
D. Extracorporeal membrane oxygenation

169. When reviewing cardiac enzyme results to rule out myocardial infarction, the nurse knows that which laboratory value would be most helpful?
A. Total creatine kinase (CK)
B. Aspartate aminotransferase (AST)
C. Total lactate dehydrogenase (LD)
D. Creatine kinase-MB (CK-MB)

170. A 73-year-old female patient is admitted to the hospital with exertional dyspnea, weight loss, and palpitations. Her history reveals a severe lack of medical care and medical knowledge, but she does report having rheumatic fever as a child. The nurse auscultates a grade 3/6 holosystolic murmur at the apex of the patient's heart. Based on the history and the assessment, the nurse would suspect that the patient has which valvular disorder?
A. Mitral regurgitation
B. Mitral stenosis
C. Tricuspid regurgitation
D. Aortic stenosis

171. Recognizing and treating early septic shock is critical to patient survival. The nurse should be prepared to assist by:
A. Administering antibiotics, monitoring fluid restrictions, and treating related complications, such as acidosis, respiratory failure, and cardiac failure
B. Administering antibiotics, initiating fluid resuscitation, and maintaining respiratory and cardiac function
C. Administering afterload reduction agents, initiating fluid resuscitation, and treating related complications, such as acidosis, respiratory failure, and cardiac failure
D. Administering broad-spectrum antibiotics and blood products and using a hyperthermia unit to maintain temperature

172. Which rationale best explains why broad-spectrum antibiotics are used for a patient with major renal trauma?
A. Uremia decreases the effectiveness of white blood cells to fight infection
B. The operative site predisposes the patient to pulmonary infection
C. Renal parenchyma are susceptible to infection
D. The extent of the injury predisposes the patient to septicemia

173. Which findings are likely in a patient who has been successfully treated for renal trauma?
A. Creatinine and blood urea nitrogen levels within normal limits
B. Afebrile status and normal white blood cell count
C. Clean, dry, intact wound
D. All of the above

174. During an exacerbation of asthma, a patient experiences hyperventilation, diaphoresis, and exhaustion. Which nursing intervention is most appropriate for treating these symptoms?
A. Promoting comfort
B. Relieving pain
C. Ensuring adequate hydration
D. Administering oxygen

175. The critical care nurse would tell a patient with non-Q wave myocardial infarction (MI) that:
A. Patients with non-Q wave MI have higher hospital mortality but lower mortality at 1 year than patients with Q-wave MI
B. Patients with non-Q wave MI have lower hospital mortality but the same mortality at 1 year as patients with Q-wave MI
C. Patients with non-Q wave MI have equal mortality in the hospital and at 1 year as patients with Q-wave MI
D. It is inappropriate for the nurse to discuss mortality outcomes with the patient

176. Specific nursing interventions for a patient with infectious endocarditis may include:
A. Obtaining blood cultures, assessing for positive Homan's sign, and monitoring cardiac output and cardiac index
B. Obtaining blood cultures, limiting visiting hours to provide rest periods, and monitoring blood pressure
C. Monitoring systemic vascular resistance and checking oxygen saturation via pulse oximetry
D. Providing small but frequent meals, limiting visiting hours, and restricting the patient to bed rest

177. The nurse is caring for a patient recently diagnosed with adult respiratory distress syndrome. The patient is being mechanically ventilated at the following settings: assist-control mode, 11 breaths/minute; tidal volume, 900 ml; positive end-expiratory pressure, 5 cm H_2O; and FIO_2, 80%. During the assessment, the nurse notes that the patient's respiratory rate is 42 breaths/minute and the ventilator alarm registers with each breath. The patient is otherwise hemodynamically stable, and his pulmonary catheter pressure readings are within normal limits. Which intervention is most appropriate?
A. Increasing the respiratory rate on the ventilator
B. Decreasing the respiratory rate on the ventilator
C. Sedating and pharmacologically paralyzing the patient
D. Infusing dopamine and nitroprusside to reduce preload and afterload

178. A 25-year-old female is brought to the emergency department after being stabbed in the mid-chest region. Chest expansion is equal bilaterally, with the chest X-ray film showing pneumomediastinum, subcutaneous air, and possible pleural effusion. The patient complains of substernal chest pain. Vital signs are blood pressure, 100/50 mm Hg; heart rate, 160 beats/minute; respirations, 35 breaths/minute; and temperature, 100.4° F (38° C). Oxygen saturation is 94% on 35% oxygen via face mask. This patient is exhibiting signs and symptoms of:
A. Tracheobronchial injury
B. Bronchial injury
C. Esophageal injury
D. Tracheal injury

179. Which combination of drugs usually is prescribed for a patient with angina?
A. Captopril (Capoten) and nitroglycerin patches
B. Procainamide (Procan SR) and ranitidine (Zantac)
C. Diltiazem (Cardizem) and isosorbide dinitrate (Isordil)
D. Captopril (Capoten) and propranolol (Inderal)

180. A 56-year-old female with unstable angina is admitted to the cardiac care unit. She has a 2-year history of angina and frequently uses Mylanta at home for heartburn but with no relief. As part of the cardiovascular admission assessment, the nurse should obtain the following information from the patient:
A. Description of epigastric pain
B. Description of any discomfort
C. Description of chest pain
D. Educational level

181. A patient is admitted to the hospital to rule out myocardial infarction. Assessment of the admitting 12-lead ECG reveals significant Q waves in leads V_1 and V_2. The nurse suspects:
A. Acute inferior wall myocardial infarction
B. Prinzmetal's angina
C. Noncardiac pathology
D. Lateral wall necrosis

182. In a patient with a dissecting aortic aneurysm who experiences a hypertensive crisis, blood pressure should be lowered to:
A. Half the systolic value
B. Half the diastolic value
C. 160 to 180 mm Hg systolic
D. Normal level

183. A patient in cardiogenic shock would have all of the following signs and symptoms *except:*
A. Hypocalcemia
B. Hyperglycemia
C. Increased blood urea nitrogen level
D. Normal serum creatinine level

184. The effects of hypertension on the kidneys can be assessed by monitoring:
A. Blood urea nitrogen and creatinine levels
B. Serum catecholamine level
C. Renal compensation via serial arterial blood gas analyses
D. Serum drug levels

185. The following arrhythmia is representative of:

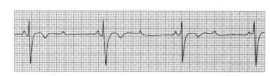

    A. Second-degree atrioventricular (AV) block, Mobitz type I
    B. Second-degree AV block, Mobitz type II
    C. Third-degree AV block
    D. AV dissociation

186. A patient has aspiration pneumonia in the middle and lower lobes of the right lung. To ensure the best ventilation-perfusion ratio, the nurse would position the patient:
    A. Right-side down
    B. Left-side down
    C. Supine
    D. Prone

187. Which of the following is a complication associated with infectious endocarditis?
    A. Systemic embolization
    B. Fever
    C. Decreased cardiac output
    D. All of the above

188. A patient with ventricular tachycardia receives an I.V. bolus of bretylium followed by a bretylium I.V. infusion. What are the most common adverse effects of bretylium therapy?
    A. Hypotension, nausea, and vomiting
    B. Prolonged QT interval, nausea, and vomiting
    C. Hypotension and prolonged QT interval
    D. Heart block, nausea, and vomiting

189. Before and during the I.V. administration of a potent vasodilator, such as nitroprusside, the nurse would check for:
    A. Correlation of cuff and arterial line blood pressures
    B. Adequate central venous or right atrial pressure
    C. Orthostatic hypotension
    D. Peripheral edema

190. A 75-year-old male patient with asthma is given I.V. aminophylline. The patient subsequently complains of nausea, tremors, and heart palpitations. Which aminophylline serum level would most likely correlate with aminophylline toxicity?
    A. 2 µg/ml
    B. 8 µg/ml
    C. 15 µg/ml
    D. 22 µg/ml

191. The nurse is planning to teach an asthmatic patient about the importance of using a spacing device. What is the primary reason that a spacing device is used with an inhaler?
    A. It increases deposition of medication in the lungs
    B. It facilitates the use of an inhaler
    C. It ensures better compliance
    D. It is more portable than an inhaler

192. Nursing care differs for patients with aortic regurgitation and those with aortic stenosis based on which of the following statements?
    A. Aortic regurgitation is a pressure overload problem
    B. Aortic regurgitation is a fluid volume overload problem
    C. Aortic regurgitation is treated with nitrate therapy only
    D. Aortic regurgitation is treated with calcium channel blockers

193. The nurse evaluates the neurologic status of a choking victim after resuscitation is performed. Because the choking incident was not witnessed, the nurse is concerned about anoxic injury. Within how many minutes after choking can anoxic injury result in death?
    A. 3 to 5 minutes
    B. 4 to 6 minutes
    C. 5 to 8 minutes
    D. 6 to 8 minutes

194. Which intervention is the first priority for a nurse who suspects that a ventilated patient has aspirated a tube feeding?
A. Notifying the physician
B. Increasing the oxygen concentration on the ventilator
C. Hyperoxygenating and suctioning the patient
D. Drawing a sample for arterial blood gas analysis

195. Complications of using an oropharyngeal airway include:
A. Increased coughing ability
B. Increased oxygen requirements
C. Vomiting and aspiration
D. Carbon dioxide retention

196. Which of the following vasopressor agents is most appropriate for a patient in cardiogenic shock?
A. Dopamine
B. Norepinephrine
C. Isoproterenol
D. Phenylephrine

197. Which finding associated with endotracheal tube suctioning is conclusive for acute gastric acid aspiration?
A. Heme-positive secretions
B. Heme-negative secretions
C. Basic pH
D. Acidic pH

198. A 25-year-old male is brought to the emergency department after a motor vehicle accident. During the assessment, the nurse notes that the patient's right chest falls on inspiration and rises on expiration. This finding is a sign of:
A. Tension pneumothorax
B. Hemothorax
C. Flail chest
D. Hemopneumothorax

199. The nurse would expect all of the following symptoms in a patient with tracheobronchial injury *except:*
A. Severe dyspnea
B. Hypotension
C. Negative Hamman's sign
D. Subcutaneous crepitation

200. A patient with multiple rib fractures and diminished expansion on the left side may benefit from all of the following ventilator settings *except:*
A. Pressure support with synchronized intermittent mandatory ventilation (SIMV)
B. SIMV and positive end-expiratory pressure
C. SIMV and sighs
D. Pressure support and sighs

Answer Sheet

	A B C D		A B C D		A B C D		A B C D
1.	○ ○ ○ ○	26.	○ ○ ○ ○	51.	○ ○ ○ ○	76.	○ ○ ○ ○
2.	○ ○ ○ ○	27.	○ ○ ○ ○	52.	○ ○ ○ ○	77.	○ ○ ○ ○
3.	○ ○ ○ ○	28.	○ ○ ○ ○	53.	○ ○ ○ ○	78.	○ ○ ○ ○
4.	○ ○ ○ ○	29.	○ ○ ○ ○	54.	○ ○ ○ ○	79.	○ ○ ○ ○
5.	○ ○ ○ ○	30.	○ ○ ○ ○	55.	○ ○ ○ ○	80.	○ ○ ○ ○
6.	○ ○ ○ ○	31.	○ ○ ○ ○	56.	○ ○ ○ ○	81.	○ ○ ○ ○
7.	○ ○ ○ ○	32.	○ ○ ○ ○	57.	○ ○ ○ ○	82.	○ ○ ○ ○
8.	○ ○ ○ ○	33.	○ ○ ○ ○	58.	○ ○ ○ ○	83.	○ ○ ○ ○
9.	○ ○ ○ ○	34.	○ ○ ○ ○	59.	○ ○ ○ ○	84.	○ ○ ○ ○
10.	○ ○ ○ ○	35.	○ ○ ○ ○	60.	○ ○ ○ ○	85.	○ ○ ○ ○
11.	○ ○ ○ ○	36.	○ ○ ○ ○	61.	○ ○ ○ ○	86.	○ ○ ○ ○
12.	○ ○ ○ ○	37.	○ ○ ○ ○	62.	○ ○ ○ ○	87.	○ ○ ○ ○
13.	○ ○ ○ ○	38.	○ ○ ○ ○	63.	○ ○ ○ ○	88.	○ ○ ○ ○
14.	○ ○ ○ ○	39.	○ ○ ○ ○	64.	○ ○ ○ ○	89.	○ ○ ○ ○
15.	○ ○ ○ ○	40.	○ ○ ○ ○	65.	○ ○ ○ ○	90.	○ ○ ○ ○
16.	○ ○ ○ ○	41.	○ ○ ○ ○	66.	○ ○ ○ ○	91.	○ ○ ○ ○
17.	○ ○ ○ ○	42.	○ ○ ○ ○	67.	○ ○ ○ ○	92.	○ ○ ○ ○
18.	○ ○ ○ ○	43.	○ ○ ○ ○	68.	○ ○ ○ ○	93.	○ ○ ○ ○
19.	○ ○ ○ ○	44.	○ ○ ○ ○	69.	○ ○ ○ ○	94.	○ ○ ○ ○
20.	○ ○ ○ ○	45.	○ ○ ○ ○	70.	○ ○ ○ ○	95.	○ ○ ○ ○
21.	○ ○ ○ ○	46.	○ ○ ○ ○	71.	○ ○ ○ ○	96.	○ ○ ○ ○
22.	○ ○ ○ ○	47.	○ ○ ○ ○	72.	○ ○ ○ ○	97.	○ ○ ○ ○
23.	○ ○ ○ ○	48.	○ ○ ○ ○	73.	○ ○ ○ ○	98.	○ ○ ○ ○
24.	○ ○ ○ ○	49.	○ ○ ○ ○	74.	○ ○ ○ ○	99.	○ ○ ○ ○
25.	○ ○ ○ ○	50.	○ ○ ○ ○	75.	○ ○ ○ ○	100.	○ ○ ○ ○

	A	B	C	D		A	B	C	D		A	B	C	D		A	B	C	D
101.	○	○	○	○	126.	○	○	○	○	151.	○	○	○	○	176.	○	○	○	○
102.	○	○	○	○	127.	○	○	○	○	152.	○	○	○	○	177.	○	○	○	○
103.	○	○	○	○	128.	○	○	○	○	153.	○	○	○	○	178.	○	○	○	○
104.	○	○	○	○	129.	○	○	○	○	154.	○	○	○	○	179.	○	○	○	○
105.	○	○	○	○	130.	○	○	○	○	155.	○	○	○	○	180.	○	○	○	○
106.	○	○	○	○	131.	○	○	○	○	156.	○	○	○	○	181.	○	○	○	○
107.	○	○	○	○	132.	○	○	○	○	157.	○	○	○	○	182.	○	○	○	○
108.	○	○	○	○	133.	○	○	○	○	158.	○	○	○	○	183.	○	○	○	○
109.	○	○	○	○	134.	○	○	○	○	159.	○	○	○	○	184.	○	○	○	○
110.	○	○	○	○	135.	○	○	○	○	160.	○	○	○	○	185.	○	○	○	○
111.	○	○	○	○	136.	○	○	○	○	161.	○	○	○	○	186.	○	○	○	○
112.	○	○	○	○	137.	○	○	○	○	162.	○	○	○	○	187.	○	○	○	○
113.	○	○	○	○	138.	○	○	○	○	163.	○	○	○	○	188.	○	○	○	○
114.	○	○	○	○	139.	○	○	○	○	164.	○	○	○	○	189.	○	○	○	○
115.	○	○	○	○	140.	○	○	○	○	165.	○	○	○	○	190.	○	○	○	○
116.	○	○	○	○	141.	○	○	○	○	166.	○	○	○	○	191.	○	○	○	○
117.	○	○	○	○	142.	○	○	○	○	167.	○	○	○	○	192.	○	○	○	○
118.	○	○	○	○	143.	○	○	○	○	168.	○	○	○	○	193.	○	○	○	○
119.	○	○	○	○	144.	○	○	○	○	169.	○	○	○	○	194.	○	○	○	○
120.	○	○	○	○	145.	○	○	○	○	170.	○	○	○	○	195.	○	○	○	○
121.	○	○	○	○	146.	○	○	○	○	171.	○	○	○	○	196.	○	○	○	○
122.	○	○	○	○	147.	○	○	○	○	172.	○	○	○	○	197.	○	○	○	○
123.	○	○	○	○	148.	○	○	○	○	173.	○	○	○	○	198.	○	○	○	○
124.	○	○	○	○	149.	○	○	○	○	174.	○	○	○	○	199.	○	○	○	○
125.	○	○	○	○	150.	○	○	○	○	175.	○	○	○	○	200.	○	○	○	○

Answers and Rationales

1. CORRECT ANSWER—**C.** The patient's blood pressure must be rapidly but safely lowered to avoid aneurysm rupture. Nitroprusside would be the most effective agent because of its instant onset of action. Methyldopa and enalapril have an onset of action of 20 to 30 minutes and 15 minutes, respectively. Hydralazine's onset occurs in 5 to 10 minutes when administered intravenously.
Nursing process step: Implementation
Cognitive level: Application

2. CORRECT ANSWER—**B.** The use of elastic bandages on dependent areas limits the amount of edema and bleeding and helps the graft to take. Maximum-absorption bandages should be avoided because these bulky dressings limit the patient's mobility. However, the nurse should use enough bandages to absorb any drainage while maintaining maximum mobility. Extremities generally are wrapped from the distal to proximal end, and strict sterile technique should be used throughout the dressing change.
Nursing process step: Implementation
Cognitive level: Comprehension

3. CORRECT ANSWER—**D.** Thrombocytosis, which is an increase in the number of platelets, occurs routinely after splenectomy. Splenectomy is not associated with an increased risk of thrombotic complications, and treatment is not required. Persistent leukocytosis after splenectomy is not a routine complication and may be a sign of intraperitoneal sepsis. Leukopenia may be caused by an adverse drug reaction, radiation poisoning, or other pathologic conditions affecting the white blood cells. Leukopenia is not a complication of splenectomy.
Nursing process step: Planning
Cognitive level: Evaluation

4. CORRECT ANSWER—**C.** The patient's signs and symptoms are indicative of superior mesenteric artery occlusion. The irregular pulse suggests possible atrial fibrillation, a known causative factor of potential mural emboli, which could result in superior mesenteric artery occlusion. Because of the patient's advanced age, the nurse would not suspect appendicitis or Crohn's disease, which are common in younger patients; these conditions also most commonly produce right lower quadrant pain. Bloody diarrhea usually is not associated with bowel obstruction, acute appendicitis, or Crohn's disease. Blood pressure decreases with bowel infarction, not bowel obstruction, because of fluid losses that occur secondary to large accumulations of fluid in the bowel lumen.
Nursing process step: Assessment
Cognitive level: Evaluation

5. CORRECT ANSWER—B. Because the patient's problem involves occlusion of the mesenteric artery, surgery is indicated. A laparotomy with embolectomy typically is performed to remove the clot and resect any nonviable ischemic bowel. A permanent ileostomy usually is not required, although a temporary ileostomy may be necessary, depending on the area and amount of ischemic bowel tissue removed. A Miller-Abbott tube is an intestinal decompression tube used in cases of bowel obstruction. The patient does not have appendicitis, so an appendectomy is unnecessary.
Nursing process step: Implementation
Cognitive level: Comprehension

6. CORRECT ANSWER—D. Bowel infarction results in intestinal ischemia and loss of fluid caused by intraluminal bowel fluid shifts (the bowel becomes edematous) and diarrhea. The ischemia also may cause necrosis and perforation with resultant peritonitis and sepsis. Initially, nursing care is aimed at restoring and maintaining homeostasis. Secondary nursing goals include relieving pain, ensuring adequate nutrition, and maintaining skin integrity.
Nursing process step: Planning
Cognitive level: Knowledge

7. CORRECT ANSWER—D. Hemodialysis is the most effective means of lowering the potassium level and also has the most lasting effect. Sodium polystyrene sulfonate (Kayexalate) can decrease the potassium level, but this treatment is fairly slow. Glucose and insulin, as well as sodium bicarbonate, are short-acting therapies that give Kayexalate time to work or the health care team time to initiate dialysis.
Nursing process step: Planning
Cognitive level: Comprehension

8. CORRECT ANSWER—A. Pneumococcal pneumonia is associated with the highest mortality rate in the elderly. *Streptococcus pneumoniae* often travels to the bloodstream and causes sepsis. The Pneumovax 23 vaccine can protect against pneumococcal pneumonia; elderly and chronically ill persons should be encouraged to receive the vaccine. *Staphylococcus aureus* and *Klebsiella* pneumonias are associated with alcoholism and chronic disease. *Legionella* pneumonia is associated with a low mortality rate in the elderly.
Nursing process step: Planning
Cognitive level: Knowledge

9. CORRECT ANSWER—C. Bubbling within the water-seal and suction-control chambers is expected as air is removed from the pleural space. These are the only areas within the chest tube drainage system in which bubbling should occur.
Nursing process step: Assessment
Cognitive level: Analysis

10. CORRECT ANSWER—D. Emergency abdominal surgery, especially when there is insufficient time for the stomach to empty after a meal, places the patient at risk for aspiration. Surgical anesthesia alone will depress the reflex response to aspiration. A cuffed endotracheal tube, which is used intraoperatively and postoperatively to ventilate the patient, can help prevent aspiration. Adenovirus pneumonia, a viral pneumonia with an insidious onset, commonly affects young adults. Fungal pneumonia is most common in immunocompromised patients. *Pseudomonas* pneumonia is more common among hospitalized patients who are immunocompromised and mechanically ventilated for prolonged periods.
Nursing process step: Planning
Cognitive level: Knowledge

11. CORRECT ANSWER—C. Because of the severe ischemia and lack of nutrients, the tissue immediately surrounding the center of the infarct is malfunctioning. During electrical systole, an abnormal electrical current called the *current of injury* flows from the healthy tissue to the injured tissue. This systolic current of injury elevates the ST segment. Injury is represented by ST-segment elevation in the leads in which the positive electrode reads across the injured or severely ischemic myocardium (leads I, III, and aV_F). ST-segment elevation is followed by T-wave inversion as the myocardial infarction evolves. Q waves are well developed after 48 hours with inferior wall infarctions and usually remain as a permanent addition to the ECG. Bradycardias, atrioventricular blocks, and intraventricular conduction disturbances, which are represented by a widened QRS complex, are common complications of inferior wall infarctions. ST-segment depression is a reciprocal change that occurs in leads I and aV_L during an acute myocardial infarction.
Nursing process step: Assessment
Cognitive level: Knowledge

12. CORRECT ANSWER—B. Many conditions predispose a patient to digoxin toxicity. These conditions include hypokalemia, hypomagnesemia, hypoxemia, active myocardial ischemia, and increased vagal tone. Depressed ST segments, hyporeflexia, and decreased peristalsis are associated with hypokalemia. Hyperkalemia, hypocalcemia, and hypermagnesemia do not predispose a patient to digoxin toxicity. Hyperkalemia is associated with skeletal muscle weakness, numbness and tingling, and abdominal cramps; hypocalcemia, with carpopedal spasm, perioral paresthesia, and muscle cramps; and hypermagnesemia, with bradycardia, diminished sensorium, and respiratory depression.
Nursing process step: Assessment
Cognitive level: Analysis

13. CORRECT ANSWER—D. The shortened PR interval evident in Wolff-Parkinson-White syndrome results from accelerated atrioventricular (AV) conduction across an accessory pathway, not involving the AV node or His-Purkinje system. The delta wave, which is an initial slurring of the QRS complex, causes the QRS complex to widen but usually not greater than 0.12 second. An inverted P wave results from retrograde conduction through the atria and is not characteristic of Wolff-Parkinson-White syndrome.
Nursing process step: Assessment
Cognitive level: Knowledge

14. CORRECT ANSWER—B. Bowel ischemia caused by decreased blood flow to the mesentery artery can lead to sepsis and death. Diarrhea in the early postoperative period is rare; in addition, the patient would be receiving I.V. fluids postoperatively, thereby preventing dehydration. Oral feedings are not an early postoperative priority. GI bleeding is identified by foul-smelling, tarry, or grossly bloody stools and does not commonly occur after abdominal aneurysm repair.
Nursing process step: Assessment
Cognitive level: Analysis

15. CORRECT ANSWER—C. This patient exhibits the classic signs of Dressler syndrome, a type of pericarditis that often follows myocardial infarction or cardiac surgery. A patient with pneumonia or influenza would have more pulmonary symptoms. Mediastinitis, as well as pneumonia and influenza, would cause a fluctuating fever and a shift-to-the-left reflected in the white blood cell differential. Wound drainage and sternal instability usually occur in mediastinitis.
Nursing process step: Assessment
Cognitive level: Evaluation

16. CORRECT ANSWER—**B.** Ibuprofen provides the anti-inflammatory action needed to treat the pericarditis and its associated pain and fever. Acetaminophen and propoxyphene hydrochloride would only treat the fever and pain; these drugs are less effective as anti-inflammatory agents. Antibiotics are not indicated for pericarditis because it is an inflammatory process, not an infection.
Nursing process step: Implementation
Cognitive level: Analysis

17. CORRECT ANSWER—**B.** Dressler syndrome, also called chronic pericarditis, is a self-limiting auto-immune response to myocardial necrosis (usually caused by myocardial infarction) or cardiac manipulation resulting from cardiac surgery; treatment is primarily symptomatic and aimed at reducing the inflammation. Positioning can help reduce the chest discomfort, but heat will have no effect; upper-extremity exercises are contraindicated for 6 to 8 weeks after sternotomy. Ibuprofen can cause stomach upset, renal dysfunction, and bleeding if used in excess. If the patient's pain does not resolve with ibuprofen, other anti-inflammatory agents, such as indomethacin or steroids, can be added.
Nursing process step: Implementation
Cognitive level: Application

18. CORRECT ANSWER—**B.** Diuretics would decrease the effects of the hypervolemic hemodilution. If the patient's blood pressure does not increase, dopamine may be ordered. The patient is unlikely to have photophobia so late after surgery, so darkening the room would not help. Urine output should increase as a result of increased cardiac output and circulating blood volume. Hemodilution decreases the hematocrit to less than 30%.
Nursing process step: Implementation
Cognitive level: Application

19. CORRECT ANSWER—**B.** Corticosteroid therapy has been shown to decrease the risk of fat emboli syndrome in susceptible patients. The benefits of steroid treatment include decreased cerebral edema, antiadhesive effect on platelets, and restoration of capillary permeability to normal level, thereby decreasing capillary leakage. The principal risk associated with steroid use is infection, which can lead to complications and possible death. Infection can be monitored by evaluating blood culture results. Corticosteroids would suppress any increase in the number of white blood cells. Monitoring the PaO_2 level would be helpful in evaluating the benefits, not the risks, associated with steroid treatment. Intracranial pressure monitoring is not considered a blood study.
Nursing process step: Evaluation
Cognitive level: Analysis

20. CORRECT ANSWER—**C.** In the immediate postoperative period, the functioning kidney produces osmotic diuresis because the normal kidney senses the osmolar load of blood urea nitrogen. This diuresis usually causes hypokalemia, hypocalcemia, and hypomagnesemia. If fluid administration is not maintained, hemoconcentration can occur and may produce hypernatremia. Hyperglycemia results from I.V. fluid administration, steroid therapy, and stress. Electrolyte values equilibrate as the kidney stabilizes; however, careful replacement therapy and constant monitoring for rejection, as evidenced by oliguria and hyperkalemia, are necessary.
Nursing process step: Assessment
Cognitive level: Comprehension

21. CORRECT ANSWER—**B.** Ranitidine is a histamine$_2$ (H_2)-receptor antagonist that blocks the action of histamine at the parietal H_2-receptor sites, thereby preventing gastric acid secretion.
Nursing process step: Implementation
Cognitive level: Comprehension

22. CORRECT ANSWER—**C.** Pyuria is not associated with renal injury. Costovertebral angle tenderness or pain, hematuria, and flank pain are signs and symptoms indicative of renal injury.
Nursing process step: Assessment
Cognitive level: Comprehension

23. CORRECT ANSWER—**C.** With inverse ratio ventilation, inspiration is prolonged to allow more time for gas exchange to occur. This causes a concomitant decrease in expiratory time. Flow rate may be decreased to allow more time for the inspiration to continue; however, the respiratory rate could not be increased because air would not be kept in the lung long enough to improve diffusion across the alveolar membrane before the next breath occurs. Minute ventilation and tidal volume are not manipulated to produce inverse ratio ventilation. Pressure support is a separate mode of ventilation regulated by pressure rather than volume. Expiratory time is decreased, not increased, with inverse ratio ventilation.
Nursing process step: Implementation
Cognitive level: Comprehension

24. CORRECT ANSWER—**C.** A patient with unstable angina typically complains of crushing chest pain that radiates to the left arm, neck, jaw, or shoulder. This patient would benefit from a calcium channel blocker, such as diltiazem hydrochloride, because it decreases the work of the heart by decreasing myocardial contractility, relaxing vascular smooth muscle, and dilating coronary arteries. A fast, racing heart may indicate an arrhythmia, which is best treated with an antiarrhythmic agent. Swollen feet may occur secondary to congestive heart failure, which may be treated with digoxin. Hunger and diaphoresis may indicate that the patient is hypoglycemic; after the patient's low blood glucose level has been confirmed, the patient would receive I.V. glucose.
Nursing process step: Assessment
Cognitive level: Analysis

25. CORRECT ANSWER—**D.** In patients with coronary or cerebral artery disease and those who have had a recent thrombotic cerebral event, lowering the blood pressure to normal level can be dangerous because it may enhance coronary or cerebral insufficiency. In such cases, safe blood pressure levels are 160 to 180 mm Hg systolic and 100 to 110 mm Hg diastolic.
Nursing process step: Planning
Cognitive level: Analysis

26. CORRECT ANSWER—**A.** The mortality rate for cardiogenic shock remains at 80% or higher despite recent advances in coronary care. The most common cause of cardiogenic shock is a large myocardial infarction involving at least 40% of the left ventricular muscle mass. Other causes include lethal arrhythmias, severe congestive heart failure, myocarditis, massive pulmonary emboli, severe valvular dysfunction, and cardiac tamponade.
Nursing process step: Implementation
Cognitive level: Knowledge

27. CORRECT ANSWER—**C.** Propranolol, nitroprusside sodium, diltiazem, and trimethaphan camsylate all reduce blood pressure. However, diltiazem is least likely to be used during the acute phase of aortic dissection and more likely to be used for control of chronic hypertension.
Nursing process step: Implementation
Cognitive level: Analysis

28. CORRECT ANSWER—**C.** Indiscriminate use of sodium bicarbonate therapy can trigger cardiovascular collapse, which is caused by arrhythmias resulting from profound hypokalemia. Sodium bicarbonate should be used in patients whose pH is less than 7.1. Metabolic acidosis does not provide a stimulus for breathing; rather, the drive to breathe is based on $PaCO_2$ and PaO_2 levels.
Nursing process step: Implementation
Cognitive level: Comprehension

29. CORRECT ANSWER—**B.** Cardiovascular signs and symptoms of hypoglycemia include tachycardia, palpitations, diaphoresis, and irritability. Central nervous (CNS) system signs of hypoglycemia include weakness, nervousness, and irritability. Because hypoglycemia stimulates the CNS, lassitude is not observed. If the hypoglycemia remains untreated, seizures, coma, and irreversible brain damage can occur.
Nursing process step: Assessment
Cognitive level: Comprehension

30. CORRECT ANSWER—**A.** The patient may have sustained a penetrating injury to a major artery in her right leg secondary to the femur fracture. In most cases of arterial trauma, there are no immediate signs of distal ischemia; consequently, the physician may have missed this diagnosis while treating the patient's splenic rupture. Studies of skeletal muscle and peripheral nerves have shown that irreversible damage occurs after 4 to 6 hours of ischemia, which qualifies this condition as an emergency. Analgesics would mask the ischemic pain, and time would be lost while they are administered. Thermal compresses and positioning are of no use in acute arterial trauma.
Nursing process step: Implementation
Cognitive level: Analysis

31. CORRECT ANSWER—**C.** Because of the splenic injury and possibility of blood loss, the nurse should closely monitor the patient's hemodynamic status to assess for hypovolemia. Neurovascular checks of the patient's leg are imperative after arterial repair and are necessary to assess for compartmental syndrome. Because of her long-bone fracture, the patient is at risk for fat embolism, and her respiratory status should be monitored. Assessing urine output and neurologic status is important, but these findings are not directly related to the patient's known injuries.
Nursing process step: Planning
Cognitive level: Evaluation

32. CORRECT ANSWER—**B.** Prolongation of the QT interval can herald the development of life-threatening arrhythmias, especially torsades du pointes, in a patient receiving procainamide. A prolonged PR interval is a rare complication of procainamide therapy. ST-segment elevation and depression are not associated with procainamide use.
Nursing process step: Assessment
Cognitive level: Comprehension

33. CORRECT ANSWER—**C.** A typical fluid restriction for a patient with SIADH is 1,000 ml per 24 hours. This amount includes fluids required for medication administration. Patients with severe hyponatremia may require a hypertonic solution.
Nursing process step: Implementation
Cognitive level: Analysis

34. CORRECT ANSWER—**A.** Cardiac output can be decreased by myocardial depressant factor, a toxin released into the circulation during shock. When a thermal injury affects more than 50% of the total body surface area, myocardial depressant factor can decrease cardiac output by as much as 30% during the first 30 minutes. Another 20% decrease in cardiac output can result from loss of circulating plasma volume. Aggressive fluid replacement, not restriction, is necessary to support cardiac function. Although vasopressors and positive inotropic agents eventually may be needed, fluids are the first line of treatment. Thermal injury increases capillary permeability and causes associated shifts in fluid and electrolytes, which can affect cardiac conduction; consequently, the patient is susceptible to arrhythmias and requires close ECG monitoring.
Nursing process step: Assessment
Cognitive level: Evaluation

35. CORRECT ANSWER—D. The differential of the percentage of each type of white blood cell in the bloodstream during infection can help predict the type of infection. Granulocytes, which are released when immature, respond to bacterial infections. Lymphocytes, which are released only when mature, respond to viral infections and allergies. An increased percentage of granulocytes (neutrophils, basophils, and eosinophils) occurs with bacterial infection and constitutes a "shift to the left" (shift toward immaturity) on the differential scale. An increased percentage of lymphocytes occurs with viral infection and represents a "shift to the right." Pernicious anemia and hepatic disease are characterized by low hemoglobin, decreased red blood cell count, and, possibly, a low white blood cell count; the differential is not affected.
Nursing process step: Assessment
Cognitive level: Analysis

36. CORRECT ANSWER—D. The blood urea nitrogen level indicates the amount of nitrogen in the blood in the form of urea. The liver normally breaks down urea, but when it cannot do so, the urea level in the blood rises. In patients with liver failure, the albumin level decreases as a result of the reduced production of albumin by the liver and increased portal pressure, which forces albumin to leak from the vessels surrounding the liver. This leakage of albumin leads to ascites. The bilirubin level increases because bilirubin cannot be broken down chemically by the liver. Serum glucose decreases because of the reduced production of carbohydrate by the liver.
Nursing process step: Assessment
Cognitive level: Evaluation

37. CORRECT ANSWER—B. A nasogastric tube should be inserted because gastric decompression reduces pressure on the injured spleen. A jejunostomy tube is inserted surgically into the jejunum to administer liquefied feedings. A Dobhoff feeding tube is inserted through the nare down to the stomach or jejunum for enteral nutrition. Neither a jejunostomy tube nor a Dobhoff tube is indicated at this point because the priority is to decrease pressure on the injured spleen, not to provide nutrition. A cecostomy tube, which is inserted into the cecum to allow fecal drainage, is used for patients with intestinal obstructions.
Nursing process step: Implementation
Cognitive level: Analysis

38. CORRECT ANSWER—C. In hemothorax, free-flowing fluid collects in the lower chest while air collects in the upper chest. Therefore, hemothorax is best drained by placing a chest tube at the eighth or ninth intercostal space on the affected side.
Nursing process step: Planning
Cognitive level: Comprehension

39. CORRECT ANSWER—B. The lowest acceptable range of negative pressure for weaning a patient from a ventilator is −20 to −25 cm H_2O. Pressures lower than −20 cm H_2O indicate that the patient is unable to move the volume of air necessary to maintain ventilation. A pressure of −20 cm H_2O or higher indicates that the patient is ready for extubation.
Nursing process step: Evaluation
Cognitive level: Evaluation

40. CORRECT ANSWER—**B.** Although the total creatine kinase (CK) is slightly elevated, the creatine kinase-MB (CK-MB) is within normal limits. Total CK may be increased for several reasons, including skeletal muscle damage, I.M. injections, brain injury, muscular or neuromuscular disease, vigorous exercise, trauma, or surgery. The CK-MB is a more sensitive and specific indicator of myocardial damage. Lactate dehydrogenase (LD) is useful if CK has not been measured within 24 hours of an acute myocardial infarction (MI); the LD level peaks 2 to 5 days after an acute MI has occurred. An elevated LD level also may occur in severe shock, renal disease, leukemia, pulmonary infarction, tumor, and hepatic disease.
Nursing process step: Evaluation
Cognitive level: Application

41. CORRECT ANSWER—**A.** Digitalis glycosides, such as digoxin, are indicated for atrial fibrillation, atrial flutter, paroxysmal atrial tachycardia, and congestive heart failure. Amrinone is a positive inotropic agent used to treat refractory congestive heart failure. Dobutamine, a synthetic catecholamine, stimulates beta$_1$-adrenergic receptors and is used in patients with refractory heart failure and pulmonary congestion. The antihypertensive captopril can be used to treat heart failure that does not respond to conventional therapies.
Nursing process step: Implementation
Cognitive level: Knowledge

42. CORRECT ANSWER—**C.** Autonomic dysreflexia requires immediate treatment. The resulting hypertension (not hypotension) can lead to stroke if it is not controlled. Poor autonomic function prevents vasodilation in response to the hypertension. Chest pain may occur, but arrhythmias are not common.
Nursing process step: Assessment
Cognitive level: Comprehension

43. CORRECT ANSWER—**B.** Diabetes insipidus results from the decreased release of antidiuretic hormone (ADH) that may occur after head trauma. It is associated with high urine output and elevated serum sodium level and elevated serum osmolality. Syndrome of inappropriate antidiuretic hormone (SIADH) results from excessive ADH activity. The patient's clinical history is not consistent with high-output renal failure. The laboratory data are consistent with hypovolemia, not hypervolemia.
Nursing process step: Planning
Cognitive level: Analysis

44. CORRECT ANSWER—**D.** A patient with diabetes insipidus typically loses an excessive amount of urine; therefore, an equal volume of I.V. fluid must be administered to prevent circulatory collapse. Pulmonary artery catheters generally are not necessary in young patients with diabetes insipidus; such patients have low central pressures, necessitating fluid replacement. To prevent aspiration, oral fluids are contraindicated in patients who have a decreased level of consciousness.
Nursing process step: Implementation
Cognitive level: Analysis

45. CORRECT ANSWER—**C.** Because diabetes insipidus causes a deficiency of circulating antidiuretic hormone (also called vasopressin), vasopressin is the definitive treatment. Although potassium chloride may be needed to replenish urine losses of potassium, it would not treat the underlying diabetes insipidus. Diuretics (furosemide and ethacrynic acid) are contraindicated because the goal of therapy is to replace intravascular fluid.
Nursing process step: Implementation
Cognitive level: Analysis

46. CORRECT ANSWER—**A.** Alcohol temporarily decreases antidiuretic hormone secretion, and volume replacement is necessary. The patient's hemoglobin level is not indicative of blood loss. Diuretic abuse is unlikely in a 27-year-old man. Extravasation of fluid secondary to bilateral femur fractures does not cause hemodynamically significant hypovolemia.
Nursing process step: Evaluation
Cognitive level: Analysis

47. CORRECT ANSWER—**C.** Occasionally, bullets are not surgically retrieved if they are located outside the vascular tree and away from vital organs or if they do not cause symptoms. When there is no identifiable exit wound or the bullet cannot be located, the surgeon must search for the bullet because of the high morbidity associated with embolization of foreign bodies that travel to the lungs, heart, and brain. Bullets are no more likely to embolize from the groin or chest than from other parts of the body. Embolization secondary to high activity is likely only if the bullet enters the vascular tree.
Nursing process step: Evaluation
Cognitive level: Comprehension

48. CORRECT ANSWER—**A.** The goal of therapy in patients with chronic atrial fibrillation is to control the ventricular rate and prevent embolization of thrombi from the atrium. Digoxin commonly is used for heart rate control; a calcium channel blocker, such as verapamil or diltiazem, often is added if needed. Warfarin is used to prevent thrombus formation in the atrium. The antihypertensive hydralazine would be used only if the patient's blood pressure was elevated.
Nursing process step: Implementation
Cognitive level: Analysis

49. CORRECT ANSWER—**B.** Early nutritional support is essential to prevent complications, including sepsis resulting from translocation of bacteria from the colon. Although many patients with spinal cord injuries have initial ileus, early parenteral nutrition prevents catabolism and later enteral nutrition preserves the mucosal barrier, which also decreases the risk of catabolism. Metoclopramide hydrochloride can prevent aspiration and may help resolve ileus, but it does not prevent catabolism. Caloric intake typically is increased in patients with spinal cord injuries because of stress and the need to rebuild traumatized tissue. Early mobilization helps prevent venous stasis and loss of muscle strength in nonparalyzed muscles, but it will not prevent the negative nitrogen balance created by catabolism.
Nursing process step: Implementation
Cognitive level: Analysis

50. CORRECT ANSWER—**B.** Temporary pacing wires are indicated for any patient who exhibits second-degree atrioventricular (AV) block, Mobitz type II, because of the origin of the block. A type II block is a high-grade AV block that occurs below the level of the bundle of His. Not all impulses from the atria are conducted to the ventricles, and the patient is at risk for complete heart block or ventricular standstill. Because the risk is so great, the nurse must intervene rather than just monitor for progression of the block. Other characteristics of a Mobitz type II AV block include regular atrial rhythm, more P waves than QRS complexes, and PR intervals that remain consistent whenever P waves are conducted. Mobitz type II AV block is most often associated with extensive anterior wall damage. Although advanced cardiac life support guidelines discuss the use of such drugs as dopamine and epinephrine, this patient is asymptomatic and pacing wires would be inserted prophylactically. An intra-aortic balloon pump would not help a patient who suffers complete heart block. If complete heart block existed, the patient would need a temporary sequential pacemaker.
Nursing process step: Implementation
Cognitive level: Application

51. CORRECT ANSWER—D. Hepatic encephalopathy may be caused by an accumulation of sedatives, which are detoxified by the liver. It also can result from hypoxia, which increases central nervous system sensitivity to any substance. Because constipation can increase production and absorption of ammonia from the gut, stool softeners may decrease the ammonia level. Hypokalemia predisposes patients to metabolic alkalosis, which favors the conversion of ammonium to ammonia. Because ammonia cannot be broken down by the diseased liver, it accumulates in the blood and travels unchanged to the brain, causing symptoms indicative of hepatic encephalopathy.
Nursing process step: Planning
Cognitive level: Analysis

52. CORRECT ANSWER—C. Serum creatinine, a waste product of muscle metabolism, is highly sensitive to changes in the glomerular filtration rate. Blood urea nitrogen can be influenced by other sources, such as hydration, catabolism, tissue breakdown, and medication. Serum potassium is affected by oral intake and acid-base status. Urine creatinine is useful for evaluating renal status in relation to the serum creatinine, but it is not the best indicator of renal failure.
Nursing process step: Assessment
Cognitive level: Evaluation

53. CORRECT ANSWER—A. When a patient is known to have ingested a caustic substance, an abdominal X-ray film can help rule out gastric or intestinal perforation. A patient who has ingested a caustic agent must not be given syrup of ipecac because vomiting of the caustic agent would occur, thereby damaging the esophagus and oropharynx. Because the patient has been stabilized, an airway would have been established and oxygen already administered. Obtaining blood drug levels would not provide immediately useful information.
Nursing process step: Planning
Cognitive level: Analysis

54. CORRECT ANSWER—C. All patients with burn injuries, including those who are undernourished, should receive enteral feedings as soon as bowel sounds are heard. All burn patients typically require up to 4,000 calories daily, and protein mass must be maintained. Aggressive nutritional support improves survival, reduces the risk of infection, and prevents Curling's ulcers. Formulas are available that contain appropriate amounts of calories and protein to prevent depletion of protein mass and maintain a positive nitrogen balance. Because patients with burn injuries often are subjected to various therapies and surgeries, obtaining adequate nutrition from oral intake is difficult.
Nursing process step: Implementation
Cognitive level: Analysis

55. CORRECT ANSWER—A. As the tumor gradually compresses portions of the spinal cord, weakness or sensory losses and pain occur. Although paralysis may occur later, weakness, pain, and sensory loss usually are seen initially. Anterior cord syndrome and Brown-Séquard syndrome are incomplete spinal cord injuries associated with certain degrees of motor and sensory function loss.
Nursing process step: Assessment
Cognitive level: Comprehension

56. CORRECT ANSWER—B. A fourth heart sound results from atrial contraction and reverberation of the contraction against a distended, stiff ventricle, as occurs in restrictive cardiomyopathy. An S_3 gallop is associated with elevated left ventricular filling pressures and would be expected in a patient with acute congestive heart failure, as would crackles and jugular vein distention.
Nursing process step: Assessment
Cognitive level: Evaluation

57. CORRECT ANSWER—**D.** Because the patient is known to have severe coronary artery disease, catheterization would define the coronary anatomy and identify any reversible lesion. A stress test is appropriate, but the patient is too ill for a treadmill exercise test. Endomyocardial biopsy is used to help diagnose transplant rejection and occasionally to diagnose autoimmune causes of cardiomyopathy. Electrophysiologic studies are reserved for patients who have demonstrated symptomatic ventricular arrhythmias.
Nursing process step: Planning
Cognitive level: Comprehension

58. CORRECT ANSWER—**D.** The decrease in pulmonary artery pressure and systolic pressure after the administration of unloading agents indicates hypovolemia. The nitroprusside infusion rate should be temporarily decreased to maintain an adequate systolic pressure while fluid is cautiously infused, using changes in pulmonary artery pressure as a guide. Increasing the dobutamine or nitroprusside infusion rates would exacerbate the hypotension. With an ejection fraction of 15%, the patient probably would not tolerate rapid infusion of I.V. fluids.
Nursing process step: Implementation
Cognitive level: Analysis

59. CORRECT ANSWER—**B.** Many of the medications the patient would be receiving, such as digoxin, have a narrow therapeutic index and can easily reach toxic levels in a patient with renal dysfunction. Dopamine increases renal blood flow at rates of 3 to 5 mcg/kg/minute but decreases renal perfusion at rates exceeding 10 mcg/kg/minute. Cautious I.V. fluid challenges or a furosemide infusion might be appropriate, but the nurse does not have enough information at this time to implement such measures.
Nursing process step: Implementation
Cognitive level: Analysis

60. CORRECT ANSWER—**A.** Clinical indicators of right-sided heart failure include jugular vein distention, hepatojugular reflux, hepatomegaly, splenomegaly, ascites, nausea, vomiting, abdominal distention, anorexia, peripheral edema, weight gain, and elevated central venous pressure and right arterial pressure. Isolated right ventricular failure can result from right ventricular infarction; if left untreated, it will progress to global heart failure. Symptoms of left ventricular failure include pulmonary congestion, tachycardia, hypotension, atrial and ventricular gallops, decreased cardiac output, and low urine output. In compensated heart failure, the body responds to the heart failure with compensatory mechanisms, which should effectively overcome symptoms of congestive heart failure. These symptoms include sodium and water retention, increased cardiac output, increased heart rate, and hypertrophy of the ventricle in response to increased afterload and filling volumes. Hepatomegaly is not initially seen in acute heart failure.
Nursing process step: Assessment
Cognitive level: Knowledge

61. CORRECT ANSWER—**B.** Nitroglycerin given by the sublingual route usually rapidly relieves chest pain caused by ischemia. If the ischemia is not alleviated, the myocardium continues to be hypoxic. In this case, the nurse should suspect myocardial infarction and perform a 12-lead ECG. Unstable angina would be relieved by nitroglycerin tablets. Congestive heart failure and ventricular septal defects could lead to myocardial infarction; however, they are not usually associated with crushing chest pain.
Nursing process step: Assessment
Cognitive level: Analysis

62. CORRECT ANSWER—**C.** The patient is experiencing ventricular tachycardia, as indicated by wide, bizarre QRS complexes at a rate of 187 beats/minute and no discernible P waves. The patient is symptomatic with this rhythm, as evidenced by his dizziness and decreased blood pressure. Immediate cardioversion is required in any clinically symptomatic patient with tachycardia at a rate greater than 150 beats/minute. A patient experiencing asystole or ventricular fibrillation would not have a blood pressure. The rhythm strip cannot differentiate between pulseless ventricular tachycardia and ventricular tachycardia accompanied by a pulse; however, perfusion is occurring because a blood pressure reading has been obtained. A patient with supraventricular tachycardia may have P waves, but because the origin of the impulse is above the ventricles, the QRS complex is not as wide or bizarre-looking as in ventricular tachycardia.
Nursing process step: Implementation
Cognitive level: Application

63. CORRECT ANSWER—**D.** Dyspnea is a symptom, not a pathophysiologic mechanism. All the other options are correct.
Nursing process step: Evaluation
Cognitive level: Comprehension

64. CORRECT ANSWER—**A.** Right-sided endocarditis can produce a thrombus that breaks loose, enters the pulmonary circulation, and subsequently causes shortness of breath and hypoxia. A decreased level of consciousness and right-sided paralysis are symptoms of cerebral embolism. A cold, mottled left arm without pulses indicate the presence of an arterial embolism in the left upper arm. Urine output of less than 30 ml/hour for 4 hours indicates compromised perfusion to the kidneys, which would occur with a renal artery embolism. Cerebral embolism, peripheral arterial embolism, and abdominal organ arterial embolism commonly occur with vegetations on valves situated on the left side of the heart, namely, the mitral and aortic valves.
Nursing process step: Assessment
Cognitive level: Analysis

65. CORRECT ANSWER—**B.** Hyperosmolar non-ketotic syndrome (HNKS) typically develops in patients older than age 50 who have type II, not type I, diabetes mellitus. A patient with well-controlled diabetes is not susceptible to HNKS. Patients receiving steroids, diuretics, or total parenteral nutrition who have a history of diet-controlled diabetes are at risk for HNKS. However, a patient with only transiently elevated glucose levels is not at risk.
Nursing process step: Assessment
Cognitive level: Knowledge

66. CORRECT ANSWER—**B.** A high percentage of patients with hyperosmolar nonketotic syndrome (HNKS) have gastric stasis and ileus. These patients typically experience nausea, vomiting, and discomfort, all of which can be alleviated via nasogastric tube suctioning. Gastric lavage, intestinal intubation, and enema or laxative therapy are not used to manage HNKS.
Nursing process step: Implementation
Cognitive level: Analysis

67. CORRECT ANSWER—**B.** Thrombosis accounts for 50% of all acute arterial occlusions. Systemic factors contributing to thrombosis formation include dehydration, fever, infection, thrombocytosis, disseminated intravascular coagulation, and polycythemia vera. Fluid tends to sequester in the affected extremity in patients with venous occlusion, not arterial occlusion. Myoglobinuria and subsequent renal failure are potential sequelae of crushing injuries to large muscle groups. Lactic acid has no diuretic activity.
Nursing process step: Implementation
Cognitive level: Analysis

68. CORRECT ANSWER—**D.** When assessing the abdomen, the nurse should proceed sequentially with inspection, auscultation, percussion, and palpation. Abdominal auscultation must be performed before percussion and palpation because these two techniques could alter intestinal activity and bowel sounds.
Nursing process step: Assessment
Cognitive level: Knowledge

69. CORRECT ANSWER—**B.** Distended neck veins are caused by obstructed blood flow through the chest cavity due to increased intrapleural pressure. Breath sounds are absent in the affected or collapsed lung fields. Because of the disruption in the pleural cavity, air rushes in and replaces the normally negative pressure with positive pressure; the positive pressure pushes the trachea and mediastinal contents in the opposite direction.
Nursing process step: Assessment
Cognitive level: Evaluation

70. CORRECT ANSWER—**D.** Ongoing surveillance of sputum smears for presence of acid-fast bacilli is needed to detect and prevent multidrug-resistant tuberculosis. Second-line drugs may be necessary in patients with atypical mycobacterial disease or drug-resistant tuberculosis. These second-line drugs, which include aminosalicylic acid (which can produce severe GI distress) and cycloserine (which can result in neurotoxicity), are more toxic than the first-line agents isoniazid and rifampin. The length of treatment is no guarantee that the patient is not infectious.
Nursing process step: Implementation
Cognitive level: Knowledge

71. CORRECT ANSWER—**C.** Hyperkalemia in a patient with cardiac failure is caused by decreased perfusion, not cellular breakdown. Crush trauma, burns, and acidosis all lead to cellular destruction and potassium release.
Nursing process step: Assessment
Cognitive level: Analysis

72. CORRECT ANSWER—**B.** Turner's sign is ecchymosis along a patient's flank. Cullen's sign is ecchymosis in the periumbilical area and indicates blood in that region. Homan's sign is pain on dorsiflexion of the foot and is a possible sign of thrombophlebitis. Kernig's sign is a symptom of meningitis evidenced by pain and resistance when attempting to completely extend the leg after flexing the thigh upon the abdomen.
Nursing process step: Assessment
Cognitive level: Comprehension

73. CORRECT ANSWER—**C.** Treatment for acute pancreatitis is more palliative than curative. Ice chips must be avoided because they can stimulate pancreatic enzyme secretion. Administering histamine$_2$-receptor antagonists, aspirating gastric secretions via nasogastric (NG) tube suctioning, and reducing physical activity suppress pancreatic secretions. These interventions provide pain relief and pancreatic rest until the autodigestive process subsides. NG tube suctioning has the additional benefit of decreasing abdominal distention and vomiting.
Nursing process step: Implementation
Cognitive level: Analysis

74. CORRECT ANSWER—**A.** Malignancies commonly seen in patients with acquired immunodeficiency syndrome (AIDS) are Kaposi's sarcoma and lymphoid disorders, such as lymphocytic leukemia and lymphoma. Other cancers that may be associated with AIDS include small-cell lung cancer, anal cancer, and head or neck cancer. Gastric carcinoma, spinal neoplasm, and malignant melanoma commonly are not associated with AIDS.
Nursing process step: Planning
Cognitive level: Comprehension

75. CORRECT ANSWER—**A.** Induced emesis is recommended only for patients who are alert, have an intact gag reflex, and have not ingested a caustic substance. A patient having seizures does not have a protected airway, which contraindicates induced vomiting. Inducing emesis in infants under age 9 months has not been proved safe. The patient who has ingested an overdose of tricyclic antidepressants is susceptible to rapid decompensation in level of consciousness and would be unable to protect her airway.
Nursing process step: Assessment
Cognitive level: Analysis

76. CORRECT ANSWER—**A.** Dobutamine and amrinone can be used to enhance inotropic action in acute heart failure. Calcium channel blockers (such as diltiazem) and beta-blockers (such as propranolol) generally are not used in the acute phase of heart failure because of their negative inotropic effects on the myocardium. Although digoxin is used to manage chronic heart failure, its use early in the acute phase generally is not supported. Digoxin is most effective in patients with marked ventricular dilatation resulting from chronic heart failure.
Nursing process step: Assessment
Cognitive level: Evaluation

77. CORRECT ANSWER—**C.** Although cardiac output can be used to assess a patient's response to therapy, any value indexed to the body surface area provides a more accurate indication of function. Because cardiac index is a more precise indicator of tissue perfusion, it is the more useful guide in evaluating circulatory status and response to therapy. A normal cardiac index ranges from 2.5 to 4.2 liters/minute/m^2. Right atrial pressure and pulmonary capillary wedge pressure can be affected by cardiac output, but they are more indicative of a patient's fluid status.
Nursing process step: Evaluation
Cognitive level: Evaluation

78. CORRECT ANSWER—**D.** Pentamidine isethionate is becoming more widely used in the treatment of pneumocystic pneumonia. This antiprotozoal agent may work by inhibiting dihydrofolate reductase, interfering with aerobic glycolysis, and inhibiting oxidative phosphorylation and nucleic acid synthesis. Pentamidine's major adverse effects include low platelet count, hypotension, and hypoglycemia. Blood pressure and the results of blood glucose fingerstick tests should be monitored closely. Pentamidine also may decrease the calcium, not sodium, level. Although liver enzyme levels may be elevated, increased prothrombin time has not been reported with pentamidine use. A patient with renal impairment requires lower parenteral doses of this potentially nephrotoxic drug.
Nursing process step: Evaluation
Cognitive level: Evaluation

79. CORRECT ANSWER—**A.** A temperature of 102.2° F (39° C) increases metabolism and carbon dioxide production. Weaning under these conditions would not be successful. The increased heart rate and blood pressure most likely are adverse effects of the patient's fever; however, they could further compromise the patient's cardiovascular status by increasing myocardial oxygen consumption. The patient may not be initiating breaths because she is adequately ventilated at the current ventilator settings.
Nursing process step: Assessment
Cognitive level: Evaluation

80. CORRECT ANSWER—**B.** Replacing the endotracheal tube with a tracheostomy tube will lower airway resistance by decreasing the length of the artificial airway. Compliance, elasticity, and functional residual capacity are not affected by airway size.
Nursing process step: Implementation
Cognitive level: Analysis

81. CORRECT ANSWER—**D.** Magnesium and calcium are essential for nerve impulses to be transmitted appropriately, and phosphate is essential for production of the adenosine triphosphate that muscle can use for energy. These electrolytes help strengthen the diaphragmatic muscle. Although sodium, chloride, and potassium play an important role in fluid and acid-base balance (and thus kidney function), the patient can be weaned if an imbalance in any of these three electrolytes exists. Sodium, chloride, and potassium may affect weaning and need to be monitored.
Nursing process step: Implementation
Cognitive level: Analysis

82. CORRECT ANSWER—**C.** Effective treatment of hypernatremia is indicated by a serum sodium level of 135 to 145 mEq/liter and a serum osmolarity between 280 and 295 mOsm/liter.
Nursing process step: Evaluation
Cognitive level: Evaluation

83. CORRECT ANSWER—**B.** Hepatitis is not considered a complication of pancreatitis. Patients with pancreatitis are on bed rest, which can lead to pulmonary emboli if preventive measures, such as antiembolism stockings, are not used. Prolonged bed rest and reduced physical activity also can lead to atelectasis and pneumonia. Pulmonary edema, with or without cardiac failure, is one of the most serious complications of acute pancreatitis. Pulmonary edema usually occurs 3 to 7 days after the onset of pancreatitis in patients who have received large volumes of fluid to maintain blood pressure and urine output. Other complications of pancreatitis include hypotension, shock, and hypocalcemia.
Nursing process step: Planning
Cognitive level: Analysis

84. CORRECT ANSWER—**D.** Within the first 30 days after allogenic bone marrow transplantation, a patient is at risk for three major, potentially life-threatening complications: rejection in the form of graft-versus-host disease, failure to engraft accompanied by aplastic anemia or thrombocytopenia, and infection resulting from aplasia. Bacterial infections (both gram-positive and gram-negative types) occur within the first 30 days after the procedure, but viral infections typically occur later (that is, more than 50 days after surgery). Cytomegalovirus infection may develop in immunosuppressed patients and in those who have received a transplanted organ. Although pneumonia may develop in these patients, it does not commonly occur in the first 30 days after transplantation. Other hematologic complications associated with engraftment difficulties include hemolytic-uremic syndrome, bleeding disorders (such as pulmonary hemorrhage), hyperammonemia, and hepatic veno-occlusive disease.
Nursing process step: Planning
Cognitive level: Evaluation

85. CORRECT ANSWER—**D.** The PaO_2 of 60 mm Hg suggests that the patient is not receiving enough oxygen at the cellular level; this requires immediate intervention. The FIO_2 needs to be increased and the cause of the hypoxia investigated by means of chest X-ray films, continued auscultation of breath sounds, and vigorous pulmonary toilet to treat atelectasis. The patient is not hyperventilating, and there is no evidence of lactic acid production with a base excess of +5 and an HCO_3^- of 32 mm Hg. The patient is in respiratory acidosis with metabolic compensation; the increased base excess and the increased HCO_3^- reflect the body's metabolic compensatory actions to retain bicarbonate and return the pH to normal. His breathing is being mechanically assisted, and his ventilatory rate or tidal volume may need to be increased if the $PaCO_2$ is increased because of sedation or because the patient is not taking adequate spontaneous breaths. The patient may require assist-control mode for mechanical ventilation or the addition of pressure support to mechanical ventilation for increased respiratory support. The work of the respiratory muscles is increased because of the artificial airway and the ventilator circuit; adding to or increasing the pressure support will decrease the work of breathing.
Nursing process step: Implementation
Cognitive level: Analysis

86. CORRECT ANSWER—**A.** Although all the goals listed are appropriate for a patient in septic shock, the most important nursing goal is to promote adequate tissue perfusion and support the patient's ventilation, oxygenation, and hemodynamic stability. These measures are crucial to sustaining the patient's life; the other options focus on treating potential complications and providing comfort.
Nursing process step: Planning
Cognitive level: Evaluation

87. CORRECT ANSWER—**C.** After a patient undergoes surgery for arteriovenous malformation, the head of the bed should be elevated and the patient's head and neck kept in straight alignment to help the drainage of venous blood from the head. Purposeful hypotension helps reduce the risk of cerebral edema caused by hyperemia and decreases the risk of hemorrhage by normalizing cerebral perfusion pressure in the area of the resection. Mannitol and furosemide are administered during surgery, and doses of these drugs would not be repeated unless symptoms of cerebral swelling occur. Because the patient is extubated, hyperventilation cannot be provided as it requires mechanical ventilation.
Nursing process step: Implementation
Cognitive level: Analysis

88. CORRECT ANSWER—**C.** During a water deprivation test, fluids are withheld from the patient and body weight, serum and urine osmolalities, and urine specific gravity are measured hourly. The most serious adverse effect of the test is severe dehydration. Given the rigors of the test, the nurse must provide emotional support. Close assessment of vital signs also is necessary to prevent hypovolemic shock.
Nursing process step: Implementation
Cognitive level: Evaluation

89. CORRECT ANSWER—**B.** Pulses distal to the acute occlusion would be absent. Because the femoral artery is proximal to the popliteal artery, a femoral pulse should be present. A popliteal pulse may be present, depending on the location of the occlusion in the popliteal artery. The popliteal artery trifurcates to form the anterior tibial, posterior tibial, and peroneal arteries; no pulses distal to the knee would be expected.
Nursing process step: Assessment
Cognitive level: Comprehension

90. CORRECT ANSWER—**A.** Thrombolytic agents, such as urokinase, generally are administered in conjunction with an I.V. heparin infusion to prevent further thrombus formation. Subcutaneous heparin effectively prevents deep vein thrombosis associated with bed rest, but subcutaneous injections are contraindicated in patients receiving thrombolytic agents because of the potential for subcutaneous bleeding. Also, obtaining therapeutic anticoagulation with subcutaneous heparin is difficult. Dipyridamole and warfarin sodium may be administered once the thrombus is lysed, but they are not part of acute therapy.
Nursing process step: Planning
Cognitive level: Analysis

91. CORRECT ANSWER—**C.** In a patient with hypertrophic cardiomyopathy, the ventricular septum is disproportionately large compared with the rest of the ventricle, causing the left ventricle to be abnormally shaped. A patient with dilated (congestive) cardiomyopathy has a uniformly enlarged, distended heart. A stiff, noncompliant ventricle wall is seen in restrictive cardiomyopathy. The characteristics described in option D do not apply to any particular group of patients.
Nursing process step: Evaluation
Cognitive level: Comprehension

92. CORRECT ANSWER—**C.** Abdominal ultrasonography is a noninvasive, fairly inexpensive method of identifying an abdominal aneurysm. A computed tomography scan of the chest, cardiac catheterization, and echocardiography are used in the differential diagnosis of thoracic aneurysm.
Nursing process step: Implementation
Cognitive level: Comprehension

93. CORRECT ANSWER—**B.** A ventilator change is necessary to correct the patient's hypoxia. Because the patient is oxygenating at less than optimal capacity and already is receiving a toxic level of oxygen, increasing the positive end-expiratory pressure (PEEP) is the logical next step. The PEEP should be increased to a level that maximizes functional residual capacity while improving PaO_2. The goal is to maintain peak inspiratory pressures as low as possible while maintaining an adequate PaO_2. The nurse should continue to monitor peak inspiratory pressures with any increase in PEEP; at present, these pressures are at an acceptable level. Increasing the tidal volume would increase peak inspiratory pressures and increase the risk of barotrauma and pneumothorax. The patient should be kept as dry as possible without compromising cardiac output; he also should be closely monitored for acid-base imbalances. These actions can be performed after hypoxia has been corrected.
Nursing process step: Implementation
Cognitive level: Analysis

94. CORRECT ANSWER—**A.** The patient is at risk for additional lung damage resulting from oxygen toxicity in the lung. Oxygen toxicity is caused by prolonged exposure (more than 24 hours) of lung tissue to high fractions of inspired oxygen (FIO_2). A high FIO_2 is defined as greater than .50. Decreasing the tidal volume, respiratory rate, or positive end-expiratory pressure might decrease PaO_2 (the opposite of what is desirable in this situation), while still exposing the lung to dangerous amounts of oxygen. The nurse should decrease FIO_2 as much as possible while maintaining a safe blood oxygen level.
Nursing process step: Planning
Cognitive level: Synthesis

95. CORRECT ANSWER—**B.** Heparin increases the partial thromboplastin time (PTT), and the therapeutic level of heparin is obtained by controlling the PTT. Heparin-induced thrombocytopenia is a life-threatening adverse reaction to heparin therapy; this complication can be identified by monitoring the platelet count. Heparin does not affect the prothrombin time or fibrinogen count.
Nursing process step: Implementation
Cognitive level: Analysis

96. CORRECT ANSWER—**A.** A Minnesota tube is used to control bleeding from esophageal varices. The esophageal balloon is inflated to 20 to 40 mm Hg and clamped; it should be released periodically to prevent necrosis. The gastric balloon is inflated with 200 to 400 cc of air. The esophageal balloon must be deflated before the gastric balloon is decompressed to prevent airway obstruction. Traction on the tube, which is achieved with overbed traction and 2 pounds of weights, provides additional pressure against the blood vessels in the distal esophagus.
Nursing process step: Implementation
Cognitive level: Knowledge

97. CORRECT ANSWER—**A.** Warfarin sodium affects the prothrombin time. The therapeutic level of warfarin varies according to the desired response and physician preference. Generally, a therapeutic response is indicated by a prothrombin time between 16 and 22 seconds. Warfarin usually does not affect the partial thromboplastin time, fibrinogen count, or platelet count.
Nursing process step: Evaluation
Cognitive level: Evaluation

98. CORRECT ANSWER—**A.** Ingestion of paint chips can lead to lead poisoning, which is treated with the antidote succimer. After oral administration, succimer forms water-soluble complexes with lead and increases lead excretion in the urine. Iron overdose is treated with sodium bicarbonate before absorption occurs; iron reacts with sodium bicarbonate to form iron bicarbonate. Acute iron intoxication also is treated with the chelating agent deferoxamine mesylate, which binds to iron ions. Aspirin overdose is not treated with an antidote. Excess vitamin C is not considered harmful because the excess is excreted by the kidneys.
Nursing process step: Implementation
Cognitive level: Comprehension

99. CORRECT ANSWER—**B.** Kussmaul's respirations occur in response to metabolic acidosis as the body seeks to remove carbonic acid by exhaling carbon dioxide. This respiratory pattern is not triggered by hyperglycemia, nor is it evoked in hypovolemic states.
Nursing process step: Assessment
Cognitive level: Evaluation

100. CORRECT ANSWER—**C.** ECG changes in a patient with cardiac contusion mimic those of acute myocardial infarction, including ST-segment and T-wave changes. Serial ECGs are required because the initial ECG often is normal. Continuous rhythm monitoring is necessary to document and treat contusion-induced arrhythmias, which are most commonly observed 48 to 72 hours after the trauma. Enzyme studies are difficult to interpret because the patient often has multiple injuries with large amounts of skeletal muscle damage. Chest wall pain, which may be similar to anginal pain, is not a reliable assessment tool. Although the heart rate in a patient with cardiac contusion may increase as a compensatory mechanism, other factors, such as pain and fear, also can trigger tachycardia. Therefore, tachycardic response is not the most effective tool for evaluating cardiac contusion.
Nursing process step: Assessment
Cognitive level: Evaluation

101. CORRECT ANSWER—A. Cerebral perfusion pressure (CPP) is calculated as mean arterial pressure (MAP) minus intracranial pressure (ICP); therefore, CPP increases if MAP increases or ICP decreases. If ICP increases, MAP increases in an effort to maintain CPP. If MAP does not increase in response to increased ICP or the CPP is not maintained at 50 mm Hg or higher, cerebral perfusion will be compromised.
Nursing process step: Implementation
Cognitive level: Analysis

102. CORRECT ANSWER—A. The patient has a cerebral embolus in the left frontal lobe, the area of the brain that controls motor speech and movement of the right side of the body. A lesion in the right frontal lobe would affect the left side of the body. The left temporal lobe controls receptive speech and hearing and autonomic responses. The right parietal lobe is responsible for sensory function on the left side of the body.
Nursing process step: Assessment
Cognitive level: Comprehension

103. CORRECT ANSWER—C. Patients at risk for mural thrombi in the atria sometimes are prescribed anticoagulants to reduce the occurrence of emboli. Digoxin can help control the atrial fibrillation but would not affect the clot formation common in patients with atrial fibrillation. Sequential compression devices reduce the risk of deep vein thrombosis and decrease the number of pulmonary emboli, not arterial emboli. Dextran reduces platelet cohesiveness and is beneficial after vascular surgery, but it is not commonly used to reduce the risk of mural thrombi.
Nursing process step: Implementation
Cognitive level: Analysis

104. CORRECT ANSWER—C. The oxyhemoglobin dissociation curve is a graphic expression of the affinity between oxygen and hemoglobin, or the amount of oxygen chemically bound to the hemoglobin in the blood as a function of oxygen pressure. Variables that affect the affinity of hemoglobin for oxygen include pH, temperature, and carbon dioxide pressure. A shift to the left, in which red blood cells hold onto oxygen, can occur with alkalosis, hypothermia, and a decreased level of carbon dioxide. A shift to the right, in which red blood cells release oxygen, can occur with acidosis, fever, and an increased carbon dioxide level. This patient is bordering on hypoxia; if he were to become hypothermic, even less oxygen would be available at the tissue level because of the resulting shift to the left.
Nursing process step: Implementation
Cognitive level: Comprehension

105. CORRECT ANSWER—B. A patient who has undergone liver transplantation requires a continuous I.V. infusion of insulin to counteract hyperglycemia, which occurs along with good graft function. Some compromised liver function is likely in the postoperative patient, along with reaccumulation of ascites, pleural effusions, and coagulopathy. Therefore, intermittent platelet transfusions may be necessary, and diuretics, such as furosemide, may be administered based on the patient's fluid status. Metabolic alkalosis indicates liver function as the citrate from blood replacements is broken down into bicarbonate. Continuous or intermittent antiemetic therapy is not routinely administered to liver transplant patients.
Nursing process step: Implementation
Cognitive level: Knowledge

106. CORRECT ANSWER—B. Airway inflammation and bronchoconstriction are pathophysiologic changes that occur in patients with asthma. Only I.V. corticosteroids help decrease this inflammation. Beta$_2$-agonists, epinephrine, and aminophylline are bronchodilators.
Nursing process step: Implementation
Cognitive level: Analysis

107. CORRECT ANSWER—A. Measuring the decrease in systolic blood pressure that occurs during inspiration, or "pulsus paradoxus," provides objective evidence of the degree of airflow obstruction. During expiration, an asthmatic patient generates great positive pleural pressure that decreases venous return to the right atrium. During vigorous inspiration, the pressure falls and venous return to the right atrium increases. Increased pressure on the right side of the heart impairs left ventricular filling. Patients with an acute exacerbation of asthma may not be dehydrated initially but can quickly become dehydrated as a result of the increased work of breathing and insensible fluid losses. Aminophylline and diuretics potentiate hypotension, not hypertension.
Nursing process step: Evaluation
Cognitive level: Evaluation

108. CORRECT ANSWER—C. Development of the balloon-tipped, flow-directed pulmonary artery catheter in 1970 now allows bedside assessment of left ventricular function in addition to pulmonary artery systolic and diastolic pressures. The pulmonary artery catheter also provides data that can be used to monitor fluid status and to differentiate cardiogenic from noncardiogenic causes of pulmonary edema. An indwelling urinary (Foley) catheter is an indirect method of monitoring a patient's fluid status. Blood pressure monitoring via an arterial line or blood pressure cuff also provides an indirect measure of fluid status and can be affected by many other factors. An intra-aortic balloon pump is inserted to treat patients with cardiac failure; it is not used to assess fluid status.
Nursing process step: Planning
Cognitive level: Analysis

109. CORRECT ANSWER—D. To avoid errors in treatment, the nurse should confirm the asystole on an ECG by checking two leads' results. Asystole, the absence of organized activity in the heart, is indicated by a flattened, almost straight baseline, whereas fine ventricular fibrillation manifests as a slight, wavy baseline. A 12-lead ECG is not necessary to confirm asystole. If asystole is present, advanced cardiac life support (ACLS) measures, including the administration of epinephrine and atropine and the insertion of a pacemaker, must be implemented. The ACLS algorithm for asystole does not include the administration of lidocaine or isoproterenol.
Nursing process step: Implementation
Cognitive level: Analysis

110. CORRECT ANSWER—B. Negative inspiratory force measures how effectively a patient can move a volume of air sufficient to maintain adequate ventilation. A negative inspiratory pressure greater than -20 cm H_2O indicates a sufficient ability of the respiratory muscles to breathe spontaneously. All the other options are incorrect.
Nursing process step: Assessment
Cognitive level: Knowledge

111. CORRECT ANSWER—D. On the oxyhemoglobin dissociation curve, an oxygen saturation of 90% correlates with a PaO_2 of 60 mm Hg. Factors that affect the release of oxygen at the cellular level include temperature, pH, $PaCO_2$, and 2,3-diphosphoglycerate (2,3-DPG) level.
Nursing process step: Planning
Cognitive level: Comprehension

112. CORRECT ANSWER—B. The treatment of choice for flail chest is internal stabilization of the chest wall with a volume-controlled mechanical ventilator. The patient is experiencing acute respiratory failure resulting from the combination of the flail chest, splinting, and pain medication. He has respiratory acidosis and hypoxia, both of which require immediate intubation and ventilation to prevent further complications. Discontinuing the morphine would only worsen the splinting and cause the patient to become more hypoxic and hypercapnic. A chest X-ray film can wait until the patient is stabilized.
Nursing process step: Implementation
Cognitive level: Knowledge

113. CORRECT ANSWER—C. Turning the patient during sclerotherapy enhances distribution of the medication across the pleural cavity and ensures that the pleura is properly sealed. The sclerosing agent is not meant to be absorbed; after instillation and rotation, the medication is drained via a chest tube. Sclerotherapy often is a painful procedure, and the patient may be given numbing agents and opioid analgesics. Turning the patient will not decrease the pain. Chest tube drainage, rather than turning the patient frequently, is used to empty the pleural cavity of the sclerosing agent.
Nursing process step: Implementation
Cognitive level: Analysis

114. CORRECT ANSWER—B. Positioning the patient with the unaffected side down improves the ventilation-perfusion ratio, which increases oxygenation. With the patient positioned on the unaffected lung, gravity promotes blood flow to well-ventilated areas of the lung.
Nursing process step: Implementation
Cognitive level: Evaluation

115. CORRECT ANSWER—B. Bronchial or tubular breath sounds are normal when heard over the area of the manubrium. The presence of bronchial breath sounds anywhere else is pathologic and indicates lung consolidation or compression of lung tissue. A major airway must be patent to transmit the bronchial breath sound; if the airways are blocked, breath sounds are decreased or absent. Fremitus is increased over a consolidation. Egophony is present when a whispered word sounds loud because of increased transmission of sound through a solid or liquid rather than through air. Crackles, wheezes, and rhonchi are nonspecific findings. A friction rub is heard when the pleura is inflamed.
Nursing process step: Assessment
Cognitive level: Evaluation

116. CORRECT ANSWER—C. Acute prerenal failure results from decreased perfusion to the kidneys secondary to hypovolemia or heart failure. All interventions are aimed at correcting the cause of the hypovolemia. Depending on the specific situation, administering fluids or a positive inotropic agent, such as dobutamine, would be appropriate to increase the patient's cardiac output. Low-dosage dopamine dilates renal vessels, which increases perfusion to the kidneys. Diuretic therapy is not first-line therapy for patients with prerenal failure because diuretics can exacerbate the hypovolemia and hypoperfusion of the kidneys.
Nursing process step: Planning
Cognitive level: Analysis

117. CORRECT ANSWER—A. Bleeding in the upper GI tract produces swift, severe, arterial blood losses that requires massive red blood cell replacement. However, red blood cells do not replenish the coagulation proteins and platelets lost through exsanguination. After an exchange transfusion (approximately 10 units within 24 hours), clotting factors must be replaced. Provided the patient is stable, blood products should be given in the same order as they are used by the body for clotting—platelets, clotting factors (plasma), factor VIII (destroyed by cooling plasma), and red blood cells.
Nursing process step: Implementation
Cognitive level: Evaluation

118. CORRECT ANSWER—A. Patients receiving immunosuppressant therapy often have an increased appetite, as well as fluid volume excess related to sodium and water retention. Therefore, weight gain is common and must be monitored. Immunosuppressed patients are at high risk for infectious complications and should be informed of how to detect infection, when to report infection, and the potential consequences of not following up on symptoms of infection. Because the inflammatory and immune responses are suppressed, the patient must be taught to recognize the few symptoms of infection that are present, frequently only fever. The degree of immunosuppression cannot be directly measured, but it does correlate with the specific agent, dosage, and duration of therapy; follow-up visits are necessary to monitor the effects of the immunosuppressant treatment.
Nursing process step: Implementation
Cognitive level: Evaluation

119. CORRECT ANSWER—A. The Rule of Nines is the most commonly used method of assessing the extent of a burn injury and determining fluid resuscitation requirements. An easy system, the Rule of Nines divides the body into nine sections and assigns a specific percentage of the total body surface area to each section. It does not take into account age-related size differences and therefore is inaccurate in children. The palmar method, which is considered inaccurate, is used to assess small burn wounds. This method involves assigning one palm to equal 1% of the total body surface area. The Lund and Browder method, which is the most accurate means of determining the size of a burn, allows for age-related size differences; however, this method is time-consuming.
Nursing process step: Evaluation
Cognitive level: Analysis

120. CORRECT ANSWER—C. Hypoglycemia can occur suddenly in a patient with insulin-dependent diabetes mellitus, often during the peak action of insulin. The nurse must treat the patient immediately or permanent brain damage or death may result. Ideally, the nurse would check the patient's serum glucose level, then administer a 50% dextrose solution to a diabetic patient. Sodium chloride solution, insulin, or mannitol would not correct the hypoglycemia.
Nursing process step: Implementation
Cognitive level: Evaluation

121. CORRECT ANSWER—C. Pulmonary disease can falsely elevate the central venous pressure (CVP) reading. In patients with pulmonary disease, a pulmonary artery catheter may be necessary for reliable and accurate assessment of fluid status. The CVP is a useful tool in patients with chronic renal failure, hypovolemia secondary to indirect fluid loss, and head trauma.
Nursing process step: Assessment
Cognitive level: Comprehension

122. CORRECT ANSWER—B. ECG changes are the most reliable means of monitoring myocardial damage caused by cardiac contusion and should guide the nurse in initiating progressive activity. Ambulation started too early can injure the heart. The patient's interest in increasing activity may occur long after it is hemodynamically and musculoskeletally safe to do so.
Nursing process step: Implementation
Cognitive level: Evaluation

123. CORRECT ANSWER—D. Meningitis, a common complication of an abscess, causes nuchal rigidity, headache, and irritability. A decreased level of consciousness results from increased intracranial pressure. If the abscess acts as a space-occupying lesion, the patient's respiratory pattern may change, but hypertension and respiratory alkalosis are more likely to occur. Although photophobia is associated with meningitis, status epilepticus is not.
Nursing process step: Assessment
Cognitive level: Knowledge

124. CORRECT ANSWER—C. A craniotomy is the most likely course of treatment because the large lesion is causing increased intracranial pressure and focal neurologic deficits. The craniotomy also allows diagnosis of the infecting organism, which probably is toxoplasmosis. Antibiotics can be given once the organism is positively identified. Steroids, not diuretics, may be used before and after surgery to reduce swelling. Because the patient has not specifically requested supportive care and has not requested that no drugs be administered, the health care team would act aggressively to reduce the increased intracranial pressure.
Nursing process step: Implementation
Cognitive level: Analysis

125. CORRECT ANSWER—B. ST-segment elevation indicates myocardial ischemia resulting from coronary artery disease. The blood volume necessary to prime the dialysis tubing and filter causes a significant loss of circulating blood volume, thus triggering the ischemia. Hypovolemia alone would not cause ECG changes. Pericarditis and pulmonary embolus would produce ECG changes that do not resolve.
Nursing process step: Implementation
Cognitive level: Evaluation

126. CORRECT ANSWER—B. Injection sclerotherapy can stop acute variceal bleeding in 80% of cases. Inserting a quadruple-lumen Minnesota tube, administering I.V. vasopressin, and surgically decompressing portal hypertension are less effective treatment options. Variceal bleeding often recurs after balloon tamponade with tubes, such as the Minnesota tube, is discontinued.
Nursing process step: Planning
Cognitive level: Evaluation

127. CORRECT ANSWER—B. The beta blocker propranolol can lower portal pressure. The usual dosage is 20 to 80 mg twice daily. Vasopressin may be administered into the superior mesenteric artery or via an I.V. drip to temporarily stop bleeding; however, patients receiving vasopressin therapy must be monitored in the intensive care unit. Vitamin K would be administered to promote formation of active prothrombin and help decrease the bleeding. Furosemide is a diuretic often used to treat hypertension and pulmonary edema.
Nursing process step: Assessment
Cognitive level: Comprehension

128. CORRECT ANSWER—**A.** Airway pressure can be decreased through measures that increase the elasticity of the lung or decrease resistance to flow into the lung. Increasing the pressure within the endotracheal cuff will not decrease airway pressure. Bronchodilators can increase the diameter of constricted airways. Suctioning the endotracheal tube can remove mucus plugs or the accumulation of secretions. Humidification loosens secretions within the lungs.
Nursing process step: Implementation
Cognitive level: Analysis

129. CORRECT ANSWER—**C.** An open pneumothorax is defined by the communication between the external atmosphere and the pleural space. Gunshot wounds, knife wounds, and motor vehicle accidents that result in open chest trauma are common causes of open pneumothoraces.
Nursing process step: Assessment
Cognitive level: Analysis

130. CORRECT ANSWER—**C.** Equal chest expansion and bilateral breath sounds are evidence of lung reexpansion and indicate successful chest tube therapy. Arterial blood gas studies and pulse oximetry are indicators of lung expansion and the diffusion capacity of the lung, but are not accurate indicators of the full extent of lung expansion. A chest tube placed for a pneumothorax is unlikely to have significant amounts of drainage; therefore, drainage is an inappropriate indicator of therapeutic success. Bubbling in the water-seal chamber indicates an air leak.
Nursing process step: Evaluation
Cognitive level: Analysis

131. CORRECT ANSWER—**B.** Severe pulmonary disease produces low voltage (amplitude) in all components of an ECG. Right-axis deviation occurs secondary to right ventricular hypertrophy, a common finding in patients with severe chronic obstructive pulmonary disease (COPD) or cor pulmonale. A large amplitude in the ECG leads usually occurs in very thin patients or from mechanical manipulation of the gain. Left-axis deviation is caused by left ventricular hypertrophy, which is not commonly associated with COPD.
Nursing process step: Assessment
Cognitive level: Evaluation

132. CORRECT ANSWER—**A.** A left-sided fourth heart sound (S_4) is caused by vibrations of the atria after contraction and can be heard by placing the bell of the stethoscope at the apex of the heart during expiration. Called an atrial or presystolic gallop, S_4 usually is a sign of disease, such as myocardial infarction or impending heart failure from another cause. A physiologic S_4 may be heard in infants, children, and adults over age 50. An S_4 gallop is created by atrial contraction and cannot be heard in patients with atrial arrhythmias, such as atrial fibrillation or atrial flutter.
Nursing process step: Evaluation
Cognitive level: Evaluation

133. CORRECT ANSWER—**A.** The earlier thrombolytic therapy is initiated, the greater the amount of salvaged myocardium. It is widely believed that little myocardial salvage can occur if more than 6 hours have passed after the initial insult.
Nursing process step: Planning
Cognitive level: Comprehension

134. CORRECT ANSWER—B. This rhythm indicates failure of the pacemaker to capture. When capture does not occur, the pacing spike appears at the appropriate time but a QRS complex does not follow. Failure to capture can result from catheter movement, scarring at the contact site, battery failure, or catheter fracture. The nurse can respond to a failure to capture in several ways. These include placing the patient on the left side, increasing the pacemaker output, and checking all connections in the pacing system. Changing the pacing mode from paced to fixed or increasing the paced rate will not resolve the problems associated with failure to capture. If the nurse's actions do not correct the situation and the patient is symptomatic, then advanced cardiac life support (ACLS) protocol should be initiated.
Nursing process step: Evaluation
Cognitive level: Application

135. CORRECT ANSWER—B. Cardiogenic shock is characterized by acute myocardial infarction pattern on a 12-lead ECG; systolic blood pressure less than 80 mm Hg, or less than 90 mm Hg if the patient was previously hypertensive; pulse rate greater than 100 beats/minute, unless an atrioventricular block is present; urine output less than 30 ml/hour; symptoms of peripheral collapse; increased respiratory rate and pulmonary congestion; central nervous system changes; cardiac output of less than 4 to 7 liters/minute; and cardiac index of less than 1.8 liters/minute/m^2.
Nursing process step: Assessment
Cognitive level: Comprehension

136. CORRECT ANSWER—C. Basilar skull fractures are seldom detected radiographically; the diagnosis usually is made by clinical examination. Clinical signs of basilar skull fracture include periorbital ecchymosis (raccoon eyes), mastoid ecchymosis (Battle's sign), rhinorrhea (leakage of cerebrospinal fluid or blood from the nose), otorrhea (leakage of cerebrospinal fluid or blood from the ears), hematotympanum, and conjunctival hemorrhage without evidence of direct trauma. Unequal pupils (difference of approximately 1 mm in diameter) occur in approximately 17% of healthy persons and are not associated with basilar skull fractures.
Nursing process step: Assessment
Cognitive level: Knowledge

137. CORRECT ANSWER—D. In patients with encephalitis, metabolism increases secondary to the infectious organism, often resulting in hyperthermia, not hypothermia. All the other nursing diagnoses are appropriate for a patient with encephalitis.
Nursing process step: Implementation
Cognitive level: Analysis

138. CORRECT ANSWER—B. Salicylates (aspirin) inhibit platelet aggregation through irreversible pathways that interfere with thromboxane A$_2$ production, which is necessary for platelet clumping. A patient who takes an overdose of salicylates is at high risk for hemorrhage, hypoglycemia, compensatory metabolic acidosis, and hearing loss. Constipation and infections are not complications of salicylate toxicity.
Nursing process step: Evaluation
Cognitive level: Evaluation

139. CORRECT ANSWER—C. Clotting mechanisms are triggered when the body perceives an injury. The three principal stimuli for clotting are vessel injury, which stimulates platelet aggregation and clot formation; tissue injury, which activates thromboplastin and the extrinsic pathway; and the presence of a foreign body in the bloodstream, which triggers a humoral immune response and subsequent clotting. Vasodilation itself does not stimulate clotting, although several inflammatory mediators that also cause vasodilation can precipitate thromboxane production and clotting.
Nursing process step: Assessment
Cognitive level: Knowledge

140. CORRECT ANSWER—C. The cardinal sign of pheochromocytoma is persistent or paroxysmal hypertension. Common clinical effects of pheochromocytoma include palpitations, tachycardia, headache, diaphoresis, pallor, excitation, blurred vision, anxiety, and abdominal pain; these symptoms frequently occur when any pressure is exerted on the abdomen (such as from heavy lifting or exercise). The cause of pheochromocytoma may be a tumor on the adrenal medulla that causes oversecretion of the catecholamines epinephrine and norepinephrine. A diagnosis of pheochromocytoma is confirmed by the symptomatology, a 24-hour urine collection of catecholamine and its metabolites, and a computed tomography (CT) scan identifying an intra-adrenal lesion. Appendicitis presents with abdominal pain that becomes progressively worse and is accompanied by an elevated white blood cell count. Pancreatitis is accompanied by intense epigastric pain that radiates to the back and is aggravated by eating fatty foods. Although a CT scan may identify the presence of pancreatic cysts, a urine collection would not be helpful in the diagnosis of pancreatitis. Characteristic symptoms of Crohn's disease include fatigue, fever, abdominal pain, and diarrhea. Tests use to confirm a diagnosis of Crohn's disease include barium enema, sigmoidoscopy, and a biopsy of the colon.
Nursing process step: Assessment
Cognitive level: Analysis

141. CORRECT ANSWER—C. Second-degree atrioventricular (AV) block, Mobitz type II indicates a serious problem in the AV node and often progresses to complete heart block. First-degree heart block, second-degree AV block Mobitz type I, and sinus bradycardia are less likely to progress to more serious heart blocks.
Nursing process step: Planning
Cognitive level: Analysis

142. CORRECT ANSWER—A. An epidural hematoma is a rapidly expanding, space-occupying lesion. The resulting arterial bleeding increases intracranial pressure and can lead to early herniation of brain tissue and death. Immediate surgery is required and must not be delayed until the morning. Because of the increased intracranial pressure, lumbar puncture would lead to herniation of the brain stem and possible cardiac or respiratory arrest.
Nursing process step: Implementation
Cognitive level: Analysis

143. CORRECT ANSWER—B. Ranitidine increases microenzyme activity in the liver, which may lower plasma levels of anticonvulsants, especially carbamazepine. Ranitidine does not affect the potassium level.
Nursing process step: Assessment
Cognitive level: Knowledge

144. CORRECT ANSWER—C. Placing a pillow, blanket, or jacket under the patient's head can prevent injury if the head hits the floor or another object. A patient suffering a seizure cannot be restrained, and attempts to do so could cause more harm. Nothing should be forced into the patient's mouth. Intubation is not a priority; the nurse must first protect the patient from injury and attempt to stop the seizure by administering ordered medications.
Nursing process step: Implementation
Cognitive level: Knowledge

145. CORRECT ANSWER—**A.** A major burn is defined as a second-degree burn covering more than 25% of the total body surface area or a third-degree burn covering more than 10% of the total body surface area. Fourth-degree burns are the most severe; they extend through deeply charred subcutaneous tissue into the muscle and bone. First-degree burns are limited to the epidermis and cause erythema and pain. Second-degree burns involve the epidermis and part of the dermis, producing blisters and moderate pain and edema. Third-degree burns involve the epidermis and dermis; they are characterized by visible thrombosed vessels, absence of blisters, and white, brown, or leathery black tissue. Although third-degree burns may be painless, this patient has suffered a combination of second- and third-degree burns.
Nursing process step: Planning
Cognitive level: Analysis

146. CORRECT ANSWER—**D.** Hypokalemia increases myocardial excitability or irritability; it does not directly depress myocardial function. Arrhythmias associated with hypokalemia include premature ventricular beats, paroxysmal atrial tachycardia, and ventricular tachycardia. Hypokalemia can predispose a patient to digitalis toxicity. Because of their potency, loop diuretics can cause profound diuresis and water and electrolyte depletion. As alkalosis is corrected, the kidneys begin to retain potassium as they excrete excess hydrogen ions.
Nursing process step: Implementation
Cognitive level: Evaluation

147. CORRECT ANSWER—**C.** An upright, not supine, chest X-ray film provides the best visualization of vascular injuries and free-floating fluid within the chest cavity. However, the physician must rule out cervical spine injury before this film is obtained, and the thoracic and lumbar spine must be evaluated for possible problems. Although left lateral and right lateral films provide views of thoracic structures, the preferred view is a full frontal chest film, with the patient in an upright position.
Nursing process step: Planning
Cognitive level: Knowledge

148. CORRECT ANSWER—**C.** An FIO_2 greater than .50 damages the alveolar-capillary membrane, worsening the patient's condition. Changes in FIO_2 do not cause barotrauma or affect the ease of ventilation. Decreasing FIO_2 decreases PaO_2.
Nursing process step: Assessment
Cognitive level: Comprehension

149. CORRECT ANSWER—**D.** Positive end-expiratory pressure causes overdistention of the compliant alveoli remaining in the lung, thereby compressing the alveolar-capillary bed and decreasing blood flow to these areas. Increased pressure within the thoracic cavity compresses the great vessels and squeezes the heart, which decreases cardiac output and possibly blood pressure. The patient may be able to compensate for decreased blood volume with an increase in heart rate. A decreased heart rate also may occur as the baroceptors in the aortic arch and carotid body respond to the increase in intrathoracic pressures.
Nursing process step: Evaluation
Cognitive level: Evaluation

150. CORRECT ANSWER—A. Positive end-expiratory pressure increases the risk of tension pneumothorax. The patient's signs and symptoms are consistent with tension pneumothorax, as is the sounding of the pressure alarm with each inspiratory cycle. A ruptured pulmonary artery would be indicated by blood in the endotracheal tube secretions. Cardiac tamponade and esophageal tear would not cause the high-pressure alarm to sound.
Nursing process step: Assessment
Cognitive level: Analysis

151. CORRECT ANSWER—B. In patients in the early stage of septic shock, compensatory mechanisms are activated as fluids are shunted into the interstitial space and hypovolemia develops. The increased sympathetic response increases heart rate, vasoconstriction, and myocardial contractility. However, the patient quickly becomes unable to compensate and progresses to cardiogenic shock with increased myocardial oxygen demands. Symptoms of late septic shock include cold and clammy skin, oliguria leading to anuria, and changes in mental status. These symptoms are related to decreased organ perfusion. Ultimately, the patient succumbs to cardiac, respiratory, and renal failure.
Nursing process step: Evaluation
Cognitive level: Evaluation

152. CORRECT ANSWER—C. In the early stage of septic shock, peripheral vasodilation occurs, so drugs such as nitroprusside and dobutamine, which promote vasodilation, would not be useful. Dopamine at low dosages promotes renal perfusion; at moderate to high dosages, it has vasoconstrictive effects. Dopamine and oxygen administered together are appropriate for patients in early septic shock; these patients have an increased metabolic rate and oxygen depletion at the cellular level. Before any vasoactive drug—including nitroprusside, dobutamine, dopamine, and norepinephrine—is added to the patient's medication regimen, appropriate fluid volume replacement is required. In the later stages of sepsis, norepinephrine and dobutamine may be used to support the patient's blood pressure and cardiovascular function if fluid resuscitation is not effective. Procainamide, an antiarrhythmic, would be inappropriate. This drug commonly is prescribed for atrial arrhythmias, but ventricular arrhythmias are seen in the late stages of septic shock.
Nursing process step: Implementation
Cognitive level: Analysis

153. CORRECT ANSWER—A. Kernig's sign is characterized by pain in the lower back and resistance when, after flexing the leg at the hip and knee, the leg is extended while the thigh is flexed on the abdomen. A positive Brudzinski's sign is pain in the neck when flexing the neck forward and involuntary flexion of the arm, hip, and knee when passively flexing the neck. Both signs are symptoms of meningeal irritation. Cerebral thrombosis, viral encephalitis, and status epilepticus do not cause meningeal irritation.
Nursing process step: Assessment
Cognitive level: Knowledge

154. CORRECT ANSWER—D. Adult respiratory distress syndrome can result from multiple blood transfusions and shock. Transfusion reactions usually occur during actual transfusion of the blood product. A febrile nonhemolytic transfusion reaction is most common; it develops when cytotoxic or agglutinating antibodies in the recipient plasma attack antigens on transfused lymphocytes, granulocytes, or plasma cells. Immediate signs and symptoms of transfusion reaction occur within a few minutes or hours of the transfusion. Delayed hemolytic reactions, which are less common, can occur up to several weeks after a transfusion. The hepatitis B antigen can be detected approximately 30 days after a transfusion. Hypovolemia, not hypervolemia, might occur as a result of third-space fluid shifting and continued blood loss.
Nursing process step: Evaluation
Cognitive level: Evaluation

155. CORRECT ANSWER—B. Dopamine at high dosages (10 mcg/kg/minute or higher) stimulates alpha-adrenergic receptors, causing increased renal vasoconstriction, increased systemic vascular resistance, and profound tachycardia. At low to moderate dosages (2 to 9 mcg/kg/minute), dopamine stimulates $beta_1$ and dopamine receptors, enhancing renal blood flow and producing mild tachycardia. Dopamine does not affect pulmonary capillary wedge pressure.
Nursing process step: Planning
Cognitive level: Knowledge

156. CORRECT ANSWER—A. The first priority in treating cardiogenic shock is to expand the circulating blood volume with I.V. fluids, using either the pulmonary capillary wedge pressure, pulmonary artery end-diastolic pressure, or central venous pressure as a guide. For many years, cardiogenic shock was treated primarily with sympathomimetic amines to increase blood pressure through vasoconstriction. Today, I.V. fluids and oxygen are considered first-line therapy. A pacemaker may be used if the patient has persistent bradycardia or heart block. A critically ill patient who does not respond to first-line treatment may require an intra-aortic balloon pump or ventricular assist device to maintain cardiac output. Any changes in level of consciousness must be evaluated, but such an assessment is not the first priority.
Nursing process step: Planning
Cognitive level: Evaluation

157. CORRECT ANSWER—D. Family visits can contribute to or mitigate a patient's stress and anxiety and should be carefully monitored for these effects. Assessing the patient *before and after* all visits helps the nurse establish a baseline for evaluating the patient's response to family visits. Based on these assessments, the nurse should establish visiting guidelines that meet the needs of both the patient and family members.
Nursing process step: Implementation
Cognitive level: Synthesis

158. CORRECT ANSWER—D. The nurse must monitor for complications associated with extracorporeal membrane oxygenation (ECMO). A patient receiving ECMO typically is given heparin, necessitating meticulous monitoring to detect signs of bleeding. Infection also is a concern because invasive cannulas are used during ECMO. The invasive nature of ECMO necessitates pharmacologic paralysis, making the patient hard to turn and susceptible to complications related to immobility secondary to the low-flow state of the cardiovascular system. To prevent these complications, the patient should be placed on a low-air-loss mattress. Only health care professionals trained in the mechanics of ECMO, such as perfusionists, should adjust the ECMO settings. Evaluating daily chest X-ray films is important, but not a direct nursing responsibility.
Nursing process step: Implementation
Cognitive level: Analysis

159. CORRECT ANSWER—C. In patients suffering from carbon monoxide poisoning, oxygen is administered as a dispositional antagonist because it hastens the breakdown of carboxyhemoglobin and increases the availability of oxygen at the tissue level. Calcium precipitates fluoride and is the recommended antidote for fluoride poisoning. Sodium bicarbonate and ethanol are common antidotes for methanol poisoning; sodium bicarbonate offsets the acidosis common with methanol poisoning, and ethanol slows the formation of the toxic products of methanol. Naloxone is used for narcotic overdoses because it displaces the narcotic from the receptor sites.
Nursing process step: Implementation
Cognitive level: Comprehension

160. CORRECT ANSWER—A. Common signs of infection in younger patients, including elevated temperature, increased white blood cell count, and tachycardia, may not be seen in elderly patients. Consequently, the most commonly observed signs and symptoms of infection in elderly patients include altered mental status and afebrile temperature. Infections do not affect the albumin or sodium level.
Nursing process step: Assessment
Cognitive level: Comprehension

161. CORRECT ANSWER—A. Inhalation of gastric acid causes gastric pneumonitis, with signs and symptoms evident 2 to 4 hours after aspiration. Signs of respiratory compromise resulting from gastric aspiration include dyspnea, bronchospasm, wheezing, fever, leukocytosis, and frothy, nonpurulent sputum. The severity of the lung injury increases as the pH falls below 2.5.
Nursing process step: Assessment
Cognitive level: Analysis

162. CORRECT ANSWER—C. Aspiration of small particles can cause severe subacute pulmonary inflammation and hemorrhagic pneumonia. Signs and symptoms of aspiration include increased $PaCO_2$ and increased intrapulmonary shunting. Bronchospasm as evidenced by decreased compliance occurs in the aspiration of gastric contents.
Nursing process step: Evaluation
Cognitive level: Knowledge

163. CORRECT ANSWER—**B.** A Denver shunt is a surgically positioned tube that allows continuous reinfusion of ascitic fluid into the venous system. The tube runs from the abdominal cavity through the peritoneum, under the subcutaneous tissue, and into the jugular vein or superior vena cava. Portosystemic shunts, such as the portacaval shunt, are used to treat esophageal varices (not a Denver shunt). These shunts decrease portal hypertension by diverting some of the blood flow away from the liver. Because the Denver shunt diverts ascitic fluid only, it is not useful for hepatic encephalopathy. This condition is treated by helping the body excrete ammonia. Treatment for hepatorenal syndrome consists of albumin administration, water restriction, and diuretic therapy because this syndrome involves renal failure secondary to liver failure, which also must be treated.
Nursing process step: Implementation
Cognitive level: Comprehension

164. CORRECT ANSWER—**B.** Several events occur in the early stage of septic shock. Cellular toxins are released and damage cells. Complement stimulates the release of vasoactive proteins and activates factor XII of the coagulation cascade. Vasoactive kinins promote peripheral vasodilation and increase capillary permeability. The peripheral vasodilation decreases systemic vascular resistance, thereby reducing afterload and increasing cardiac output.
Nursing process step: Assessment
Cognitive level: Comprehension

165. CORRECT ANSWER—**A.** Traumatic valvular injury is rare, but should be suspected when a new murmur develops after chest trauma. In most cases, the aortic valve is affected, and regurgitation can be auscultated as a diastolic murmur over the aortic valve at the second right interspace. Mitral valve regurgitation produces a holosystolic murmur. A continuous murmur, in which the separate components of the cardiac cycle cannot be differentiated, can be auscultated in patients with a large ventricular septal defect and left-to-right shunting. Murmurs are not associated with aortic dissection unless the aortic valve is involved.
Nursing process step: Assessment
Cognitive level: Analysis

166. CORRECT ANSWER—**A.** The turbulent blood flow generated by arterial branching encourages the formation of atherosclerotic plaques. The plaques originate in the intima of the arterial wall as fatty streaks.
Nursing process step: Assessment
Cognitive level: Comprehension

167. CORRECT ANSWER—**C.** Echocardiography is a noninvasive means of studying structural abnormalities and blood flow dynamics. During echocardiography, a transducer is placed on the patient's chest. The transducer produces high-frequency sound waves that bounce off the heart and great vessels, eventually returning through the transducer to the monitor to produce an echocardiogram. Cardiac catheterization is an invasive test used to determine the extent of valvular disease and its effect on cardiac output. An ECG and chest X-ray film are noninvasive methods of assessing the effects of valvular heart disease; however, they provide no specific data on structural abnormalities or blood flow dynamics.
Nursing process step: Planning
Cognitive level: Evaluation

168. CORRECT ANSWER—C. A patient with severe hemodynamic impairment and clinical evidence of acute heart failure can benefit most from mechanical assistance, which may include insertion of an intra-aortic balloon pump. Because the left side of the heart is failing, the patient probably is hypotensive and is unlikely to benefit from diuretic therapy or semi-Fowler's positioning. Extracorporeal membrane oxygenation is indicated for patients with life-threatening hypoxia, such as in severe adult respiratory distress syndrome, who have not responded to conventional treatment.
Nursing process step: Implementation
Cognitive level: Analysis

169. CORRECT ANSWER—D. Analysis of the creatine kinase-MB (CK-MB) isoenzyme is preferable to that of creatine kinase (CK), aspartate aminotransferase (AST), and lactate dehydrogenase (LD) isoenzyme because of the high specificity and sensitivity of CK-MB for myocardial damage. Serum CK, AST, and LD can be increased by many other causes, including renal impairment, liver disease, and skeletal muscle damage. When admission to the hospital has been delayed for 48 hours or more after onset of symptoms, LD isoenzyme analysis is more helpful in differentiating unstable angina from myocardial infarction.
Nursing process step: Assessment
Cognitive level: Knowledge

170. CORRECT ANSWER—A. Although mitral regurgitation, mitral stenosis, tricuspid regurgitation, and aortic stenosis may be caused by rheumatic fever, the important assessment finding in this situation is the holosystolic murmur heard at the apex of the heart that is most characteristic of mitral regurgitation. The patient also is exhibiting other symptoms commonly associated with mitral regurgitation. The murmur of mitral stenosis is a loud, opening snap and a diastolic murmur heard at the apex of the heart along the left sternal border or at the base of the heart. Tricuspid regurgitation produces a holosystolic murmur heard best over the lower left sternal border. Murmurs associated with aortic stenosis are systolic murmurs best auscultated over the second right intercostal space.
Nursing process step: Assessment
Cognitive level: Analysis

171. CORRECT ANSWER—B. Initial interventions for early septic shock focus on replacing fluids, typically in the form of colloids to increase osmotic pressure and to hold fluid in the intravascular space; blood products also may be administered, if indicated. Usually two broad-spectrum antibiotics are administered intravenously to increase the likelihood of destroying the causative organism. Treating actual or potential complications related to acidosis or respiratory or cardiac failure is essential; however, respiratory alkalosis is more prevalent in the early stage of septic shock, whereas metabolic acidosis occurs in the late stage. Other interventions include administering inotropic agents, vasopressors, and corticosteroids to inhibit the effects of endotoxins or complement by decreasing pulmonary vascular resistance. Afterload reduction is not a goal of therapy in the initial stage of shock because systemic vascular resistance already is low during this stage. During early septic shock, the patient is hyperthermic and may require treatment with a hypothermia unit and antipyretic agents. In the late stage of septic shock, the patient's temperature may be normal or hypothermic.
Nursing process step: Implementation
Cognitive level: Application

172. CORRECT ANSWER—C. Major renal trauma increases the susceptibility of renal parenchyma to infection because of hematuria, ischemia, and urinary extravasation. Uremia is not necessarily present unless renal failure occurs after the trauma. Pulmonary infection can be prevented with respiratory maintenance therapy, such as coughing and deep-breathing exercises. Septicemia is not associated with major renal trauma and is not a reason for using broad-spectrum antibiotics.
Nursing process step: Implementation
Cognitive level: Evaluation

173. CORRECT ANSWER—D. In the successful treatment of renal trauma, the nurse would expect to see evidence of normal renal function as indicated by normal creatinine and blood urea nitrogen levels. Absence of infection as indicated by normothermia and a normal white blood cell count also are useful evaluation criteria. Evidence of wound healing is a sign of a successful patient outcome.
Nursing process step: Planning
Cognitive level: Evaluation

174. CORRECT ANSWER—C. During an exacerbation of asthma, a patient can become dehydrated from hyperventilation, increased temperature, and increased metabolic demands. Therefore, the nurse must ensure that the patient is adequately hydrated. Pain is unlikely, but the patient may suffer extreme anxiety; an antianxiety medication should be administered if indicated. A patient with an exacerbation of asthma should receive oxygen; however, oxygen does not treat the problems associated with decreased hydration.
Nursing process step: Implementation
Cognitive level: Analysis

175. CORRECT ANSWER—B. Studies have shown that patients with non-Q wave MI have lower hospital mortality but the same mortality at 1 year as patients with Q-wave MI. The nurse should provide this information so the patient can obtain appropriate medical follow-up after discharge. It is the nurse's responsibility to educate and be honest with all patients.
Nursing process step: Implementation
Cognitive level: Synthesis

176. CORRECT ANSWER—A. Nursing interventions for a patient with infectious endocarditis are aimed at identifying the infectious organism by drawing blood samples for cultures at appropriate times and assessing for signs of systemic embolization and valvular dysfunction. Systemic embolization may be indicated by a positive Homan's sign, signifying thrombophlebitis. Cardiovascular function should be monitored to detect decreases in cardiac output or cardiac index, which can occur with infectious endocarditis and related valvular dysfunction. A patient with infectious endocarditis needs adequate rest, including bed rest initially; however, visiting hours need not be restricted: The patient is at risk for complications related to valvular dysfunction; these complications are best identified by monitoring cardiac output, cardiac index, and pulmonary artery pressures, not by monitoring systemic vascular resistance. Monitoring breathing patterns, oxygen saturation, and arterial blood gas results will alert the nurse to signs of hypoxia, which may be related to decreased cardiac output and valvular dysfunction. The patient must receive nothing by mouth (NPO status) until surgery is no longer an option.
Nursing process step: Implementation
Cognitive level: Analysis

177. CORRECT ANSWER—C. Hypoxemia is characteristically severe in a patient with adult respiratory distress syndrome, primarily because blood is shunted through the poorly ventilated lung. This shunting may result from perfusion of atelectatic or fluid-filled alveoli. A patient in this condition compensates by increasing his respiratory rate. The ventilator alarm is sounding because the patient is breathing at a high rate and not allowing for complete alveolar emptying before delivering the next breath. Sedating and pharmacologically paralyzing the patient enables the nurse to control the respiratory rate. Pharmacologic paralysis also eliminates skeletal muscle activity, thereby decreasing the patient's oxygen demand. Any patient given a paralyzing agent also should receive a sedative because the effects of paralysis can be disturbing. Paralyzing agents, specifically neuromuscular blockers, should not be administered continuously for long periods, especially if steroids are administered concurrently; this places the patient at increased risk for prolonged muscle weakness after treatment is discontinued. The patient's hemodynamic status does not warrant preload or afterload reduction. Increasing the respiratory rate will exacerbate the problem as there would be less time for alveolar emptying between breaths. Decreasing the respiratory rate set on the ventilator will not work because it is set on assist-control mode; with assist control, the patient's respiratory efforts will trigger the ventilator and, if the patient's respiratory rate is 42 breaths/minute, the ventilator will cycle with every inspiratory effort.
Nursing process step: Implementation
Cognitive level: Evaluation

178. CORRECT ANSWER—C. Esophageal injuries can occur with blunt or penetrating trauma. A patient with an esophageal injury typically is acutely ill, with substernal chest pain, fever, and shock. Mediastinitis, which results from contamination of the mediastinum with saliva and gastric contents, is the principal cause of morbidity and mortality in such patients. Chest X-ray findings in esophageal injuries typically include pneumomediastinum, hydropneumothorax, pleural effusion, and evidence of subcutaneous air from the communication between the esophagus and mediastinum. Patients with tracheobronchial injury usually complain of dyspnea, cough, and localized chest pain. Bronchial injuries cause a higher level of respiratory compromise. Signs and symptoms of tracheal injuries include increased hemoptysis, airway obstruction, and respiratory compromise.
Nursing process step: Assessment
Cognitive level: Comprehension

179. CORRECT ANSWER—C. The most effective drug regimen for a patient with angina is a calcium channel blocker, such as diltiazem, combined with nitrate therapy, such as isosorbide dinitrate or nitroglycerin. Nitrates act primarily as vasodilators of smooth muscle. They decrease preload by dilating veins and decrease afterload by dilating arteries. Nitrates also promote coronary artery autoregulation, thereby improving blood flow to ischemic areas and decreasing blood flow to unaffected areas. Calcium channel blockers decrease contractility, which, in turn, decreases the workload of the heart, and vasodilate coronary arteries, which helps prevent further ischemic episodes. Captopril, an angiotensin-converting enzyme inhibitor, may be added to control hypertension. Procainamide would be given to correct atrial or ventricular arrhythmias. Ranitidine, a histamine$_2$-receptor antagonist, is used for patients at risk for ulcers. Propranolol is a class II antiarrhythmic and may be prescribed for its antihypertensive and antianginal effects.
Nursing process step: Implementation
Cognitive level: Knowledge

180. CORRECT ANSWER—**B.** The nurse must determine how the anginal pain manifests itself. The PQRST system often is helpful in obtaining this information. In this documentation system, P = provoke (what activities provoke the angina attacks?); Q = quality (is the pain burning, crushing, or stabbing?); R = radiation/region (where is the pain located and where does it radiate?); S = severity (how severe is the pain on a scale of 1 to 10?); and T = timing (how long has the episode of pain lasted?). The patient may not have "chest pain" in the literal sense. In this case, the patient is experiencing anginal pain in the form of heartburn. After assessing the patient's symptoms, the nurse can effectively treat the patient. Although knowing the patient's education level will help direct later patient-teaching efforts, obtaining information about the patient's discomfort is more important during the initial assessment.
Nursing process step: Implementation
Cognitive level: Comprehension

181. CORRECT ANSWER—**C.** With certain physiologic or positional variants, ventricular depolarization proceeds in a left to right fashion, and large Q waves may be normal in leads V_1, V_2, aV_L, and I. One example of a noncardiac cause of significant Q waves is left-sided pneumothorax, in which the right side of the heart is accentuated on the ECG. Acute inferior wall myocardial infarction can cause ST-segment and T-wave changes in leads II, III, and aV_F. Prinzmetal's angina is represented on the ECG by ST-segment elevations. Q waves in leads V_1 and V_2 may indicate posterior wall necrosis, not lateral wall necrosis.
Nursing process step: Assessment
Cognitive level: Knowledge

182. CORRECT ANSWER—**D.** In patients with acute dissecting aneurysm of the aorta or a pheochromocytoma and in those who have been taking monoamine oxidase (MAO) inhibitors, the systolic blood pressure can be lowered to a normal level of 110 to 120 mm Hg during a hypertensive crisis. Similarly, if renal function is normal and there is no history of cerebral or coronary artery disease, blood pressure can be lowered to normal level.
Nursing process step: Implementation
Cognitive level: Knowledge

183. CORRECT ANSWER—**B.** In patients in cardiogenic shock, the serum glucose level usually is increased by the release of epinephrine, which occurs in response to physiologic stress. Electrolyte imbalances occur if the patient has been taking diuretics, which increase the potential for hypokalemia. The blood urea nitrogen level may rise as a result of poor kidney perfusion; however, the serum creatinine level remains normal unless the patient has underlying renal dysfunction. Although hypocalcemia may occur in cardiogenic shock, it is not a presenting symptom.
Nursing process step: Evaluation
Cognitive level: Analysis

184. CORRECT ANSWER—**A.** Renal involvement may not occur in the early stages of hypertension. However, over time, renal function tests can become abnormal. Such tests include measurements of serum blood urea nitrogen and creatinine, urine and serum osmolality, urine specific gravity, and urine sodium level. Urinalysis is used to check for glomerulonephritis as indicated by presence of protein, red blood cells, and white blood cells in the urine. I.V. pyelography also is a useful diagnostic tool in patients with renal disease. The serum catecholamine level is not used to assess kidney damage. Renal compensation as determined by serial arterial blood gas analyses indicates the ability of the kidneys to correct a respiratory or metabolic process. Serum drug levels are obtained in patients with questionable kidney function who are taking drugs excreted by the kidneys; these levels are used to prevent toxic effects and adjust drug dosages. Serum drug levels do not provide information about renal function.
Nursing process step: Assessment
Cognitive level: Comprehension

185. CORRECT ANSWER—**B.** ECG signs of second-degree atrioventricular (AV) block, Mobitz type II, include constant, normal PR intervals when P waves are conducted (however, many P waves are not conducted); more P waves than QRS complexes; and regular atrial rhythm. Mobitz type II AV blocks are clinically different from Mobitz type I AV blocks; they may worsen when atropine is given and may improve with carotid sinus massage. A Mobitz type II AV block indicates a pathologic condition or blockage in the bundle of His. Because this type of block commonly is associated with a bundle branch block, the QRS complex may be widened (> 0.12 second).
Nursing process step: Assessment
Cognitive level: Application

186. CORRECT ANSWER—**B.** Patient positioning should be based on the effect of gravity on the lung fields. Perfusion is greatest in the dependent lung or the dependent portions of the lungs. The healthy portion of the lung should be dependent and receive the greatest amount of perfusion. In this case, the left lung is healthy, and the patient should be positioned with the left-side down. The frequency of position changes is determined by the patient's pulmonary parameters after a position change, mobilization of secretions, and hemodynamic assessment.
Nursing process step: Implementation
Cognitive level: Evaluation

187. CORRECT ANSWER—**D.** In patients with infectious endocarditis, systemic embolization can occur as the valves of the heart become cluttered with infective material that breaks free and enters the systemic circulation. Fever is caused by the presence of the causative organism. Cardiac output is decreased by valvular dysfunction, congestive heart failure, or fluid volume excess.
Nursing process step: Evaluation
Cognitive level: Knowledge

188. CORRECT ANSWER—**A.** The most common adverse reactions to bretylium are hypotension, nausea, and vomiting. A prolonged QT interval is associated with procainamide and quinidine therapy. Heart blocks are a potential adverse effect of all antiarrhythmic medications, but are not particularly common with bretylium.
Nursing process step: Evaluation
Cognitive level: Comprehension

189. CORRECT ANSWER—B. Hemodynamic parameters, which include central venous or right atrial pressure, blood pressure, and cardiac output, must reflect adequate filling volumes and pressures when a patient is given a vasodilator. If a volume-depleted patient receives a vasodilating medication, problems can result from a labile and often too low blood pressure. Correlation of cuff and arterial line blood pressures is important, especially when a patient receives medications that directly affect blood pressure; however, assessment of the patient's volume status before vasodilator administration is essential. A patient treated with a vasodilator must remain supine to prevent orthostatic hypotension. The presence of peripheral edema is not relevant to vasodilator therapy.
Nursing process step: Evaluation
Cognitive level: Knowledge

190. CORRECT ANSWER—D. Aminophylline is a theophylline compound; theophylline has a narrow therapeutic range of 10 to 20 µg/ml. Symptoms of low-level toxicity, including nausea, vomiting, anorexia, agitation, insomnia, and tremors, are common reasons for drug intolerance in the elderly. Even a less than therapeutic level can cause signs of toxicity in elderly patients.
Nursing process step: Assessment
Cognitive level: Comprehension

191. CORRECT ANSWER—A. Spacing devices, also known as spacers or extenders, double the deposition of inhaled medication in the lungs. More than half of asthmatic patients use their inhaler incorrectly. The spacing device helps decrease problems with inhaler use. It also enhances the effectiveness of the inhaler, although it may not make the inhaler easier to use nor does it ensure better compliance. The spacing device is no more portable than an inhaler.
Nursing process step: Implementation
Cognitive level: Evaluation

192. CORRECT ANSWER—B. Aortic regurgitation is a fluid volume overload problem that can be treated with diuretics, vasodilators (such as nitrates), and agents that reduce both preload and afterload. Aortic stenosis is a pressure overload problem best treated by removing the obstruction to outflow. Calcium channel blockers decrease contractility but do not directly decrease preload or afterload.
Nursing process step: Implementation
Cognitive level: Analysis

193. CORRECT ANSWER—B. A patient who is choking and in respiratory arrest must receive immediate treatment. Cellular anoxia can lead to brain damage and death within 4 to 6 minutes.
Nursing process step: Assessment
Cognitive level: Comprehension

194. CORRECT ANSWER—C. A ventilated patient suspected of aspirating a tube feeding should be hyperoxygenated with 100% inspired oxygen, then suctioned to remove any possible aspirated contents to decrease the risk of aspiration pneumonia. Glucose and pH testing can help determine whether the patient aspirated the tube feeding. Any tube feeding that may have been aspirated must be immediately removed to prevent aspiration pneumonia. The physician should be notified after this has been done. Increasing the oxygen delivery rate on the ventilator is inappropriate until further assessment results are obtained. Arterial blood gas analysis can help determine whether ventilation or oxygenation has been compromised; however, this intervention is not the first priority for this patient, and would be appropriate only after the patient has been suctioned.
Nursing process step: Implementation
Cognitive level: Evaluation

195. CORRECT ANSWER—C. An oropharyngeal airway helps maintain a patent airway and ventilation by holding the tongue anteriorly. Because the airway device stimulates the gag reflex, vomiting and aspiration are common complications, especially in a patient who is awake. Coughing ability is determined by the patient's ability to close the glottis and increase intra-abdominal pressure, which is not enhanced by the oropharyngeal airway. An oropharyngeal airway does not increase oxygen requirements or cause carbon dioxide retention.
Nursing process step: Implementation
Cognitive level: Knowledge

196. CORRECT ANSWER—A. In addition to its vasoconstrictive properties, dopamine at low dosages helps maintain renal and mesenteric blood flow. At moderate dosages, dopamine stimulates beta$_1$-adrenergic receptor sites, which increases heart rate and contractility and improves cardiac output. At high dosages, dopamine stimulates alpha-adrenergic receptor sites and causes peripheral vasoconstriction, thus raising blood pressure. High dosages of dopamine should be used only for short periods and after the patient has received adequate volume replacement. Norepinephrine is an alpha-adrenergic agonist that also should be used only for short periods because of its intense vasoconstrictive effects, which can cause capillary stasis and leakage of fluid from the intravascular compartment to the extracellular space. When these conditions develop, the patient becomes unresponsive to the drug, which worsens the state of shock and may lead to death. Isoproterenol should be used only after the hypovolemia is corrected. The use of isoproterenol in a patient in cardiogenic shock resulting from acute myocardial infarction can stress the myocardium by increasing myocardial oxygen consumption. Phenylephrine, like norepinephrine, is a potent alpha-adrenergic agonist and should be used only for short periods in patients in extremely hypotensive states.
Nursing process step: Implementation
Cognitive level: Analysis

197. CORRECT ANSWER—D. Acidic endotracheal tube secretions are a positive sign of gastric acid aspiration. Aspiration of gastric acid often is accompanied by hypoxemia, normal or low PaCO$_2$, and infiltrates in dependent lung segments. Heme-positive endotracheal secretions are not related to acute gastric acid aspiration. However, 6 hours after aspiration, endotracheal secretions may be heme-positive because of subacute inflammatory pulmonary processes and hemorrhagic pneumonia.
Nursing process step: Assessment
Cognitive level: Evaluation

198. CORRECT ANSWER—C. After any accident that causes multiple rib fractures, the continuity of the thorax may be destroyed, resulting in a flail chest. In patients with flail chest, the rib cage no longer moves in unison with the respiratory muscles. Instead, the thorax moves as changes in intrapleural pressures occur. With flail chest, the chest wall collapses inward on inspiration and expands on expiration, which compromises effective ventilation. In patients with tension pneumothorax, hemothorax, or hemopneumothorax, the lung is collapsed, resulting in minimal chest wall movement.
Nursing process step: Assessment
Cognitive level: Evaluation

199. CORRECT ANSWER—C. Tracheobronchial injury can cause air to accumulate throughout the thoracic cavity. Lobar atelectasis, hemoptysis, and persistent air leak syndrome are seen in patients with untreated tracheobronchial injuries. Symptoms of tracheobronchial injury include abrupt subcutaneous crepitation of the neck and anterior chest wall, severe dyspnea, hypotension, tachycardia, cyanosis, and anxiety. A positive Hamman's sign indicates a ruptured trachea or bronchi; it is defined as a loud, crushing, crunching sound synchronous with the heartbeat.
Nursing process step: Evaluation
Cognitive level: Analysis

200. CORRECT ANSWER—**B.** Multiple rib fractures and diminished lung expansion indicate an air leak disorder. Positive end-expiratory pressure (PEEP) increases intra-alveolar pressures and exacerbates air leakage, which can worsen the existing pneumothorax or cause subcutaneous emphysema or tension pneumothorax. If PEEP is required to maintain oxygenation, the patient must be closely monitored for deterioration and evaluated for possible chest tube placement. Pressure support, synchronized intermitten ventilation, and sighs support and enhance ventilation.
Nursing process step: Implementation
Cognitive level: Analysis

Appendix A: Critical Laboratory Values

Critical laboratory values represent severe pathophysiologic states that are life-threatening unless immediate corrective action is taken. The chart below lists critical limits as determined by a national survey of trauma and medical centers in the United States. The chart lists low and high critical limits, as well as the low and high ranges, for tests for clinical chemistry, blood gases and pH, and hematology; it also lists important qualitative results.

Critical values in clinical chemistry					
Test	Units	Low	Range	High	Range
Bilirubin	μmol/liter	N/A	N/A	257	86 to 513
	mg/dl	N/A	N/A	15	5 to 30
Calcium	mmol/liter	1.65	1.25 to 2.15	3.22	2.62 to 3.49
	mg/dl	6.6	5.0 to 8.6	12.9	10.5 to 14.0
Calcium, free	mmol/liter	0.78	0.75 to 0.88	1.58	1.50 to 1.63
	mg/dl	3.13	3.01 to 3.53	6.33	6.01 to 6.53
Chloride	mmol/liter	75	60 to 90	126	115 to 156
CO_2 content	mmol/liter	11	5 to 20	40	35 to 50
Creatinine	μmol/liter	N/A	N/A	654	177 to 1,326
	mg/dl	N/A	N/A	7.4	2.0 to 15.0
Glucose	mmol/liter	2.6	1.7 to 3.9	26.9	6.1 to 55.5
	mg/dl	46	30 to 70	484	110 to 1,000
Glucose, CSF	mmol/liter	2.1	1.1 to 2.8	24.3	13.9 to 38.9
	mg/dl	37	20 to 50	438	250 to 700
Lactate dehydrogenase	mmol/liter	N/A	N/A	3.4	2.3 to 5.0
	mg/dl	N/A	N/A	30.6	20.7 to 45.0
Magnesium	mmol/liter	0.41	0.21 to 0.74	2.02	1.03 to 5.02
	mg/dl	1.0	0.5 to 1.8	4.9	2.5 to 12.2
Osmolality	mmol/kg	250	230 to 280	326	295 to 375
Phosphorus	mmol/liter	0.39	0.26 to 0.65	2.87	2.26 to 3.23
	mg/dl	1.2	0.8 to 2.0	8.9	7.0 to 10.0
Potassium	mmol/liter	2.8	2.5 to 3.6	6.2 8.0 (hemolyzed)	5.0 to 8.0
Sodium	mmol/liter	120	110 to 137	158	145 to 170
Urea nitrogen	mmol/liter	N/A	N/A	37.1	14.3 to 107.1
	mg/dl	N/A	N/A	104	40 to 300
Uric acid	μmol/liter	N/A	N/A	773	595 to 892
	mg/dl	N/A	N/A	13	10 to 15

Critical values in blood gases and pH

Test	Units	Low	Range	High	Range
PCO$_2$	mm Hg	19	9 to 25	67	50 to 80
	kPa	2.5	1.2 to 3.3	8.9	6.7 to 10.7
pH		7.21	7.00 to 7.35	7.59	7.50 to 7.65
PO$_2$	mm Hg	43	30 to 55	N/A	N/A
	kPa	5.7	4.0 to 7.3	N/A	N/A
PO$_2$, newborn	mm Hg	37	30 to 50	92	70 to 100
	kPa	4.9	4.0 to 6.7	12.3	9.3 to 13.3

Critical values in hematology

Test	Units	Low	Range	High	Range
Fibrinogen	g/liter	0.88	0.5 to 1	7.75	5 to 10
Hematocrit		0.18	0.12 to 0.30	0.61	0.54 to 0.80
Hemoglobin	g/liter	66	40 to 120	199	170 to 300
Partial thromboplastin time	seconds	N/A	N/A	68	32 to 150
Platelets	$\times 10^9$/liter	37	10 to 100	910	555 to 1,000
Prothrombin time	seconds	N/A	N/A	27	14 to 40
White blood cell count	$\times 10^9$/liter	2.0	1.0 to 4.0	37	10.0 to 100.0

Critical qualitative findings

Hematology	• blasts on blood smear • new diagnosis or findings of leukemia • sickle cells (or aplastic crisis)
Microbiology and parasitology	• positive culture or Gram stain from blood, CSF, or body cavity fluid • positive antigen detection for *Cryptococcus,* group b streptococci, *Haemophilus influenzae* b, or *Neisseria meningitidis* • positive acid-fast bacillus or culture • *Salmonella, Shigella,* or *Campylobacter* on stool culture • malarial parasites
Microscopy and urinalysis	• elevated white blood cell count in CSF • malignant cells, blasts, or microorganisms in CSF or body fluids • positive results for glucose or ketones in urine • pathologic crystals on urinalysis
Blood blank and immunology	• incompatible crossmatch • positive test for syphilis

Source: Kost, Gerald J. "Critical Limits for Urgent Clinician Notification at U.S. Medical Centers," *JAMA* 263(5):704-707, February 2, 1990.

Appendix B: Hemodynamic Monitoring

Invasive hemodynamic monitoring is widely used in the critical care setting. Various monitoring devices allow health care personnel to diagnose a patient's hemodynamic status and to evaluate the effectiveness of treatments. The chart below lists the normal values for certain hemodynamic parameters.

Hemodynamic variable	Definition	Normal value
Pulmonary artery systolic (PAS) pressure	Peak pressure of the right ventricle	20 to 30 mm Hg
Pulmonary artery diastolic (PAD) pressure	Lowest pressure produced in the pulmonary artery; also an indirect measurement of the left atrial pressure (LAP)	10 to 15 mm Hg
Mean pulmonary artery pressure	Average of the systolic and diastolic pulmonary artery pressures; also known as mean pulmonary artery pressure	10 to 20 mm Hg
Pulmonary capillary wedge pressure (PCWP)	Indirect measurement of LAP and left ventricular end diastolic pressure (LVEDP)	4 to 12 mm Hg
Cardiac output (CO)	Volume of blood ejected from the left ventricle per minute	4 to 6 liters/minute
Cardiac index (CI)	Cardiac output per unit time divided by patient's body surface area	2.5 to 4.2 liters/minute/m^2
Systemic vascular resistance (SVR)	Measurement of left ventricular afterload	900 to 1,200 dynes/second/cm^{-5}
Pulmonary vascular resistance (PVR)	Measurement of right ventricular afterload, that is, the total resistance to blood flow in the pulmonary circulation	20 to 120 dynes/second/cm^{-5}

Selected
References

Alspach, J.G., ed. *AACN's Core Curriculum for Critical Care Nursing*, 4th ed. Philadelphia: W.B. Saunders Co., 1991.

Baer, C., and Williams, B. *Clinical Pharmacology and Nursing*, 3rd ed. Springhouse, Pa.: Springhouse Corp., 1996.

Bartlett, J.G. *Pocketbook of Infectious Disease Therapy*. Baltimore: Williams & Wilkins Co., 1994.

Brody, G.M. "Diabetic ketoacidosis and hyperosmolar hyperglycemic nonketotic coma." *Topics in Emergency Medicine*, 14(1): 12-22, March 1992.

Cardona, V.D., Hurn, P.D., Bastnagel-Mason, P.J., Scanlon, A.M., and Veise-Berry, S.W., eds. *Trauma Nursing: From Resuscitation Through Rehabilitation*, 2nd ed. Philadelphia: W.B. Saunders Co., 1994.

Catalano, J.T. *Guide to ECG Analysis*. Philadelphia: J.B. Lippincott Co., 1993.

Cernaianu, A., DelRossi, A., et al. "Continuous venous oximetry for hemodymanic and oxygen transport stability post cardiac surgery." *Journal of Cardiovascular Surgery*, 33(1): 14-20, January/February 1992.

Clochesy, J.M., Breu, C., Cardin, S., Rudy, E.B., and Whittaker, A.A., eds. *Critical Care Nursing*. Philadelphia: W.B. Saunders Co., 1993.

Conover, M. *Understanding Electrocardiography: Arrhythmias and the 12-Lead ECG*, 6th ed. St Louis: Mosby, Inc., 1992.

Daily, E.K., and Schroeder, J.S. *Techniques in Bedside Hemodynamic Monitoring*, 5th ed. St Louis: Mosby, Inc., 1994.

Daleiden, A. "Clinical manifestations of blunt cardiac injury: A challenge to the critical care practitioner." *Critical Care Nursing Quarterly*, 17(2): 13-23, August 1994.

Dossey, B.M., Guzzetta, C.E., and Kenner, C.V. *Critical Care Nursing*, 3rd ed. Philadelphia: J.B. Lippincott Co., 1992.

Dunham, C.M., and Cowley, R.A., eds. *Shock Trauma/Critical Care Manual*. Rockville, Md.: Aspen Publications, 1991.

Gardner, R.M., et al. "Fundamentals of physiologic monitoring." *AACN Clinical Issues in Critical Care Nursing*, (4)1: 11-24, February 1993.

Hickey, J.V. *The Clinical Practice of Neurological and Neurosurgical Nursing*, 3rd ed. Philadelphia: J.B. Lippincott Co., 1992.

Hudak, C.M., and Gallo, B.M. *Critical Care Nursing: A Holistic Approach*, 6th ed. Philadelphia: J.B. Lippincott Co., 1994.

Jacobs, D.S., Kasten, B.L., DeMott, W.R., and Wolfson, W. *Laboratory Test Handbook*, 3rd ed. Baltimore: Williams & Wilkins, 1994.

Kinney, M., Packa, D., Dunbar, S.B., et al. *AACN's Clinical Reference for Critical-Care Nursing*, 3rd ed. St Louis: Mosby, Inc., 1993.

Neff, J., and Kidd, P. *Trauma Nursing: The Art and Science.* St Louis: Mosby, Inc., 1993.

Norton, M., Leizia, M., and Jenrich, J.A. "Right ventricular infarction vs. left ventricular infarction: Review of pathophysiology, medical treatment, and nursing care." *Medsurg Nursing,* 2(3): 203-209, 220, June 1993.

Responding to Patients in Crisis. Advanced Skills Series. Springhouse, Pa.: Springhouse Corp., 1993.

Swearingen, P.J., and Keen, J.H. *Manual of Critical Care,* 3rd ed. St Louis: Mosby, Inc., 1995.

Thelan, L.A., et al. *Critical Care Nursing: Diagnosis and Management,* 2nd ed. St Louis: Mosby, Inc., 1994.

Wright, J.E., and Shelton, B.K., eds. *Desk Reference for Critical Care Nursing.* Boston, Jones and Bartlett, 1993.

Index